Quality

Quality

Second Edition

KATE MCCORMICK
Devon, United Kingdom

JANET H. SANDERS
East Carolina University, Greenville, NC, United States

 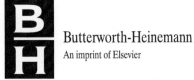

Butterworth-Heinemann
An imprint of Elsevier

ELSEVIER

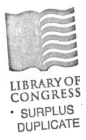

Butterworth-Heinemann is an imprint of Elsevier
The Boulevard, Langford Lane, Kidlington, Oxford OX5 1GB, United Kingdom
50 Hampshire Street, 5th Floor, Cambridge, MA 02139, United States

ISBN: 978-0-323-90815-3

For Information on all Butterworth-Heinemann publications
visit our website at https://www.elsevier.com/books-and-journals

Publisher: Susan Dennis
Acquisitions Editor: Anita Koch
Editorial Project Manager: Howi M. De Ramos
Production Project Manager: Bharatwaj Varatharajan
Cover Designer: Matthew Limbert

Typeset by MPS Limited, Chennai, India

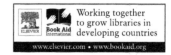

Working together
to grow libraries in
developing countries

www.elsevier.com • www.bookaid.org

Contents

Acknowledgments

Thanks are due to all the people who have helped in the research and writing of this book, in particular Bruce Davis of Global Consulting, Dominic Parry of Inspired Pharma Training Ltd, Allen Pfitzenmaier of Bryllan LLC, and Marianne Bock of ISPE. I am grateful to Anita Koch and Howell Angelo De Ramos of Elsevier for their patience and guidance. Special thanks to my coauthor, Janet Sanders, without whom this second edition would never have been written. Working on this project with her has been a delight. And finally, my thanks as always to Michael McCormick for advice, support, tea, and chocolate.

Kate McCormick

First of all, I must thank the folks at Elsevier for responding to my email and reaching out to Kate McCormick about my inquiry to write a follow-up to her original Quality book and for giving us the opportunity to write this book. Next, I must thank Kate for accepting my call and for trusting that I could deliver my promise to help update the content. It has been a pleasure coauthoring this book with her even though we are in different parts of the world. I must also thank my former and current department chairs at East Carolina University for helping me to expand my knowledge in the pharmaceutical area by requiring me to teach the courses, conduct research, and do industry outreach with local companies. I thank the pharmaceutical companies that I worked with for allowing me to share my expertise with them and for opening their doors to share their processes with me. Finally, I must thank my family for being so supportive. It was challenging to coauthor a book while working full-time and be a good wife and mother. I couldn't have completed this project without the support of my husband, Steve Hardy, and my wonderful children, AJ, Janae, and Jasmine.

Janet H. Sanders

Abbreviations

Abbreviation	Definition
AAPS	American Association of Pharmaceutical Scientists
ABS	Acrylonitrile butadiene styrene
ADME	Absorption, distribution, metabolism, and elimination
ADR	Adverse drug reaction
AERS	Adverse Event Reporting System
ANDA	Abbreviated New Drug Application
ANVISA	Brazilian Health Regulatory Agency
AP	Authorized person
API	Active pharmaceutical ingredient
APS	Aseptic process simulation
ASQ	American Society for Quality
BOD	Biological oxygen demand
BS	British Standard
C&E	Cause and effect
CA	Corrective action
CAPA	Corrective and preventive action
CBER	Center for Biologics Evaluation and Research
CBRNE	Chemical, biological, radiological, nuclear, and high-yield explosives
CDE	Center for Drug Evaluation (China)
CDER	Center for Drug Evaluation and Research
CEDI	Continuous electrodeionization
CEN	European Committee for Standardization
CFDA	China Food and Drug Administration
CFDI	Center for Food and Drug Inspection (China)
CFR	Code of Federal Regulations
CFU	Colony forming units
CGMP	Current good manufacturing practice
CHMP	Committee for Medicinal Products for Human Use (EMA)
CI	Continuous improvement
CIOMS	Council for International Organizations of Medical Sciences
CIP	Clean-in-place
COD	Chemical oxygen demand
COPQ	Cost of poor quality
COQ	Cost of quality
CPD	Continuing professional development
CPMP	Committee for Proprietary Medicinal Products
CPP	Critical process parameter
CQA	Critical quality attribute
CRO	Contract research organization

CT	Concentration x time
CTA	Clinical trial approval
CTC	Clinical trial certificate
CTN	Clinical trial notification
CTX	Clinical trial exemption
DFSS	Design for six sigma
DIA	Drug Information Association
DMADV	Define, measure, analyze, design, and verify/validate
DMAIC	Define, measure, analyze, improve, and control
DPMO	Defects per million opportunities
DQ	Design qualification
DSC	Differential scanning calorimetry
DTA	Differential thermal analysis
EC	European Commission
EDI	Electrodeionization
EDQM	European Directorate for the Quality of Medicines
EFPIA	European Federation of Pharmaceutical Industries and Associations
EFTA	European Free Trade Association
EIPG	European Industrial Pharmacists Group
EMA	European Medicines Agency
EMEA	European Medicines Evaluation Agency
EN	European Standards
ENCePP	European Network of Centres for Pharmacoepidemiology and Pharmacovigilance
ETO	Ethylene oxide
EU	European Union
EUA	Emergency Use Authorization
FD&C Act	Federal Food, Drug, and Cosmetic Act
FDA	Food and Drug Administration
FEFO	First expired, first out
FIH	First-in-human studies
FIM	First-in-man studies
FMEA	Failure mode and effects analysis
FSMA	Food Safety Modernization Act
GCLP	Good control laboratory practice
GCP	Good clinical practice
GDP	Good distribution practice
GLP	Good laboratory practice
GMP	Good manufacturing practice
GQP	Good quality practices (Japan)
GRP	Glass reinforced plastic
GSP	Good storage practice
HEPA	High Efficiency Particulate Air
HHS	Department of Health and Human Services
HPFB	Health Products and Food Branch (Canada)
HR	Human resources

ICH	International Council for Harmonisation of Technical Requirements for Pharmaceuticals for Human Use
ICMRA	International Coalition of Medicines Regulatory Authorities
IEC	Independent Ethics Committee
IFPMA	International Federation of Pharmaceutical Manufacturers and Associations
IMP	Investigational medicinal product
IND	Investigational new drug
IQ	Installation qualification
IRB	Institutional Review Board
ISO	International Organization for Standardization
ISoP	International Society of Pharmacovigilance
ISPE i	International Society for Pharmacoepidemiology
ISPE ii	International Society for Pharmaceutical Engineering
ITS	International Temperature Scale
JPMA	Japan Pharmaceutical Manufacturers Associations
JUSE	Union of Japanese Scientists and Engineers
K-T	Kepner-Tregoe
LCL	Lower control limit
LIMS	Laboratory Information Management System
LSS	Lean Six Sigma
LVP	Large volume parenteral
MD	Managing Director
MEP	Manufacturing Extension Partnership
MHLW	Ministry of Health, Labour and Welfare (Japan)
MHRA	Medicines and Healthcare products Regulatory Agency (United Kingdom)
MNC	Multinational company
MTD	Maximum tolerated dose
NCE	New chemical entity
NDA	New drug application
NDE	New drug entity
NDS	New drug submission (Canada)
NGT	Nominal group technique
NIFDC	National Institutes for Food and Drug Control (Japan)
NOAEL	No-observed-adverse-effect level
OECD	Organisation for Economic Co-operation and Development
OQ	Operational qualification
OTC	Over the counter
PA	Preventive action
PAFSC	Pharmaceutical Affairs and Food Sanitation Council (Japan)
PAL	Pharmaceutical Affairs Law (Japan)
PASS	Post-authorisation safety studies
PAT	Process analytical technology
PDCA	Plan-Do-Check-Act
PDSA	Plan-Do-Study-Act
PFSB	Pharmaceutical and Food Safety Bureau (Japan)
Ph. Eur.	European pharmacopoeia

PhRMA	Pharmaceutical Research and Manufacturers of America
PIC/S	Pharmaceutical Inspection Convention/Pharmaceutical Inspection Co-operation Scheme
PIL	Patient information leaflet
PMA	Pharmaceutical Manufacturers Association
PMD Act	Pharmaceuticals and Medical Devices Act (Japan)
PMDA	Pharmaceuticals and Medical Devices Agency (Japan)
POS	Potential operating space
PPQ	Process performance qualification
PQ	Performance qualification
PSI	Per square inch
PTFE	Polytetrafluoroethylene
PV	Process validation
PVC	Polyvinyl chloride
PVDF	Polyvinylidene fluoride
QA	Quality assurance
QbD	Quality by design
QC	Quality control
QMS	Quality management system
QP	Qualified person
QRM	Quality risk management
QTPP	Quality target product profile
R&D	Research and Development
RCA	Root cause analysis
RFS	Release for supply (Australia)
RO	Reverse osmosis
RP	Responsible person
RPN	Risk priority number
RTRT	Real-time release testing
SA	South Africa
SAHPRA	South African Health Products Regulatory Authority
SI	International System of Units
SIP	Steam-in-place
SMED	Single minute-exchange of die
SOP	Standard operating procedure
SPC	Statistical process control
SQC	Statistical quality control
SVP	Small volume parenteral
TC	Technical Committee
TGA i	Thermogravimetric analysis
TGA ii	Therapeutic Goods Administration (Australia)
TOC	Total organic carbon
TPD	Therapeutic Products Directorate (Canada)
TPS	Toyota Production System
TQM	Total quality management
UCL	Upper control limit

UMC	Uppsala Monitoring Centre
UNICEF	United Nations International Children's Emergency Fund
US	United States
US FDA	United States Food and Drug Administration
USP	United States pharmacopoeia
UV	Ultraviolet
VICH	Veterinary International Conference on Harmonization
VMP	Validation master plan
WECO	Western Electric Company
WFI	Water for injection(s)
WHO	World Health Organization
WHO-PIDM	WHO Program for International Drug Monitoring
WMA	World Medical Association

CHAPTER 1

Product life cycle

1.1 Introduction

Within the pharmaceutical industry, quality is the key issue to be addressed. Hence, so many regulations, guidelines, and controls are required. This volume deals with the quality from a broad perspective. It includes a review and discussion of domestic and international guidelines and regulations; international quality systems such as the ISO 9000 and ISO 14000 series of standards; generic quality approaches such as total quality management (TQM), the cost of quality (COQ), Lean Six Sigma (LSS), and corrective and preventive action (CAPA) which are applicable across all industries; industry-specific topics such as good clinical practice (GCP), good laboratory practice (GLP), and good manufacturing practice (GMP); and lesser discussed topics such as validation, calibration, technology transfer, and good distribution practice (GDP).

In this chapter, an overview of quality at all the stages of the pharmaceutical life cycle is presented. Quality considerations relating specifically to the drug development process, including GLP and GCP are discussed. Additionally, the mechanisms in place to ensure only pharmaceuticals of the appropriate quality are distributed to the patient, in Europe, Japan, and the United States, are discussed. Brief mention is made on the quality considerations relating to manufacturing, although GMP is a large enough topic to be covered in a standalone chapter (see Chapter 2). Similarly, the quality considerations relating to logistics and distribution are briefly reviewed in this chapter, but GDP is fully covered elsewhere (see Chapter 14).

1.2 The drug development process

Before a new drug can be marketed, there are several lengthy processes that must be completed, which may be described as the Drug Development Process. This section summarizes the processes, which are essentially the same in Europe, Canada, Japan, and the United States, and typically take between 8 and 10 years for a completely new molecule, although as the COVID-19 global pandemic has demonstrated, timescales can be greatly reduced by modifying the approach in an emergency. Fig. 1.1 shows the typical life cycle for drug development and approval.

The figure shows that the development of a pharmaceutical is a stepwise process and the typical period from discovery to patient use is several years; however, the time span could vary. The timeline from development to distribution could be a fraction of

Quality
DOI: https://doi.org/10.1016/B978-0-323-90815-3.00006-2

1

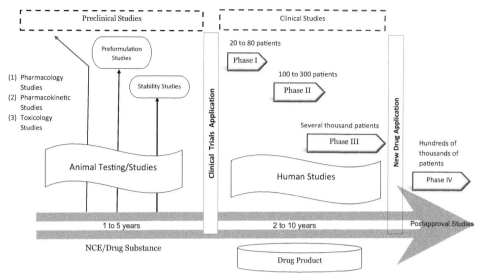

Figure 1.1 The drug development timeline.

the typical timeline when an emergency use declaration is enacted (see Section 1.5). This development process involves the evaluation of both animal and human efficacy as well as the safety of the product.

1.3 Preclinical studies

In the early development stage of the product cycle when a new chemical entity (NCE) is discovered, the NCE must undergo a series of clinical trials prior to being transformed into a drug product. These trials are typically described as preclinical research studies and are required worldwide by regulatory bodies. The goals of these studies include a characterization of toxic effects on target organs, dose dependence, and exposure limits. The information gained from these trials is used to help estimate initial ranges of safe starting doses for the human trials and to identify potential adverse effects that should be monitored during the clinical trials, because very few drugs can be said to cause no adverse reactions.

The three largest regions for drug development, that is, Europe, Japan, and the United States, have continuously worked together in an effort to unify the regulations for preclinical studies, which is published through the International Council for Harmonization (ICH) compendium of guidances. Prior to the ICH and modern general toxicology planning, it was not uncommon for a drug developer to primarily conduct acute to chronic GLP studies prior to entry into the clinical phase. In the United States, these preclinical studies are referred to as Investigational New Drug (IND) enabling studies. After the IND is submitted to the United States Food and Drug Administration (US FDA), the Sponsor must wait 30 calendar days before initiating any clinical trials.

Preclinical research includes pharmacological studies of the NCE and its effects on toxicity, carcinogenicity, mutagenicity, and reproductive development. The goal of the pharmacological studies is to get data on the safety and effectiveness of the NCE. These studies include an analysis the pharmacodynamics, pharmacokinetics, and toxicology. Pharmacodynamics focuses on the actions of the drug on the target, that is, the dose-response effect. Its studies measure the effects of a drug on some particular response, such as heart rate, enzyme levels, or muscle relaxation/contraction. In contrast, pharmacokinetics focuses on the actions of the body on the drug. Toxicology focuses on the safety aspects of the potential drug.

1.3.1 Pharmacodynamic/Pharmacology studies

The pharmacodynamic studies may include a battery of screening tests of the NCE to determine its effects on various physiological systems in animals. These studies may be conducted as part of the safety pharmacology studies. The safety pharmacology studies investigate the potential and undesirable pharmacodynamic effects on the physiological functions of vital organs, such as the cardiovascular, respiratory, and central nervous systems. Both *in vitro* and *in vivo* methods are used to determine whether the NCE has the potential to cause serious harm. *In vitro* testing is done in a lab using a glass (or plastic) vessel, tube, or dish. The *in vitro* evaluation is typically followed by *in vivo* testing. *In vivo* is done in the body of a living organism such as plants, animals, or humans. Safety pharmacology studies may not be needed for dermal or ocular agents or where the pharmacology of the NCE is well characterized and where systemic exposure or distribution to other organs or tissues is low.

1.3.2 Pharmacokinetic studies

As part of the process of finalizing the dosage form, it is necessary to carry out pharmacokinetic studies to ensure a sufficient concentration of the drug reaches the part of the body where it is required and is maintained at the right concentration for the right period of time. Pharmacokinetics includes identification of the appropriate dosage levels and frequency. This study of how the human body deals with the drug after it has been administered and the transportation of the drug to the correct body part is expressed as the kinetics of absorption, distribution, metabolism, and elimination (ADME). The ADME terms are defined as follows:

- **Absorption:** The way in which the drug enters the body and reaches the bloodstream. The concentration of the drug in the bloodstream over time is affected by the method in which the drug is administered, that is, oral, rectal, intramuscular, transdermal or topical, inhalation, or intravenous. The amount of drug reaching the bloodstream, and the speed at which it takes place is called its *bioavailability*.

- **Distribution:** The way in which the drug travels through the body and is distributed to various tissues in the body.
- **Metabolism:** The way in which the drug is changed by the body.
- **Elimination (Excretion):** The way in which the drug leaves the body. Drugs are excreted from the body by the kidneys, lungs, intestine and colon, or the skin.

1.3.3 Toxicology studies

Toxicology studies are typically initiated after the completion of the pharmacology and pharmacokinetic studies. The toxicological investigation focuses on the safety aspects of the potential drug. The global effort to standardize preclinical toxicology programs began in the 1990s. The ultimate goal of toxicology studies is to translate animal responses to a drug into an understanding of the risk to humans. Even after a successful drug candidate for a disease or illness is identified, it still faces challenges. Many drugs fail in this stage of drug development because of their unacceptable toxicity. Furthermore, safety issues are the leading cause of failure at all stages of the drug development process.

A judgment must be made as to whether the benefits of a drug outweigh the potential side effects. Therefore, depending on the type of drug, several different types of toxicology studies must be conducted. These studies (categorized by the duration of exposure) may include some or all of the following:

- **Acute (Single Dose) toxicity:** Studies are conducted to evaluate the acute effects, defined as those occurring rapidly. These studies determine the short-term adverse (or unintended) effects of a drug when administered in a single dose during a 24-hour period. A single dose or multiple doses are administered for up to 2 weeks in two mammalian species (one rodent and one nonrodent) to determine the maximum tolerated dose (MTD) that will result in mortality (death) or morbidity (illness). In Japan, a 4-week rodent trial may be required. The results from this study could be useful to predict the consequences of human overdose.
- **Subacute (Repeated Dose) toxicity:** Studies are conducted to evaluate a drug's potential adverse effects following a treatment period from 2 to 4 weeks. These studies help to determine if the drug is tolerable at multiples of a potential clinically relevant dose. Since the drug is administered over a longer dose period, the studies help to further develop the MTD toxicity profile and determine the no-observed-adverse-effect level (NOAEL). The NOAEL implies the effects are considered not to be a side effect, are not biologically relevant, and/or are within estimations of background historical data.
- **Subchronic toxicity:** Studies are conducted over 13 weeks (90 days) with rodents, from 20 to 25 animals per sex. Nonrodents may also be tested. These studies build on the toxicological data obtained thus far and provide toxicological and toxicokinetic data for longer exposure periods.

- **Chronic (Cumulative toxicity) toxicity:** Studies are conducted from 6 to 12 months in a rodent and nonrodent to evaluate the same toxicological parameters monitored in the 13-week study, but over a longer period of time.
- **Genotoxicity:** Studies are conducted to detect compounds that induce genetic damage directly or indirectly by various mechanisms. The recommended tests include a test for gene mutation (mutagenic toxicity) in bacteria (Ames test), an *in vitro* test with cytogenetic evaluation of chromosomal damage with mammalian cells or an *in vitro* mouse lymphoma TK assay and an *in vivo* test for chromosomal damage using rodent hematopoietic cells.
- **Carcinogenicity studies:** These studies are recommended for NCEs if there is concern about the carcinogenic potential of the drug or if it will be used in the treatment of chronic or recurrent conditions. These studies are not required until registration, for postapproval commitment, or not at all.
- **Reproductive toxicity:** Studies are conducted to evaluate the occurrence, causes, manifestations, and ramifications of adverse effects of exogenous agents on fertility or reproduction. The studies should be conducted as is appropriate for the female and/or male population to be exposed to the NCE.

This stage of the drug development process can take several years and must be completed before a company can obtain approval to carry out clinical studies. The duration of these tests may change in response to Phase I or II testing requirements, reference ICH M3, ICH S4A, and ICH S6(R1).

1.3.4 Preformulation studies

These studies constitute an important part of early chemical and pharmaceutical drug development activities as they evaluate the physical and chemical properties of the drug prior to the compounding process. The primary objective of the preformulation phase is to lay the foundation for transforming the new drug entity (NDE) into a pharmaceutical formulation that can be administered correctly, in the correct amount, and that hits the correct targets. Another objective of the studies conducted in this phase is to identify the long-term stability of the formulation and to evaluate its performance. Additionally, these studies are conducted to determine the physicochemical characteristics of the molecule and the most appropriate dosage forms that can be used. The studies will include some or all of the following evaluations of the physical characteristics and pharmaceutical properties of the NDE:

- **Solubility:** The amount of the drug that dissolves in a given solvent to produce a saturated solution at constant temperature and pressure. A drug's solubility is determined by the physical properties such as its crystalline characteristics, temperature, pH, complexation, and molecular structure.
- **Crystallinity:** Characterized by regular repetitious spacing of atoms and molecules in a three-dimensional structure. This form is very stable.

- **Polymorphism:** Amorphous form characterized by randomly formed atoms and molecules. This form has higher solubility and dissolution rates in comparison to the crystalline forms.
- **Particle size characterization:** Particle size may affect a drug's formulation and product efficacy including the drug dissolution rate, content uniformity, solubility, bioavailability, texture, stability, flow characteristics, and sedimentation rates.
- **Hygroscopicity (hydrolysis):** Refers to the drug's tendency to absorb atmospheric moisture, also known as water absorption.
- **Oxidation:** Refers to the exposure of a molecule to atmospheric oxygen. Oxidation can also be initiated by the presence of light or elevated temperatures. Oxidation can be controlled by avoiding exposure to lights and storage at controlled temperatures.
- **Photolysis:** Refers to the decomposition of a molecule due to exposure to light. Exposure to light may lead to photodegradation and may trigger oxidation.
- **Density:** A measure of the ratio of mass of a substance to its volume. It greatly depends on the particle size distribution and shape. Low density can make capsule and tablet formulations difficult. It can also affect homogeneity in the formulation.
- **Thermal analysis:** Measures the heat gain or loss, as a function of temperature, which results from physical or chemical changes within a sample. Differential thermal analysis, differential scanning calorimetry, or thermogravimetric analysis may be used to detect the changes.
- **Powder flow properties:** Efficient flow of the drug substance powder is important for effective tablet formulation. The flow properties can be affected by changes in particle size and shape, density, and absorbed moisture and may affect processing and formulation.
- **Solubility analysis:** Refers to the amount of drug that dissolves in various solvents to produce a saturated solution at constant temperature and pressure. The solubility level is typically described as a range from very soluble to practically insoluble.

Once the preformulation studies have been completed, the foundation has been established for the transformation of the NCE into a safe, effective, and stable pharmaceutical formulation.

1.3.5 Stability studies

Preclinical studies of the final dosage form will extend to include stability studies. Stability studies typically start at the preclinical stage of drug development but continue through Phases I, II, and III clinical trials. According to the FDA and ICH guidance, the purpose of stability testing is to:

1. provide evidence on how the quality of a drug product or new drug formulation may vary with time under the influence of environmental factors such as temperature, humidity, and light;

2. to establish a retest period for the drug substance or shelf life for the drug product;

3. to determine the recommended storage conditions.

The ICH codes for these guidelines are as follows: Q1A, Q1B, Q1C, Q1D, Q1E, Q1F, Q5C, Q6A, and Q6B (https://www.ema.europa.eu/en/ich-q1a-r2-stability-testing-new-drug-substances-drug-products). Originally these guidelines only addressed climatic Zones I and II of the four kinetic temperature climatic Zones I, II, III, and IV (The kinetic temperature in any part of the world between Zones I to IV.) and only covered new drug formulations and products. In 1996 the World Health Organization (WHO) modified the guidelines to also address the extreme climatic conditions found in many countries and to cover established products in circulation in the WHO umbrella countries. The choice of test conditions defined in the guidance is based on an analysis of the effects of climatic conditions in the European Union, the United States, and Japan.

The types of stability studies include the following:

- **Physical stability:** These studies determine if the original physical properties such as appearance, color, dissolution, palatability, or suspendability are retained. The uniformity and release rate of the substance may be affected by its physical stability which could then affect the efficacy and safety of the product.
- **Chemical stability:** These studies evaluate the tendency of the drug substance to resist change or decomposition due to reactions caused by environmental factors like air, atmosphere, temperature, and moisture.
- **Microbiological stability:** These studies evaluate the tendency of the drug substance to resist microbiological changes, that is, growth of microorganisms, and ability of the antimicrobial agents used in the preparation to retain their effectiveness within the specified limits.
- **Therapeutic stability:** These studies evaluate whether the therapeutic effect of the drug product changes.
- **Toxicological stability:** These studies evaluate whether there is significant increase in the toxicity of the drug substance or not.

1.3.5.1 Stability testing methods

As indicated by the FDA, ICH, and WHO guidance, one of the primary purposes of stability testing is to provide assurance that the drug product will remain at an acceptable level of fitness and quality throughout the period for which the product is on the market and is available for supply to the patients. Additionally, the testing will determine if the drug product will be fit for consumption until the patient uses the last unit of the product. The stability testing procedures typically fall under the following four types:

1. Real-time stability testing: This testing is normally performed for a longer duration of the test period to allow for significant product degradation under the recommended storage conditions. Depending on the stability of the product, the test period should be long enough to clearly indicate if measurable degradation occurs. The length of the test period should also permit the ability to distinguish degradation from interassay variation. Data must be collected during the test period such that trend analysis can be conducted to distinguish instability from day-to-day ambiguity.

2. **Accelerated stability testing:** For this testing, the drug substance is stressed at several high temperatures warmer than the ambient temperature to determine the amount of heat required to cause product failure. To enhance statistical integrity, four different stress temperatures are recommended for this study. The other stress conditions included with this testing are light, moisture, agitation, pH, and gravity. With this testing, the product is subjected to stress, refrigerated after stressing, and then assayed concurrently. Since the duration of this testing is short, the likelihood of instability in the measurement system is reduced in comparison to the real-time study.

3. **Cyclic temperature stress testing:** This testing is conducted to mimic the likely conditions in the marketplace. The recommended minimum and maximum test temperatures are determined for each specific product according to the recommended storage temperature and the physical degradation properties of the product. The period of each cycle is typically 24 hours, simulating the 24-hour daily rhythm on the earth. The recommended number of cycles is 20.

4. **Retained sample stability testing:** This testing is typical for every marketed product for which stability data are required. When the product is first introduced to the market, samples from at least one batch per year are retained for storage. The number of samples can be decreased at a later stage. These samples, which help to predict the shelf life of the product, are periodically tested to determine the amount of degradation. From 2% to 5% degradation is allowed. For example, for a product with a 5-year shelf life, the conventional test intervals are the 3rd, 6th, 12th, 24th, 36th, 48th, and 60th month. Any changes in the product's physical, chemical, and microbial composition are noted and compared with the regulated permissible levels.

1.3.5.2 Stability study (guidance) protocol

In an attempt to reduce healthcare costs globally and to help accelerate drug development, different regulatory agencies began working collectively over the last decades. In the 1990s representatives from regulatory agencies in the United States, Europe, and Japan in collaboration with associated industries developed The International Conference on Harmonization of Technical Requirements for Registration of Pharmaceuticals for Human Use (https://www.ich.org/). One of the initial goals of ICH was to harmonize some of the regulatory and scientific requirements for these countries. Additionally, ICH made significant strides toward harmonizing key aspects of the drug development process by providing harmonized guidelines for safety, quality, and efficacy. It also provided recommendations for the amount of preclinical toxicity testing required to support clinical trials and market registration for a new drug. In 2015 the council changed its name to the ICH and became recognized as an independent legal entity under Swiss law. The organization has continued to evolve over the years and has changed its governance structure. It has also started new initiatives and increased its international outreach.

The stability protocols, as recommended by the WHO, FDA, and ICH, contain written guidance and key instructions for the regulation of well-controlled stability studies. Since the testing condition is based on the stability of the drug substance and drug product, the type of dosage form, and the proposed container-closure system, the protocol may differ by product. Additionally, the specific protocol depends upon whether the product is new or if it is already in the market. Up to this point in the text, the terms drug product and drug substance have been used interchangeably; however, there is a distinction between the two and they are addressed separately in the guidance. The *drug substance* refers to the unformulated active pharmaceutical ingredient (API). The therapeutic effect in the body is due to the API. On the other hand, the *drug product* is the formulated drug substance along with excipients. Excipients assist with the delivery of the API. Conversely, the *drug product* typically refers to the final marketed dosage form of the drug substance, that is, tablet, capsule, or liquid. Although the categories and criteria are nearly identical, the guidance contains dedicated protocols for a drug substance and a drug product. For a drug substance, the recommended study protocol for a well-designed stability should include the following informations:

1. **General:** This states the information on the stability of the drug substance is an integral part of the systematic approach to stability evaluation.

2. **Stress testing:** Focuses on stress testing of the drug substance to help identify the likely degradation products which in turn can help establish the degradation pathways and the intrinsic stability of the molecules. The tests will also validate the stability-indicating power of the analytical procedures used. The nature of stress testing will be determined by the individual drug substance and the type of drug product involved. Stress testing is typically completed on a single batch of the drug substance. The testing should include an analysis of the effect of temperature, humidity, oxidation, and photolysis on the drug substance.

3. **Selection of batches:** States that data from formal stability studies should be provided from at least three primary batches of the drug substance. The batches should be manufactured to a minimum of pilot-scale production and by the same routes as for full-scale production batches. Additionally, the method of manufacture and procedures must simulate the final process used for full-scale production batches, and the overall quality of batches should be the representative of the quality of the material produced at full-scale production.

4. **Container–closure system:** States that the stability studies should be conducted on the drug substance packaged in a container-closure system that is the same or similar to the packaging proposed for storage and distribution.

5. **Specification:** Focuses on the list of tests, references to analytical procedures, and proposed acceptance criteria as addressed in ICH Q3A, Q6A, and Q6B. The studies should include testing of the attributes of the drug product that are susceptible to change during storage and will likely influence the quality, safety, and/or efficacy. The testing should also cover, as appropriate, the physical, chemical, biological, and microbiological attributes.

6. **Testing frequency:** Focuses on the test frequency relative to the type of storage conditions. For drug substances with a proposed retest period of at least 12 months, the frequency of testing at the long-term storage condition should be every 3 months over the first year, every 6 months over the second year, and annually for the remainder of the test period. At accelerated storage conditions, at least three time points must be conducted, including the initial and final time periods, that is, 0, 3, and 6 months.

7. **Storage conditions:** This criterion states that the drug substance should be evaluated under the storage conditions that test its thermal stability and, if applicable, its sensitivity to moisture. The storage conditions and the length of the studies should be sufficient to cover the storage, shipment, and subsequent use relative to the climate Zone(s) in which the active substance will be stored.

8. **Stability commitment:** Focuses on the commitment to continue stability studies postapproval when available long-term stability data on primary batches do not cover the proposed retest period granted at the time of approval. A postapproval commitment is not necessary if the submission includes long-term stability data on three production batches that cover the proposed retest period. If this condition is not met, a commitment for additional stability studies should be made as outlined in the guidance.

9. **Evaluation:** Focuses on the evaluation and analysis of the stability information used to determine a retest period for all future batches of the drug substance manufactured under similar circumstances. The stability information includes, as appropriate, results of the physical, chemical, biological, and microbiological tests based on the testing of a minimum of three batches of the drug substance. The degree of variability of individual batches affects the confidence that a future production batch will remain within specification throughout the assigned retest period. Evaluation of the data should show so little degradation and so little variability that it is apparent that the requested retest period will be granted. If the degree of variability is minimal, it is normally unnecessary to go through formal statistical analysis as provided in the guidance.

10. **Statements/labeling:** Focuses on the storage statement that should be established for labeling in accordance with relevant national and/or regional requirements. The statement should be based on the stability evaluation of the drug substance. Specific instructions, where applicable, should be provided for drug substances that cannot tolerate freezing. Additionally, statements such as "ambient conditions" or "room temperature" should be avoided.

Stability studies of pharmaceutical products serve a key contribution to the drug development life cycle. Data from these studies demonstrate whether any physical, chemical, or microbiological changes affect the efficacy or integrity of a pharmaceutical product. These studies also help determine the recommended storage conditions and shelf life ensuring the medicine is safe and effective throughout its shelf life.

1.4 Clinical studies

Assuming the preclinical studies, particularly the toxicological tests, have produced acceptable results, the company will seek permission from the appropriate regulatory body to carry out clinical studies (also called clinical trials). The requirements and documentation for clinical trials differ by country. In the United States, this permission is requested by means of an IND application. In Europe the application is known as a Clinical Trial Approval (CTA) formally known as the Clinical Trial Exemption (CTX). The change was approved in April 2014 and went into effect in 2019. The new regulation replaced the directive 2001/20/EC. Australia uses the Clinical Trial Notification (CTN) and CTX. Singapore requests permission with a clinical trial certificate. Irrespective of the country, the application contains all the data accumulated from the preclinical studies, detailed information about the procedures used to manufacture the drug substance, and the methods used to assure quality.

In Japan, approval for clinical trials is requested by way of a CTN; however, the applicant must consult with the Pharmaceuticals and Medical Devices Agency (PMDA) prior to submitting the CTN. The initial CTN is approved, by default, within 30 days and 14 days for any subsequent CTN. If PMDA does not raise any concerns or request additional information, the clinical trials can begin.

In China, the length of time needed to start a clinical trial is significantly longer than it is for the United States. China's clinical trial requirements are determined by the drug category, that is, between Categories 1 to 6. The applicant must submit a CTA dossier to the China Food and Drug Administration (CFDA). Additionally, reviews must be conducted by the Center for Drug Evaluation (CDE), the Center for Food and Drug Inspection (CFDI), and the National Institutes for Food and Drug Control (NIFDC). The entire review and approval process generally take 18 months, which makes it difficult for China to join multinational clinical trials.

The clinical studies team includes doctors, nurses, and other healthcare professionals. Prior to beginning the trial, the team will conduct a verbal or written assessment and check the health of the participants to determine if they are eligible to participate. Patients who are found eligible and who agree to participate in the trials are given specific instructions, are monitored, and carefully assessed during and after completion of the trial. The studies are conducted at hospitals and research centers around the world and are generally carried out in three or four phases.

1.4.1 Phase I

Phase 1 trials are sometimes called "first-in-human studies" (FIH) or "first-in-man studies" (FIM). The primary objective of the studies is to estimate tolerability of the drug substance in humans and to characterize pharmacokinetics and pharmacodynamics. Additional goals of the trials are to determine the drug dosage, document how the drug is metabolized and excreted, identify acute side effects and evaluate the toxicity profile. Typically, a small number of healthy volunteers (between 20 and 80) are tested in Phase 1 trials. Some companies conduct this trial in two phases: 1A and 1B.

For cancer research, different models for conducting the Phase 1 trials exist; however, most of the trials begin with the administration of a small single dose of the study drug to a small number (usually three) of patients. This first dose is no more than

1/10th of the highest dose associated with no adverse effects. If no specified level of toxicity is observed, the next predefined higher dose level or double the initial dose is tested. Until unacceptable toxicity is encountered or a dose has reached the reasonable expected maximal efficacy, the doses can be doubled repeatedly. If during the escalation of doses an unacceptable toxicity is observed, the dose escalation is terminated, and the level at termination or the previous dose is declared the MTD. This phase of testing typically take from 3 to 6 months.

For companies that adopt the Phase 1A and 1B approach, the Phase 1B trials are conducted after a successful evaluation of the Phase 1A results. In the 1B trials a multiple-dose study is conducted. These trials are similar to the single-dose ascending study. 12 patients are typically evaluated—four of them will receive a placebo. The starting dose is typically equal to the highest well-tolerated dose from the single-dose study. The dose may be administered all at once on a given day or it may be divided into lower doses and administered at intervals during a given day. At the end of the study, the multiple-dose tolerance should be compared to the levels from the efficacy study in animals to determine if the maximum tolerated levels in humans achieve the blood levels associated with efficacy in animals. The Phase 1B trials typically take from 3 to 9 months to complete. After the dose and range of doses is determined, the next phase, Phase II, will evaluate if the drug has a biological effect on humans.

1.4.2 Phase II

The emphasis for Phase I trials was safety. The emphasis for Phase II trials is effectiveness. The primary objectives of these trials are as follows:
- to evaluate the drug's beneficial effects (efficacy),
- to evaluate how well the drug works at the recommended dose,
- to identify the extent of any adverse reactions or side effects,
- to develop and refine research methods for future trials with the drug.

Similar to Phase I, Phase II can be classified as IIA and IIB studies, particularly when there is no existing standard therapy for comparison. For the Phase IIA study, the drug may be used only as a single high dose, at the MTD, to determine whether the drug has anti-disease activity that warrants further investigation. Phase IIB studies will measure the drug's effectiveness and, where applicable, will include a comparison with at least one standard treatment. Several dose levels may be tested to determine the minimally effective and optimal dose relative to efficacy and safety. Depending on the drug being studied, this phase may take several months to several years (typically from 2 to 3 years) to complete.

These trials are larger and include from 100 to 300 patients who have the disease or condition that the product could potentially treat. The patients are randomly assigned into two groups—the control group and the trial group. The control group will be given either a standard treatment for the illness or, where permitted, an inactive pill, liquid, or powder that has no treatment value, called a placebo. For some studies, the control group will receive only a placebo. The trial group will receive the drug being tested. The control group provides a basis of comparison for assessing the effects of the test treatment.

The participants are assigned to the two groups by a process of *randomization*. Typically done by computer, this is a scientific method of assigning patients to different groups in a trial so that they are equally likely to be assigned to either group without bias, preferences, or other irrelevant factors. Also, randomization helps to ensure the results of the trial provide clear answers about the intervention drug being tested. The randomized groups are sometimes referred to as *arms*. In conjunction with randomization, a concept called blinding is used to ensure the patients appear identical and no one—neither doctor nor patient—can tell whether the patient is receiving the active drug or the placebo. Blinding also helps ensure bias does not distort the conduct of the trial or the interpretation of the results. The two types of blinding are as follows:

1. **Single-blind trial:** The patients do not know whether they are receiving the experimental drug, an established treatment, or a placebo; however, the clinical studies team will know which group the patient has been assigned to.
2. **Double-blind trial:** Neither the patient nor the clinical studies team knows during the trial whether the trial drug or a placebo has been administered. The patient's

doctor will be issued a computer-coded treatment pack and usually at a prespecified time during the trial, the patients will find out whether they received the test drug or the placebo.

If Phase II trials indicate the drug appears to be effective and the risks are considered acceptable relative to the observed efficacy and the severity of the disease, the drug will move forward to a long-term Phase III study for confirmatory testing of its long-term effectiveness.

1.4.3 Phase III

After preliminary evidence from Phases I and II studies support the safety and effectiveness of the drug, Phase III trials are conducted to gather additional information about the overall benefit-to-risk relationship of the drug for possible use as a new standard of treatment. Phase III trials can involve several thousands of patients with the disease and will compare the new intervention that has shown promise in Phase II trials with an existing intervention, if one is already available, or to a placebo. The large number of patients is needed to ensure detection of less frequently arising drug-related toxicities, to reveal less common side effects, and to acquire more confidence of the drug's efficacy. The trial results can also be used to provide a basis for the pack insert or drug label.

Most Phase III drug trials are conducted as randomized, double blind, and placebo-controlled studies. These clinical studies are frequently the definitive trials for providing evidence for or against a new experimental therapy and well-conducted studies are a cornerstone for gaining drug approval. The large size of these trials makes them the costliest studies for the evaluation of a new drug. This phase can last for several years—typically from 3 to 5 years.

After the Phases I, II, and III, clinical trials have been completed with acceptable results, the company may submit their application for a marketing license for the drug in question.

1.4.4 Phase IV

Phase IV trials are conducted, if required, after the drug has been licensed by the regulatory body and is on the market. The trials involve hundreds of thousands of patients and are sometimes required as a condition of licensing a new treatment. The goals of the trials are to monitor the drug's effectiveness and safety in large, diverse populations, including children. The trials should also provide additional information about the treatment's long-term risks, benefits, and optimal use; its side effects and frequency of side effects; its implications of intervention; its new uses for the intervention; and its cost effectiveness. These studies may include mail-in questionnaires and personal interviews.

1.5 Emergency use authorization

In 2004, the US congress passed the Project BioShield Act to accelerate the research, development, purchase, and availability of effective medical products against chemical, biological, radiological, nuclear, and high yield explosive (CBRNE) agents. This act provided the government with the authority and funding to develop, acquire, stockpile, and distribute the medical products needed to protect the United States against weapons of mass destruction. One of the provisions of the Project BioShield Act was authority to temporarily use medical countermeasures under the Emergency Use Authorization (EUA) authority (https://www.fda.gov/emergency-preparedness-and-response/mcm-legal-regulatory-and-policy-framework/emergency-use-authorization). The act provides authority and implementation with the Secretary of the Department of Health and Human Services (HHS) and the agencies within HHS. The HHS Secretary may issue an EUA during military, domestic, or public health emergencies, significant potential emergency, or following the identification of a material threat sufficient to affect national security. These provisions allow the HHS Secretary to temporarily allow the use of medical products that the FDA has not approved or licensed.

The EUA permits the use of unapproved medical products like drugs, biologics, and vaccines or the use of approved medical products in unapproved ways to diagnose, treat, or prevent serious diseases. This provision was used for the expedited development and distribution of the SARS-CoV-2 tests, therapeutic agents for treatment for COVID-19, and for the CIVID-19 vaccine. On February 4, 2020, the FDA issued a directive, "Policy for Diagnostics Testing in Laboratories Certified to Perform High-Complexity Testing Under CLIA prior to Emergency Use Authorization for Coronavirus Disease-2019 during the Public Health Emergency." This document provided guidance for testing laboratories that were developing SARS-CoV-2 tests for submission for emergency use authorization. On March 27, 2020, the HHS Secretary declared circumstances existed to justify the authorization of emergency use of drugs and biologics during the 2019 coronavirus disease outbreak. Several drugs—that is, Chloroquine phosphate, hydroxychloroquine sulfate, remdesivir, and peramivir—and several vaccines were approved under this provision.

The EU also has a process for emergency use called *compassionate use*. The European Medicines Agency (EMA) provides recommendations for compassionate use through the Committee for Medicinal Products for Human Use (CHMP), but the recommendations do not create a legal framework (https://www.ema.europa.eu/en/human-regulatory/research-development/compassionate-use). The CHMP plays a vital role in the authorization of medicines in the European Union. Additionally, the committee evaluates medicines authorized at a national level and referred to the EMA for a harmonized position across the European Union (EU) and it contributes to the development of medicines and medicine regulation. Compassionate use programs are coordinated and implemented by the member states, who set their own rules and procedures. The programs are only established if the medicine is expected to help patients with life-threatening, long-lasting, or seriously debilitating illnesses which cannot be treated satisfactorily with any currently authorized medicine. The compassionate use authorization was used during the 2019 COVID-19 pandemic to approve drugs and vaccines.

Other countries, for example, Japan, Canada, and several African nations, also granted emergency authorization for the use of various drugs for treatment of COVID-19 according to their respective processes.

1.6 New drug registration process

Once a company has completed all the preclinical and clinical studies, the dossier is submitted for evaluation. Typically, when a multinational company considers bringing a new drug to the market, the company initially pursues a common regulatory strategy for the United States and Europe because they represent the largest markets. Subsequently, they may pursue other countries such as Australia, Canada, New Zealand, South Africa, and Switzerland because these countries use a dossier similar to the one used by the United States and Europe. Conversely, Japan, China, India, and South Korea typically require applicants for a new drug that include data from clinical trials conducted on subjects in their country's population. All data are reviewed, including the adverse reactions that have been observed, so a benefit-to-risk assessment can be made. It is accepted no drug is without some risk, but that risk must be balanced against the potential benefits. As part of the review process, the key studies are identified, and field inspections are made of the investigators who carried out those studies to ensure the validity of the data.

1.6.1 Drug registration in the European Union

In the European Union, all medicines must be authorized before they can be placed on the market and made available to patients. There are four routes for drug registration, which were established in 1995: the centralized procedure or three options for national authorization. The drug applicant typically chooses the registration pathway from 12 to 18 months prior to submitting an application. The pathway chosen will reflect the characteristics of the product and the organization's business strategy.

1.6.1.1 Regulatory framework

The regulation of pharmaceuticals falls within the responsibility of the Enterprise and Industry Directorate General of the European Commission. It has three aims, which are: to ensure a high level of protection of public health; to bring about a single market in pharmaceuticals; and to foster a stable and predictable environment for pharmaceutical innovation. Its areas of responsibility include drafting new legislation and ensuring it is satisfactorily implemented. It facilitates the decision-making process of the Commission by drafting decisions and advising on the procedure. It also provides support to the pharmaceutical industry, with particular emphasis on innovation and competition.

The first piece of legislation was Directive 65/65/EEC. This was followed 10 years later by two further directives (75/318/EEC and 75/319/EEC) which developed the concept of mutual recognition of marketing authorizations across the member states; and set up the Committee for Proprietary Medicinal Products (CPMP), with the responsibility for ensuring products complied with the original 1965 directive. All three directives were superseded by 2001/83/EC, which was amended over the years and finally consolidated on July 26, 2019 (https://eur-lex.europa.eu/eli/dir/2001/83/2019-07-26).

Other significant pieces of legislation include Directive 89/105/EEC, relating to regulation and transparency of prices, profits and rereimbursement, and Council Regulation EEC/1768/92 (superseded by Regulation (EC) No. 469/2009 and consolidated on July 1, 2019) (https://eur-lex.europa.eu/eli/reg/2009/469/2019-07-01) that permits the extension of a patent to compensate for the time lost during the marketing authorization process.

1.6.1.2 European Medicines Agency

The European Medicines Agency (EMA), formally known as the European Agency for the Evaluation of Medicinal Products or the European Medicines Evaluation Agency (EMEA), is responsible for the scientific evaluation, supervision, and safety monitoring of medicines in the European Union.

EMA is a scientific body that advises individual member states and other bodies within the EU and uses a network of scientists from across the EU to facilitate the operation of the evaluation system. It has responsibility for the procedures to authorize pharmaceuticals, monitor them once in the marketplace, and withdraw that authorization if there is evidence of a problem. EMA also operates information sources and electronic communication to enhance the safe use of pharmaceuticals within the European Union. The CPMP is one of the arms of the EMA.

The main responsibilities of the EMA are as follows:
- To protect and promote public health by providing safe and effective medicines for human and veterinary use.
- To give patients quick access to innovative new therapies.
- To facilitate the free movement of pharmaceutical products throughout the European Union.
- To improve information for patients and professionals on the correct use of medicinal products, to improve animal health.
- To protect consumers of animal products and harmonize scientific requirements in order to optimize pharmaceutical research worldwide.

1.6.1.3 The centralized procedure

The centralized procedure is the compulsory route for the authorization of biotechnology-derived products and most innovative or high technology products. After all the relevant information from laboratory tests and clinical trials have been collected, the Scientific Committees of the EMA conduct a comprehensive evaluation of the data and provide independent recommendations on medicines for human use.

In summary, an application via the centralized procedure is assessed by the CPMP, which recommends a decision, to be taken by the Commission. Prior to the application being assessed, a CPMP rapporteur is appointed. The rapporteur maintains the role of liaison between the company and the regulatory authorities, even after the marketing authorization is granted. There are time limits for each stage of the application. The time permitted for the CPMP assessment is 210 days. However, allowing for clock stops while the applicant is responding to queries, the whole process can take more than a year from the start of primary evaluation. An overview of this process is shown in Fig. 1.2.

Presubmission	At least 210 days
Validation	13 working days
Primary evaluation	120 days
Clock stops pending response by applicant to queries	Up to 90 days
Secondary evaluation	60 days
Clock stops pending response by applicant to queries	Up to 30 days
Final evaluation	30 days
Opinion/decision	67 days

Figure 1.2 Timeline for the centralized procedure.

If EMA determines the benefits outweigh the risks, it will give the green light and recommend to the European Commission that the medicine can be marketed across the EU and in the European Economic Area.

1.6.1.4 Decentralized procedure

Most drug applications do not fall within the requirements of the centralized procedure and will be authorized by individual national agencies. When an application is made to more than one member state at the same time, the first member state to agree to evaluate the application becomes the reference member state. Applications in the other (concerned) member states are then suspended pending the outcome of the initial evaluation. Once the evaluation is completed, the report is forwarded to the concerned member states who will either agree with the conclusions or ask supplementary questions. Once all questions are resolved, the individual agencies issue marketing authorization for their respective countries.

1.6.1.5 The mutual recognition procedure

The mutual recognition procedure applies to any product to be marketed in a member state other than the one in which it was originally authorized. The original member state becomes the reference member state.

1.6.1.6 National authorization

This procedure applies when a company makes a single application to just one member state.

1.6.1.7 Control of printed packaging materials

In 1992, Directive 92/27/EEC was issued relating to the information provided on printed packaging materials, specifically labeling and packaging leaflets. It was superseded in 2001 by Directive 2001/83/EC, which was amended over the years and finally consolidated on July 26, 2019. It defines the information that must be available on the outer packaging of a pharmaceutical for the benefit of the patient.

A patient information leaflet is required for all products. It carries a summary of the product characteristics and any contra-indications.

Both the packaging leaflet and the label must be understandable to the patient as well as the doctor and/or pharmacist. The information must be printed in the language of the country in which it is being marketed. It is for this reason that many companies have national or regional packaging operations, even if they have a centralized factory for manufacturing the bulk product. In a tableting operation, for example, where the finished pack is to be distributed across the European Union, the product may be completely undifferentiated up to the point of compression, but the bulk tablets will then be filled into a variety of different packs, depending on the final destination.

1.6.1.8 Control of advertising

Also, in 1992, Directive 92/28/EEC was issued which controls the advertising of pharmaceuticals across member states. This was superseded in 2001 by 2001/83/EC, which was amended over the years and finally consolidated on July 26, 2019. There are two types of advertising permitted. For products available over the counter (OTC), advertising is permitted to the general public and hence all the normal advertising channels are available. Examples of these are the many advertisements seen on television for cough and cold remedies, particularly during the winter season.

For medicines that are only available on prescription, those which have a psychotropic or narcotic content, where the product is eligible for rereimbursement, or for certain specific therapeutic indications, advertising is only permitted to doctors and pharmacists. This is the reason why an advertisement for a novel anticancer treatment would not appear on television but might be found in professional journals or in the advertising literature provided by medical representatives.

1.6.2 Drug registration in the United States

In the United States, the regulation and control of new drugs is based on a NDA. Since 1938, the NDA process has been used for every new drug. The drug must have an approved NDA before US commercialization. The NDA application is the method through which drug sponsors formally seek approval from the FDA for a new pharmaceutical for sale or marketing. Documentation that must be submitted in the application includes: the ingredients in the drug, data and results from the clinical trials, data and results from the animal studies, details of how the drug behaves in the body, and how the drug is manufactured, processed, and packaged. Sufficient information should be provided in the NDA so the reviewers can determine:

- Whether the drug is safe and effective for its proposed use(s);
- Whether the benefits of the drug outweigh its risks;
- Whether the drug's proposed labeling is appropriate and what it should contain;
- Whether the methods used to manufacture the drug and the controls used to maintain the drug's quality are adequate to preserve the drug's quality, purity, identity, and strength.

The NDA may contain thousands of pages and could take from 2 to 3 years for the FDA to complete its review.

1.6.3 Drug registration in Canada

The new drug application process in Canada is similar to the United States' process. After acceptable results of preclinical and clinical studies have determined the potential therapeutic benefits outweigh the risks, the drug sponsor must submit a New Drug Submission (NDS) with the appropriate Health Products and Food Branch (HPFB).

The appropriate HPFB Directorate will determine if the authorization to sell the drug in Canada will be granted. A drug sponsor can submit an NDS whether the drug trials were completed in Canada or another country. The NDS must include all the data and results from the preclinical and clinical studies.

1.6.4 Drug registration in Japan

Prior to the late 1990s, the Japanese agencies required all clinical data used to support an NDA in Japan was collected from Japanese subjects in Japan; however, since the introduction of the ICH E5 guideline on "ethnic factors in the acceptability of foreign clinical data," the Japanese regulatory authority now accepts some non-Japanese clinical data in support of an application for market approval. The process for an applicant to bring a new drug to the Japanese market requires two steps: (1) obtaining marketing approval and (2) the determination of pricing and reimbursement rate. The marketing application in Japan is the J-NDA, which is submitted to the Ministry of Health, Labour and Welfare (MHLW) and then transferred to the PMDA, before being reviewed by the Pharmaceutical Affairs and Food Sanitation Council. After the review process, which may also include an oral hearing, the PMDA will generate and submit a final report to the Evaluation and Licensing Division of the Pharmaceutical and Food Safety Bureau, which then determines the drug classification for pricing.

1.6.5 Drug registration in China

The process in China for marketing a new drug is more complex. Like the clinical studies, the drug can fall under one of six categories. Categories one to five require submission of an NDA and category six requires a generic drug application. Additionally, there are separate pathways for an imported drug. The new drug registration application is submitted to the China FDA for initial examination and acceptance, then the CDE performs a technical review and the NIFDC tests drug samples. This entire review and approval process usually take seven to 15 months.

1.7 Good laboratory practice

One of the primary responsibilities of regulatory agencies around the world is to ensure the quality and safety of all healthcare products that are marketed in their respective countries. To facilitate these responsibilities, industry and regulators, with the endorsement of individual countries, have developed "good practices," sometimes referred to as GxPs, and quality systems. These two systems work in parallel to ensure the quality of pharmaceuticals. The three main type of GxP are (1) GLP, (2) GCP, and (3) GMP. These three "good practices" coincide with the various stages of drug development. GLPs cover the conduct of nonclinical laboratory testing, generally animal studies, and provide guidelines for testing and data submitted to the regulatory agencies in support of clinal trial applications and marketing applications. GCPs apply to the design, conduct, performance, monitoring, auditing, recording, analysis, and reporting of the clinical trials used to support an application for marketing. GMPs cover the manufacturing, testing, and quality assurance required to ensure a product is safe for human use. Some countries have their own version of the GxPs; however, the guidelines are similar around the world.

1.7.1 Good laboratory practice in Europe

As noted above, GLPs were enacted to reassure regulatory authorities that the nonclinical study reports submitted to support registration of a new drug accurately reflected activities during the study and that the results are accurate. The most commonly used GLPs were enacted by the US FDA (21 Code of Federal Regulations Part 58) and the Organization for Economic Co-operation and Development (OECD). GLP requirements within the EU are covered in Section I of Annex I of Council Directive 2004/10/EC and Directive 2004/9/EC of the European Parliament. Directive 2004/9/EC which replaced Directive 88/320/EEC as of March 11, 2004 establishes the obligation of EU countries to designate the authorities responsible for GLP inspections in their territory.

These Directives require the OECD Revised Guides for Compliance Monitoring Procedures for GLP and the OECD Guidance for the Conduct of Test Facility Inspections and Study Audits, be followed during laboratory inspections and study audits. Additionally, WHO, in partnership with TDR published a "Good Laboratory Practice Handbook" broadly based on the OECD principles. As with other legislation, the individual member countries develop their own measures for implementation, although these are often harmonized across the European Union. As an example of how this is applied in Europe, the next section reviews GLP legislation within the United Kingdom. Despite the United Kingdom having left the EU in January 2020, the principles remain the same.

1.7.2 Good laboratory practice in the United Kingdom

The UK GLP regulations for a GLP study as published in the "OECD Principles of Good Laboratory Practices," Directive 2004/10/EC, consists of the following ten main sections:

1. **Test facility organization and personnel:** Focuses on the management and personnel issues including job descriptions and training records.
2. **Quality assurance program:** Focuses on the requirement for an independent QA program, with personnel who are not involved in the studies, to ensure GLP compliance.

3. **Facilities:** Ensures adequate facilities are available to allow the studies to be carried out without the results being compromised in any way by lack of space or cross-contamination.
4. **Apparatus, materials, and reagents:** Covers the validation, maintenance, and storage of equipment and chemicals.
5. **Test systems:** Ensures the integrity of both the physical/chemical data and systems and biological testing systems.
6. **Test and reference items:** Focuses on the receipt, handling, sampling, and storage of all test and reference materials.
7. **Standard operating procedures (SOPs):** Lists the main areas of activity covered by SOPs, together with the change control requirements for the system.
8. **Performance of the study:** Focuses on the development, contents, and execution of a study plan.
9. **Reporting of study results:** Covers the contents and layout of the final report
10. **Storage and retention of records and materials:** Details what should be archived and how those archives should be kept.

The European Union's approach to inspecting facilities for GLP compliance is different from the United States' approach. The EU GLP guidance for the inspection and verification is detailed in a separate guideline, Directive 2004/9/EC. In the European Union, laboratories must undergo inspection and receive certification before they can conduct a GLP study. Once approval is granted to the laboratory, it is assumed any GLP study completed in that laboratory is fully GLP compliant or has the basic infrastructure to be capable of compliance.

1.7.3 Good laboratory practice in the United States

GLP regulations and guidelines in the United States were first drafted by the FDA in 1976. Like the regulations for other countries, the intent of the guidelines were: (1) to ensure investigators conducted safety and efficacy studies in a controlled, documented, and traceable manner and (2) to ensure the quality and integrity of the data necessary to support an NDA. The US GLP regulations can be found in Part 58 of the Code of Federal Regulations Title 21 (21 CFR 58). Essentially the same material is covered in the US GLP as in the EU version, but it is phrased in a different format, covering 36 different clauses. These are numbered in numerical order, but not sequentially. For example, clause 58.15 deals with inspection of a testing facility while clause 58.35 deals with the requirement for a Quality Assurance unit. In the United States, any laboratory can conduct a GLP study and assert that the study complies with the GLP regulations. A final determination of compliance is made only after the laboratory is audited by the FDA.

1.8 Good clinical practice

Clinical trials must be performed using GCP. As noted earlier every clinical trial must be approved by the regulatory authority in the respective country or region where the trial will be conducted, and the trial must be carried out in compliance with the regulatory requirements. GCP is collectively defined as an international ethical and scientific quality standard for designing, conducting, recording, and reporting clinical research that involves the participation of human subjects. Compliance with GCP provides public assurance that the rights, safety, and well-being of trial participants are respected and protected and that clinical trial data are credible.

The concept of GCP was first established during the 18th Assembly of the World Medical Association (WMA) in Finland in 1964. The protection of clinical trial subjects was first established in the WMA Declaration of Helsinki—Ethical Principles for Medical Research Involving Human Subjects (https://www.wma.net/policies-post/wma-declaration-of-helsinki-ethical-principles-for-medical-research-involving-human-subjects/). This declaration has been amended several times in different countries—Japan in 1975, Italy in 1983, Hong Kong in 1989, South Africa in 1996, Scotland in 2000, the United States in 2002, Japan in 2004, Korea in 2008, and Brazil in 2013.

The initial versions of this declaration contained 12 principles. With its numerous amendments, as of July 2018, the principles have increased to 37, organized under the following sections:
- Preamble
- General Principles
- Risks, Burdens, and Benefits
- Vulnerable Groups and Individuals
- Scientific Requirements and Research Protocols
- Research Ethics Committees
- Privacy and Confidentiality
- Informed Consent
- Use of Placebo
- Post-Trial Provisions
- Research Registration and Publication and Dissemination of Results
- Unproven Interventions in Clinical Practice

Under the various sections, specific guidance is provided for the conduct of the clinical trials.

1.8.1 International Council for Harmonization guidelines on good clinical practice

Most pharmaceutical companies intend to market their drugs in multiple countries; however, they find it difficult to adapt to the different regulatory guidelines required for product registration in the various countries. To address the discrepancies among different drug regulatory agencies around the world, the European Union, the United States, and Japan in consultation with the International Federation of Pharmaceutical Manufacturers and Associations (IFPMA) initiated a harmonization procedure. In April 1990, the ICH was founded. The six original sponsors were the European Commission (EC), the European Federation of Pharmaceutical Industries Association (EFPIA), the Japanese MHLW/PMDA, the Japanese Pharmaceutical Manufacturers Associations (JPMA), the US FDA [the Center for Drug Evaluation and Research (CDER) and the Center for Biological Evaluation and Research (CBER)], and the Pharmaceutical Research and Manufacturers of America (PhRMA). The council was reformed as a nonprofit legal entity under Swiss law in October 2015. As of November 2020, the organization contains 17 members (https://www.ich.org/page/members-observers). The primary mission of ICH is to achieve greater harmonization worldwide to ensure safe, effective, and high-quality medicines are developed and registered in the most resource-efficient manner (http://www.ich.org).

The ICH topics are divided into four guidelines—Quality, Safety, Efficacy, and Multidisciplinary. GCP falls under the Efficacy guidelines E6(R2) and E6(R3) EWG. The Efficacy guidelines focus on the design, conduct, safety, and reporting of clinical trials and contain 20 topics numbered from E1 to E20. The initial version of the ICH E6 GCP guideline, finalized in 1996, described the responsibilities and expectations of all participants in the conduct of clinical trials, including investigators, monitors, sponsors and Institutional Review Boards (IRBs). Collectively, however, GCP refers to all aspects of monitoring, reporting, and archiving essential documents from clinical trials. Therefore in 2016, the guideline was amended with an integrated addendum to encourage implementation of improved and more efficient approaches to clinical trial design, conduct, oversight, recording and reporting, while continuing to ensure human subject protection and reliability of trial results. Additionally, standards for electronic records and essential documents intended to increase the clinical trial quality and efficiency were updated.

ICH E6(R3) EWG, endorsed by ICH in June 2019 is a revision in process of E6 (R2). The revision will address the application of GCP principles to diverse trial types and data sources being employed to support regulatory and healthcare related decision-making on drugs. The revision will also provide flexibility, whenever appropriate, to facilitate the use of technological innovations in clinical trials.

The GCP guidelines are divided into eight main chapters:

1. Glossary
2. The Principles of ICH GLP
3. Institutional Review Board/Independent Ethics Committee (IRB/IEC)
4. Investigator
5. Sponsor

6. Clinical Trial Protocol and Protocol Amendment(s)

7. Investigator's Brochure

8. Essential Documents for the Conduct of a Clinical Trial

Similar to the guidelines published for GLP, WHO published a "Handbook for Good Clinical Practice" in 2002. It is based on the ICH GCP guidelines and was published as a reference and educational tool to facilitate understanding and implementation of GCP.

1.8.2 Good clinical practice in the United States

In the United States, there is no single section or subsection designated for GCPs. As a result, the US FDA adopted and issued the ICH E6 GCP guidelines. The E6(R2) ICH guideline addresses several sections of US Title 21 of the FDA Code of Federal Regulations, namely:

- Electronic records and signatures (Part 11)
- Protection of human subjects and the issue of informed consent (Part 50)
- Financial disclosure by clinical investigators (Part 54)
- Institutional Review Board, i.e., the membership and operation (Part 56)
- IND application (Part 312)
- Application for FDA approval to market a drug (Part 314)
- Bioavailability and bioequivalence requirements (Part 320)

1.8.3 Good clinical practice in Europe

Requirements for the conduct of GCP in the EU are implemented in The Clinical Trials Directive 2001/20/EC. This directive was developed within Europe over a 10-year period and was finally published in the *Official Journal of the European Communities* in May 2001, for implementation by all member states within a 3-year period. The Directive is aimed at the regulation of clinical trials, including multicenter trials carried out within the European Union. It closely reflects the content of the ICH guidelines. The principles and definitions are followed by sections on the protection of trial subjects, the commencement of a clinical trial, exchange of information, manufacture and labeling of clinical trials materials, compliance and reporting of clinical safety data.

There are a number of major implications arising out of the Clinical Trials Directive. The requirements for authorization from both the competent authority and the ethics committee are extended to cover all trials, including Phase I studies. This was not previously the case in the United Kingdom and more than 50% of the Phase I trials performed worldwide were being carried out in the United Kingdom. The time-limit in which a request for an authorization must be dealt with was reduced, so the initiation of trials was speeded up as a result. Additionally, there were a number of implications for the protection of the patient, with a strengthening of the requirements for informed consent and the reporting of adverse events and termination of studies.

From a manufacturing point of view, the most significant implication was that all clinical trials materials must be manufactured under GMP conditions. Importing clinical trials materials requires an authorization and the services of a qualified person (QP) who will keep a register of batches. For major pharmaceutical companies and those involved in manufacturing licensed products, neither of these requirements was likely to be a problem. However, for small companies producing only clinical trials materials and academic establishments carrying out Phase I trials only, this was a significant requirement that inevitably resulted in an increase in costs.

1.8.4 Good clinical practice in Japan

As noted earlier, Japan was one of the countries who helped develop ICH and the GCP guidelines to ensure clinical studies were performed with ethical considerations using a scientific approach. Since the development of the 1990 ICH guidelines, the MHLW has conducted various studies to improve the quality of clinical studies in Japan in accordance with changes in the international regulatory environment and several revisions of GCP have been issued. The most recent and current GCP was amended in January 2016 under Ordinance No. 9. The GCP Ordinance is composed of six chapters and 59 articles (https://www.pmda.go.jp/files/000152996.pdf). Additionally, GCP is divided into three parts: standards for sponsoring clinical trials; standards for management of clinical trials; and standards for conduct of clinical trials.

It can be seen from the above that GCP guidelines for various countries cover all aspects raised in the original Declaration of Helsinki and thus act as a major control of the quality of clinical studies and the protection of the human subjects.

1.9 Pharmacovigilance

In the late 1950s and early 1960s, a drug called thalidomide was prescribed as a sedative to pregnant women. During this time, there was little, if any, regulation of medicines outside the United States and the testing and development was almost entirely in the hands of the pharmaceutical companies. The manufacturer of thalidomide made unjust claims about the safety of the medicine in pregnancy. As a result, it was marketed to pregnant women as a sedative and treatment for nausea and vomiting. Later, the drug was discovered to be a teratogen, that is, "a drug or substance capable of interfering with the development of a fetus, causing birth defects" (http://www.dictionary.com). Worldwide, thousands of babies were born with limb deformities, particularly in Germany where the drug was first marketed. This incident was the catalyst for the development of legislation to ensure such a situation could not happen again. To prevent it, the need was recognized for a mechanism to license all pharmaceuticals before they can be released on to the marketplace. In 1962, the US congress passed the Kefauver-Harris Amendments specifically designed to prevent another such disaster. Also, from that point forward, all products were required to have a marketing authorization.

The layperson's definition of pharmacovigilance is the surveillance of the safety of a medicinal product during the time it is marketed. The broader definition of pharmacovigilance provided by WHO is "The science and activities relating to the detection, assessment, understanding and prevention of adverse effects or any other drug related problems" (https://www.who.int/medicines/technical_briefing/tbs/safety-rdg-prs/en/). Prior to granting a marketing authorization, all pharmaceuticals go through the clinical trial stage, during which information is gathered regarding the effectiveness and safety of the product in use by humans. Sufficient information must be gathered at this stage to ensure the benefits of the drug are not outweighed by the adverse effects it might cause. However, the information taken from the data during this stage is limited when compared to the amount of data that can be gathered once the product is released and available to the entire population.

In most cases, the results of this wider source of data will be used to reinforce the conclusions drawn as a result of the clinical studies and to confirm the marketing authorization is valid. It is possible however that the balance of benefit and risk may change in the light of wider use and systems must be in place to deal with that eventuality, including withdrawal of the marketing authorization if appropriate.

1.9.1 Responsibility for pharmacovigilance

The two main components of pharmacovigilance are harm and safety. Harm from the perspective of an adverse drug reaction to a medicine and safety from the perspective of balancing harms with benefits. Legally, the responsibility for the safety of medicinal products falls upon the manufacturer and regulatory bodies. At an industry level, companies are required to have pharmacovigilance systems in place, so that they can react to any problems identified.

There are four elements of manufacturer reporting systems:
- Adverse drug reaction (ADR) reporting
- Periodic safety update reporting
- Postauthorization safety studies (PASS)
- Risk management planning

In respect to regulatory bodies, the FDA's primary tool is its spontaneous reporting program, MedWatch, which was established in 1993. This system receives reports from the public and, when appropriate, publishes safety alerts for FDA regulated products (https://www.fda.gov/safety/medwatch-fda-safety-information-and-adverse-event-reporting-program). More recently, the FDA's requirements for postmarketing risk management have been increasing. In 2008 the FDA launched the Sentinel Initiative, a proactive electronic system for national postmarketing surveillance.

In the European Union, in response to Directive 75/319/EEC (superseded by 2001/83/EC) and Council Regulation EEC/2309/93 (superseded by Regulation (EC) No. 726/2004), each member state has set up a national pharmacovigilance center which collates adverse reaction reports and has a system for taking appropriate action. These centers evaluate the reports from the individual companies, relating to nationally authorized products. For mutually recognized products, the reference member state takes responsibility for evaluating the reports and communicating any required actions. Any issues relating to centrally authorized products are dealt with by the appropriate CPMP rapporteur.

Pharmacovigilance activities across the European Union are coordinated by the Pharmacovigilance Risk Assessment Committee. At a global level, WHO operates a collaborating center for international drug monitoring, which deals with the national centers in the individual countries.

Under the marketing authorization system, pharmacovigilance data are part of the marketing authorization dossier and must be updated at the time of application to renew the authorization.

1.9.2 European channels of communication

There are several channels set up to facilitate communications between the regulatory bodies of the member states, within the pharmaceutical industry and to the general public.

- **EudraVigilance:** Management and analysis of suspected adverse reactions to drugs authorized or within clinical studies within the European Economic Area (https://www.ema.europa.eu/en/human-regulatory/research-development/pharmacovigilance/eudravigilance).
- **EudraLex:** The body of European legislation relating to human medicines. This is a very useful information source primarily for industry, but also for the general public. It contains legislation, guidelines, Notice to applicants and other relevant documents, which can be downloaded directly via the internet (https://eur-lex.europa.eu/summary/chapter/2913.html).
- **European Medicines Agency's Good Pharmacovigilance Practice pages:** https://www.ema.europa.eu/en/human-regulatory/post-authorisation/pharmacovigilance/good-pharmacovigilance-practices.
- **European Network of Centers for Pharmacoepidemiology and Pharmacovigilance:** A network (the ENCePP partners) of public institutions and contract research organizations (CROs) involved in research in pharmacoepidemiology and pharmacovigilance (http://www.encepp.eu).

1.9.3 International approach to pharmacovigilance

Pharmacovigilance activities are conducted, in most countries, by the national regulatory authority, which is typically an organization within the government's health department. Notable exceptions are Japan, Korea, the Netherlands, and New Zealand, where the pharmacovigilance center lies outside the government regulatory body. As noted previously, the EMA addressed many differences in pharmacovigilance practice which previously existed between different member states by developing centralized and harmonized processes. In addition to a centralized database for ADR reporting, the EMA developed European guidelines on pharmacovigilance practice and expert advisory committees with representatives from all member states. Through these mechanisms, the EMA has established international collaboration into active regulatory practice. Outside of Europe, most developing nations and increasingly emerging low- and middle-income countries, have their own medicines regulatory bodies. Countries with authorities covering the largest populations that are associated with the WHO Program for International Drug Monitoring (WHO-PIDM) include some in Africa (e.g., Nigeria and Egypt), the Middle East, Asia (e.g., India, China, and Japan), Central America (e.g., Mexico), South America (e.g., Brazil) and the Russian Federation.

In 2014 the UK Medicines and Healthcare products Regulatory Agency (MHRA) and the US FDA led the discussion and development of a global regulatory authority knows as the International Coalition of Medicines Regulatory Authorities (ICMRA). This is a voluntary organization allowing the heads of national regulatory authorities around the world to develop shared strategic leadership to address current and emerging global regulatory challenges, including safety issues. The first major example of collaboration between the ICMRA and the WHO was dealing with the Ebola virus outbreak that affected many countries. The ICMRA has established many working groups to examine efficient and rapid sharing of information.

In addition to the MHRA, FDA, and the WHO-PDIM, other organizations that play an active part in international pharmacovigilance include the following:
- The Uppsala Monitoring Center (UMC) in Sweden
- WHO Collaborating Centers in Ghana, Morocco, Netherlands, Sri Lanka, Peru, Sudan, Jamaica, and Eswatini (formerly Swaziland) (http://www.who–umc.org)
- Council for International Organizations of Medical Sciences (CIOMS)
- International Council for Harmonization (ICH)
- International Society of Pharmacovigilance (ISoP)
- International Society for Pharmacoepidemiology (ISPE)
- Drug Information Association (DIA)

In conclusion, pharmacovigilance comprises international activities encouraging collaboration and communication to monitor the safety of products marketed worldwide.

While, the United States and Europe have played a major role in the regulation, research and development, other countries outside these regions are also contributing to postmarketing surveillance.

1.10 History of drug regulation in the United States

In the United States, federal controls over the drug supply began with the inspection of imported drugs in 1848. In 1862 the Bureau of Chemistry was established within the Department of Agriculture and was charged with the investigation of adulterated foods. In 1927 the Bureau of Chemistry was reorganized into two separate entities: regulatory functions were located in the Food, Drug, And Insecticide Administration, and nonregulatory research was located in the Bureau of Chemistry and Soils. In 1930 the latter organization was renamed, and the FDA was born. In 1940 it was transferred from the Department of Agriculture to the Federal Security Agency, which was converted in 1953 into the Department of Health, Education and Welfare. However, in 1968 the FDA was again moved, this time to the Public Health Service.

Finally, in 1988 the Food and Drug Administration Act established the FDA as an agency of the Department of Health and Human Services with a Commissioner of Food and Drugs appointed by the President with the advice and consent of the Senate. This Act also sets out the responsibilities of the Secretary and the Commissioner for research, enforcement, education, and information.

During the time the FDA was developing and establishing its roles and responsibilities, there was a similar development in the laws controlling the manufacture and sale of pharmaceuticals in the United States.

1.10.1 Development of American drug laws

Drug laws in the United States have roots in English law and arose from a common concern about safety and the prevention of fraud. The first national food and drug legislation in the United States, the Food and Drugs Act, passed in 1906. The law required all drugs to meet standards for strength, quality, and purity and prohibited states from buying and selling food, drinks, or drugs that had been mislabeled or tainted.

However, it was completely revised 30 years later when it was found to be inadequate. The thalidomide incident in Europe in the 1960s was an echo of a similar tragedy that occurred in the United States in the 1930s, which also precipitated a change in the way pharmaceuticals are controlled. Around 107 people died as a result of taking Elixir Sulfanilamide, which contained a poisonous ingredient. In 1938, the Food, Drug, and Cosmetic Act forced companies to be held responsible for proving the safety of a drug before it could be marketed in the United States. In addition, the concept of factory inspections was introduced.

In 1962 as a result of the thalidomide incident in Europe, the control of drugs within the United States was strengthened with the introduction of the Kefauver-Harris Drug Amendments. These amendments required that in addition to safety, the effectiveness of the drug must also be demonstrated. The requirement was retrospectively applied to all the drugs registered since 1938. At the same time, the mechanism for adverse drug reaction reporting was established.

Since the 1980s there have been a number of other changes to the law, including the definition and management of "orphan drugs" (Orphan Drug Act 1983) and measures to reduce the requirements for registration of generics, in terms of time and money involved (Drug Price Competition and Patent Term Restoration Act 1984).

In addition, there have been various changes in drug regulations, which have not involved a change in the law. These include measures to protect the rights of subjects within clinical trials (Protection of Human Subjects; Informed Consent; Standards for Institutional Review Boards 1981) and a move to short-circuit the process for getting new drugs to people with life-threatening diseases, by moving to approval after Phase II trials (Procedures for Subpart E Drugs 1988). Another significant milestone was in 1998 when the FDA introduced the Adverse Event Reporting System for pharmacovigilance. In 2011 the Food Safety Modernization Act was passed to provide the FDA with new enforcement authorities related to food safety standards and provide tools for the FDA to hold imported foods to the same standards as domestic foods. Additional details in the timeline of United States drug laws can be found on the FDA website (https://www.fda.gov/about-fda/fdas-evolving-regulatory-powers/milestones-us-food-and-drug-law-history).

1.10.2 Center for drug evaluation and research

1.10.2.1 The early years

The Center for Drug Evaluation and Research (CDER) began life as the Drug Laboratory, set up within the Bureau of Chemistry in 1902. The objectives of the laboratory were the standardization of pharmaceuticals and the unifying of analytical results. In 1908 the Drug Laboratory was reorganized for the first time. It was renamed the Drug Division, and subdivided into four laboratories: The Drug Inspection Laboratory; the Synthetic Products Laboratory; the Essential Oils Laboratory; and the Pharmacological Laboratory. Of these subdivisions, the Drug Inspection Laboratory became the main enforcement arm of the Drug Division.

Over the next 10 years, the Division of Drugs added two new elements: the Pharmacognosy Laboratory was created in 1914 with the responsibility for investigating crude drug products and the reduction of waste during manufacture; and in 1916 an office was established to investigate false and fraudulent labeling of drugs.

In 1923 the Office of Drug Control was set up as a replacement for the Division of Drugs. The Office was responsible for all pharmaceutical controls, including crude drugs, manufactured drug ingredients, drug preparations, and patent medicines. Over the next few years, the Office expanded to include chemical, medical, veterinary and pharmacology units, together with a unit for special collaborative investigations.

In 1935 the Office of Drug Control was renamed the Drug Division. At the same time, the responsibilities for pharmacology were moved to a separate office since there was an increasing need for pharmacological investigations in relation to adulteration of foodstuffs.

1.10.2.2 The Food Drug and Cosmetic Act of 1938

The Food Drug and Cosmetic Act of 1938 established the concept of the NDA by which all drugs had to be reviewed before they could be marketed. Within the first year, the Drug Division received over 1200 submissions.

In 1945 the Drug Division was renamed as the Division of Medicine. A major review of its activities in 1955 highlighted the fact that the review process needed to be speeded up and for this to happen, both manpower and budget should be significantly increased. In 1957 the Division became the Bureau of Medicine. During the same reorganization, the seven scientific divisions within the FDA were combined to form the Bureau of Biological and Physical Sciences. The Bureau of Medicine consisted of five branches with responsibility for new drugs, drugs and devices, veterinary medicine, medical antibiotics and research, and reference.

In 1961 the branch with responsibility for new drugs became a division in its own right. It contained five branches: the Investigational Drug Branch evaluated proposed clinical trials for compliance with investigational drug regulations; the Controls Evaluation Branch reviewed the manufacturing controls proposed by drugs makers; the Medical Evaluation Branch assessed safety and efficacy data in NDAs; the New Drug Status Branch consulted with manufacturers about their NDAs and proposed dosing schedules for new products; the New Drug Surveillance Branch evaluated adverse reaction reports.

Over the next 20 or so years, the bodies with responsibility for the regulation of pharmaceuticals continued to evolve in response to changes in legislation and priorities. There was a further reorganization in 1965, another (encompassing much of the FDA) in 1969 and others in 1970s and 1980s.

1.10.2.3 1980s–1990s

In 1987 the Center for Drugs and Biologics was divided into two separate entities: The Center for Drug Evaluation and Research (CDER) and the Center for Biologics Evaluation and Research (CBER). The main offices of the CDER were: Management, Compliance, Drug Standards, Drug Evaluation (I and II), Epidemiology and Biostatistics, Research Resources, Pilot Drug Evaluation, Generic Drugs, and Professional Development.

From 1995 CDER was once again reorganized. The Division of Oncology and Pulmonary Drug Products was split into two separate Divisions; and nine new Offices were established. Included in the new Offices were three additional Offices of Drug Evaluation, an Office of Training and Communication, the Office of Review Management, the Office of Pharmaceutical Science, the Office of New Drug Chemistry, the Office of Clinical Pharmacology and Biopharmaceutics, and the Office of Testing and Research.

1.10.2.4 CDER today

CDER is now the largest unit within the FDA. As of 2021, CDER was organized into 13 different primary offices and multiple suboffices. It is described on the FDA website as "The Consumer Watchdog for Safe and Effective Drugs" (https://www. fda.gov/drugs/information-consumers-and-patients-drugs/cder-consumer-watchdog-safe-and-effective-drugs). The FDA website states that CDER "performs an essential public health task by making sure that safe and effective drugs are available to improve the health of people in the United States" (https://www.fda.gov/about-fda/fda-organization/center-drug-evaluation-and-research-cder).   The   main   areas   of responsibility can be summarized as follows:

- Review of the new drug development process, both during preclinical and clinical stages.
- Review of INDs prior to granting permission for clinical trials.
- Review of NDAs prior to granting marketing authorizations.
- Review of generic drugs by means of the Abbreviated New Drug Application (ANDA), which concentrates on safety and bioequivalence, prior to granting marketing authorizations.
- Review of the safety and effectiveness of OTC drugs and prescription drugs, including biological therapeutics and generic drugs prior to granting marketing authorizations.
- A number of postapproval review activities such as postmarketing surveillance (see Section 1.9 for an explanation of pharmacovigilance); medication errors and advertising and labeling of prescription drugs.
- Miscellaneous areas of activity including orphan drugs, women's health issues, pediatric initiatives, environmental assessments, and liaison with other parties within ICH.

1.11 Unlicensed medicines

Although the majority of medicines require a marketing authorization or product license before they can be placed on the marketplace, there are some circumstances under which unlicensed medicines can be supplied for an individual patient who might have special needs that cannot be satisfied by the standard products available on the marketplace. For example, some patients may be allergic to a particular ingredient. Alternatively, some patients may be unable to tolerate the more usual dosage form: a patient with throat problems might be unable to swallow tablets or capsules and could require the medicine to be dispensed as a liquid. The responsibility of prescribing such a product lies with the patient's doctor.

In the European Union, this is referred to as compassionate use. The EMA makes recommendations via the CPMP, but these have no legal status. The individual member states manage these programs via their National Agencies.

In the United States, the FDA will permit the sales on unlicensed drugs under strictly controlled circumstances, including where healthcare professionals rely on the drug to treat serious medical conditions when there is no FDA-approved drug to treat the condition.

In the United Kingdom, such medicines are referred to as "Specials."

1.11.1 Definition and the use of "Specials"

"Specials" are unlicensed relevant medicinal products for humans, which are specially prepared by order of a doctor or a dentist for an individual patient. The control of the manufacture, distribution, and supply of such products are covered in an MCA Guidance Note No. 14 "The supply of unlicensed medicinal products." (The exemption does not apply to other unlicensed products such as herbal remedies and investigational medicinal products.)

"Specials" may only be ordered by certain groups of people:
- Doctors or dentists
- Supplementary prescribers
- Nurse independent prescribers or pharmacist independent prescribers
- Pharmacists in hospitals, health centers or pharmacies
- Licensed wholesale dealers or manufacturers supplying to one of the above

It is the responsibility of the party supplying the "special" to ensure the product is only for purposes as specified in the regulations. This includes checking on the professional status of the person buying the product and ensuring they are aware of the unlicensed status of the drug.

1.11.2 Manufacture of "Specials"

"Specials" may only be manufactured by a company or organization holding a "specials" license, which is applied for in the same way as any other manufacturer's license. The manufacturing facility will be subject to inspection by the Regulatory Authorities in the normal way.

There are major differences in the production of "specials" as opposed to licensed pharmaceuticals. The batch size is very small, the preparation time is relatively short, and the process is generally manual. Hence it is common for a number of different products to be in progress within different areas of the same room at the same time. This has particular implications for product security systems and cleaning procedures to prevent cross-contamination.

There is no requirement for QP release on a "specials" order (see Chapter 5, for a discussion of the role of a qualified person). However, the release should be carried out by an independent QC person and all records should be kept for a specified time period pending inspection or the need to review the audit trail.

Distribution of "specials" can only be carried out by licensed wholesalers and full records must be kept. A supplier of "specials" may advertise the service supplied, but not the individual products available.

Any medical practitioner who orders "specials" is restricted in the amount of liquid and solid dosage forms they may hold in stock. However, a pharmacist may hold stock of "specials" in anticipation of an expected prescription.

There is an obligation, extending to all parts of the "specials" supply chain, to keep appropriate records on sources and destination of each order. In addition, any adverse reactions must be notified to the Regulatory Authority.

1.12 Good manufacturing practice

GMP is the concept that covers the assurance of the safety and effectiveness of pharmaceuticals during all stages of manufacturing. It thus covers the identification of suppliers and purchase of all starting materials, both raw materials and packaging materials; the approval of those starting materials for use; and their use in the manufacture and packaging of finished pharmaceuticals. The requirements of GMP cover such topics as quality management, personnel, documentation, premises and equipment, materials handling, validation, contract manufacturing and self-inspections.

GMP is fully discussed in Chapter 2. No further discussion is appropriate at this point.

1.13 Good distribution practice

GDP is the concept that covers the assurance of the safety and efficacy of pharmaceuticals from the time they leave the factory gates to the point at which they are used by the patient. The requirements of GDP cover such topics as the establishment of a Quality System, personnel, documentation, premises and equipment, deliveries to customers, returns of distributed product to the warehouse, self-inspections, and the information that must be provided to the appropriate authorities.

GDP is discussed in full in Chapter 14. No further discussion is appropriate at this point.

1.14 Chapter summary

- The primary milestones of the drug development life cycle are preclinical studies and clinical studies.
- Preclinical studies must be conducted prior to clinical studies.

- Preclinical studies are conducted with animals.
- Preclinical studies include pharmacodynamics, pharmacokinetics, toxicology, preformulation, and stability studies.
- Pharmacodynamics studies determine the effects of an NCE on various physiological systems in animals. These studies may be conducted as part of the safety pharmacology studies.
- Pharmacokinetics studies determine whether a sufficient concentration of the drug reaches the part of the body where it is required and is maintained at the right concentration for the right period of time.
- Toxicology studies translate animal responses to a drug into an understanding of the risk to humans and are used to determine whether a drug has the potential to cause serious harm to humans.
- Preformulation studies help identify the long-term stability of a drug formulation and evaluate its performance.
- Stability studies evaluate the influence of environmental factors (such as temperature humidity, and light), shelf life, and storage conditions on a drug.
- Clinical studies are conducted with humans and include four phases—Phase I, Phase II, Phase III, and Phase IV.
- Phase I characteristics—test the drug with 20 to 80 healthy patients, can last a few months to 2 years
- Phase I characteristics—tests the drug with from 100 to 300 patients who have the disease or condition that the product could potentially treat, can last several years (typically from 2 to 3 years), conducted as single-blind or double-blinded trials.
- Phase 3 characteristics—tests the drug with several thousands of patients who have the disease or condition that the product could potentially treat, can last several years (typically from 3 to 5 years), conducted as single-blind or double-blinded trials.
- Phase 4 characteristics—conducted, if required, after the drug has been licensed by the regulatory body and is on the market, involves hundreds of thousands of patients, provides additional information about the long-term risks, benefits, and optimal use, side effects and frequency of side effects.
- The process for registering a new drug differs by country or nation.
- The Emergency Use Authorization permits the use of unapproved medical products like drugs, biologics, and vaccines or the use of approved medical products in unapproved ways to diagnose, treat, or prevent serious diseases.
- The process for registering a new drug differs by country or nation.
- GLP covers the conduct of nonclinical laboratory testing, generally animal studies, and provide guidelines for testing and data that is submitted to the regulatory agencies in support of clinal trial application and marketing application.
- GCP refers to the design, conduct, performance, monitoring, auditing, recording, analysis, and reporting of the clinical trials that will be used to support an application for marketing.

- GMP covers the manufacturing, testing, and quality assurance required to ensure that a product is safe for human use.
- Pharmacovigilance is the surveillance of the safety of a medicinal product during the time that it is marketed.

1.15 Questions/problems

1. What specific studies are conducted as part of preclinical studies?
2. What specific studies are conducted under clinical studies?
3. What is the difference between the type of subjects used for preclinical and clinical studies?
4. What are the differences in the number of subjects and time for the four phases of clinical study?
5. What is the difference between single-blind and double-blind trials?
6. What is the difference between a drug substance and drug product?
7. How does the process for registering a new drug differ by country or nation?
8. How does Emergency Use Authorization vary by country or nation?
9. What is the difference between GLP, GCP, and GMP?
10. What incident(s) precipitated the development of pharmacovigilance?
11. How is pharmacovigilance implemented by various countries or nations?
12. How does the ICH harmonize key aspects of the drug development process?

Further reading

Aashigari, S., Goud, G.R., Sneha, S., Vykuntam, U., Potnuri, N.R., 2019. Stability studies of pharmaceutical products. World J. Pharm. Res. 8, 1. <http://www.wjpr.net>.

Association of State and Territorial Health Officials, Project BioShield Act. <https://astho.org/Programs/Preparedness/Public-Health-Emergency-Law/Emergency-Use-Authorization-Toolkit/Project-BioShield-Act-Fact-Sheet/> (accessed 11.03.21).

Association of State and Territorial Health Officials, Section 564 of the Federal Food, Drug, and Cosmetic Act. <https://astho.org/Programs/Preparedness/Public-Health-Emergency-Law/Emergency-Use-Authorization-Toolkit/Section-564-of-the-Federal-Food,-Drug,-and-Cosmetic-Act-Fact-Sheet/#:~:text=An%20Emergency%20Use%20Authorization%20(EUA)%20under%20Section%20564,amended%20the%20FD&C%20Act,%20among%20other%20things.%203> (accessed 11.03.21).

Australian Government Department of Health, 2020. Clinical trial exemption (CTX) scheme renamed as clinical trial approval (CTA) scheme. <https://www.tga.gov.au/clinical-trial-exemption-ctx-scheme-renamed-clinical-trial-approval-cta-scheme> (accessed 02.03.21).

Australian Government Department of Health, 2020. Clinical trial exemption (CTX) scheme renamed as clinical trial approval (CTA) scheme. <https://www.tga.gov.au/clinical-trial-exemption-ctx-scheme-renamed-clinical-trial-approval-cta-scheme> (accessed 02.03.21).

Bajaj, S., Singla, D., Sakhuja, N., 2012. Stability testing of pharmaceutical products. J. Appl. Pharm. Sci. 2 (3), 129–138. Available from: http://www.japsonline.com.

Biorelevant.com, Drug substance vs. drug product. <https://biorelevant.com/learning_center/drug-substance-vs-drug-product/> (accessed 25.02.21).

Bonderman, D., et al., 2013. Riociguat for patients with pulmonary hypertension caused by systolic left ventricular dysfunction: a phase IIb double-blind, randomized, placebo-controlled, dose-ranging hemodynamic study. Circulation. 128, 5. Vol. <https://www.ahajournals.org/doi/10.1161/CIRCULATIONAHA.113.001458>.

Bott, R.F., Oliveira, W.P., 2007. Storage conditions for stability testing of pharmaceuticals in hot and humid regions. Drug. Dev. Ind. Pharm. 33, 393—401.

Brody, T., 2016. Clinical Trials - Study Design, Endpoints and Biomarkers, Drug Safety, and FDA and ICH Guidelines, second ed. Elsevier, Massachusetts.

Carter, P.I., Loy. L.A, 1999. Federal Regulation of Pharmaceuticals in the United States and Canada, 21 Rev. 215. <https://digitalcommons.lmu.edu/ilr/vol21/iss2/>.

Chaurasia, G., 2016. A review on pharmaceutical preformulation studies in formulation and development of new drug molecules. Int. J. Pharm. Sci. Res. 7 (6), 2313—2320. <https://ijpsr.com/bft-article/a-review-on-pharmaceutical-preformulation-studies-in-formulation-and-development-of-new-drug-molecules/?view = fulltext>.

Colli, A., et al., 2014. The architecture of diagnostic research: from bench to bedside - research guidelines using liver stiffness as an example. Hepatology. 60 (1), 408—418. <https://pubmed.ncbi.nlm.nih.gov/24277656/>.

Congressional Research Service, 2014. The Project BioShield Act: Issues for the 113th Congress. <https://crsreports.congress.gov/product/pdf/R/R43607> (accessed 11.03.21).

Eastman, R.T., et al., 2020. Remdesivir: a review of its discovery and development leading to emergency use authorization for treatment of COVID-19. ACS Cent. Sci. 6, 672—683. Available from: https://doi.org/10.1021/acscentsci.0c00489.

Eua-Lex, Summaries of EU legislation, public health, pharmaceuticals. <https://eur-lex.europa.eu/summary/chapter/2913.html> (accessed 30.03.21).

Eur-Lex, 2001. Consolidated text: Directive 2001/83/EC of the European Parliament and of the Council of 6 November 2001 on the Community code relating to medicinal products for human use. <https://eur-ex.europa.eu/eli/dir/2001/83/2019-07-26> (accessed 30.03.21).

Eur-Lex, 2004. Directive 2004/10/EC OF The European Parliament and of the council of 11 February 2004 on the harmonisation of laws, regulations and administrative provisions relating to the application of the principles of good laboratory practice and the verification of their applications for tests on chemical substances. <https://eur-lex.europa.eu/LexUriServ/LexUriServ.do?uri = OJ:L:2004:050:0044:0059:EN:PDF> (accessed 30.03.21).

Eur-Lex, 2004. Directive 2004/9/EC of The European Parliament and of the council of 11 February 2004 on the inspection and verification of good laboratory practice (GLP). <https://eur-lex.europa.eu/LexUriServ/LexUriServ.do?uri = OJ:L:2004:050:0028:0043:EN:PDF> (accessed 30.03.21).

Eur-Lex, 2009. Consolidated text: regulation (EC) No 469/2009 of the European Parliament and of the council of 6 May 2009 concerning the supplementary protection certificate for medicinal products. <https://eur-lex.europa.eu/eli/reg/2009/469/2019-07-01> (accessed 30.03.21).

European Medicines Agency, 1996. ICH Q5C quality of biotechnological products: stability testing of biotechnological/biological products. <https://www.ema.europa.eu/en/ich-q5c-stability-testing-biotechnologicalbiological-products#current-version-section> (accessed 12.02.21).

European Medicines Agency, 1998. Q1C stability testing for new dosage forms. <https://www.ema.europa.eu/en/documents/scientific-guideline/ich-q-1-c-stability-testing-requirements-new-dosage-forms-step-5_en.pdf> (accessed 12.02.21).

European Medicines Agency, 2007. Guideline on strategies to identify and mitigate risks for first-in-human clinical trials with investigational medicinal products. <https://www.ema.europa.eu/en/documents/scientific-guideline/guideline-strategies-identify-mitigate-risks-first-human-early-clinical-trials-investigational_en.pdf> (accessed 11.03.21).

European Medicines Agency, 2013. ICH M3 (R2) Non-clinical safety studies for the conduct of human clinical trials for pharmaceuticals. <https://www.ema.europa.eu/en/ich-m3-r2-non-clinical-safety-studies-conduct-human-clinical-trials-pharmaceuticals#current-effective-version-section> (accessed 15.01.21).

European Medicines Agency, Committee for medicinal products for human use (CHMP) <https://www.ema.europa.eu/en/committees/committee-medicinal-products-human-use-chmp> (accessed 11.03.21).

European Medicines Agency, EMA compassionate use. <https://www.ema.europa.eu/en/human-regulatory/research-development/compassionate-use> (accessed 11.03.21).

European Medicines Agency, Eudravigilance. <https://www.ema.europa.eu/en/human-regulatory/research-development/pharmacovigilance/eudravigilance> (accessed 11.03.21).

European Medicines Agency, Good pharmacovigilance practices. <https://www.ema.europa.eu/en/human-regulatory/post-authorisation/pharmacovigilance/good-pharmacovigilance-practices> (accessed 30.03.21).

European Medicines Agency, How are new medicines approved by EMA? <https://www.ema.europa.eu/en/news/how-are-new-medicines-approved-ema> (accessed 11.03.21).

European Medicines Agency, <https://www.ema.europa.eu/en> (accessed 30.03.21).

European Network of Centres for Pharmacoepidemiology and Pharmacovigilance, <http://www.encepp.eu> (accessed 30.03.21).

European Parliament, 2004. Regulation (EC) No 726/2004 of the European Parliament and of the council of 31 March 2004 laying down community procedures for the authorisation and supervision of medicinal products for human and veterinary use and establishing a European Medicines Agency. <https://ec.europa.eu/health/sites/health/files/files/eudralex/vol-1/reg_2004_726/reg_2004_726_en.pdf> (accessed 30.03.21).

Faqi, A.S. (Ed.), 2017. A Comprehensive Guide to Toxicology in Preclinical Drug Development. second ed. Elsevier, Massachusetts.

Freyr Global Regulatory Solutions & Services, What is new chemical entity (NCE)?. <https://www.freyrsolutions.com/what-is-new-chemical-entity-nce> (accessed 14.01.21).

Friedhoff, L.T., 2009. New Drugs, An Insider's Guide to the FDA's New Drug Approval Process. Pharmaceutical Special Projects Group. LLC, New York.

Friedman, L.M., Furberg, C.D., DeMets, D.F., 2010. Fundamentals of Clinical Trials, fourth ed. Spinger, New York.

Gad, S.C. (Ed.), 2009. Clinical Trials Handbook. John Wiley & Sons, Incorporated, New Jersey.

Ghosh, D., Mondal, S., Ramakrishna, K., 2019. Acute and sub-acute (30-day) toxicity studies of Aegialitis rotundifolia Roxb., leaves extract in Wistar rats: safety assessment of a rare mangrove traditionally utilized as pain antidote. Clin. Phytosci 5, 13. Available from: https://doi.org/10.1186/s40816-019-0106-2.

Government of Canada, 2017. Applications and submissions - drug products. <https://www.canada.ca/en/health-canada/services/drugs-health-products/drug-products/applications-submissions.html> (accessed 15.03.21).

Government of Canada, 2020. Interim order respecting the importation, sale and advertising of drugs for use in relation to COVID-19. <https://www.canada.ca/en/health-canada/services/drugs-health-products/covid19-industry/drugs-vaccines-treatments/interim-order-import-sale-advertising-drugs.html> (accessed 11.03.21).

Guosheng, Y., 2012. Clinical Trial Design: Bayesian and Frequentist Adaptive Methods: Bayesian and Frequentist Adaptive Methods. John Wiley & Sons, Incorporated, New Jersey.

Harrington, J.A., Hernandez-Guerrero, T.C., Basu, B., 2017. Early phase clinical trial designs - state of play and adapting for the future. Clin. Oncol. 29 (12), 770–777. <https://www.sciencedirect.com/science/article/abs/pii/S0936655517304399>.

ICH Official Website, <https://www.ich.org/> (accessed 18.03.21).

ICH, 2020. Overview of ICH. <https://admin.ich.org/sites/default/files/2020-12/OverviewOfICH_2020_1130_0.pdf> (accessed 18.03.21).

INOUE, H., 1998. Clin. Pract. Japan: Curr. Status Future Perspect. Drug. Inf. J. 32, 1213S–1215S.

Ison, M.G., Wolfe, C., Boucher, H.W., 2020. Emergency use authorization of remdesivir, the need for a transparent distribution process. JAMA 323 (23). <https://jamanetwork.com/journals/jama/fullarticle/2766216>.

Japan Pharmaceutical Manufacturers Association, 2019. Pharmaceutical administration and regulations in Japan. <http://www.jpma.or.jp/english/> (accessed 18.03.21).

Japanese Ministerial Ordinance, 2012. Ministerial ordinance on good clinical practice for drugs. <https://www.pmda.go.jp/files/000152996.pdf> (accessed 18.03.21).

Kaur, M., Kaur, G., Kaur, H., Sharma, S., 2013. Overview on stability studies. Int. J. Pharm., Chem. And. Biol. Sci. 3 (4), 1231–1241. <https://www.ijpcbs.com/files/volume3-4-2013/33.pdf>.

Kelly, W.K., Halabi, S., 2018. Oncology Clinical Trials: Successful Design, Conduct, and Analysis. Springer Publishing Company, New York.

Kerr, D.J., et al., (Eds.), 2006. Clinical Trials Explained: A Guide to Clinical Trials in the NHS for Healthcare Professionals. Blackwell Publishing Ltd, Massachusetts.

Kwong, E., 2017. Oral Formulation Roadmap from Early Drug Discovery to Development. John Wiley & Sons, Ltd, New Jersey.

Lefferts, J.A. et al., 2020. Implementation of an emergency use authorization test during an impending national. J. Mol. Diagnost. 22 (7).

Medicines and Healthcare Products Regulatory Agency, 2014. The supply of unlicensed medicinal products ("specials") MHRA guidance note 14. <https://assets.publishing.service.gov.uk/government/uploads/system/uploads/attachment_data/file/373505/The_supply_of_unlicensed_medicinal_products__specials_pdf> (accessed 30.03.21).

Mehta, S., Goyal, V., Singh, K., 2015. Phase I (first-in-man) prophylactic vaccine's clinical trials: selecting a clinical trial site. Perspect. Clin. Res. 6 (2), 77–81. Available from: http://europepmc.org/article/PMC/4394584.

Neaustaeter, B., 2020. CTV News, Health Canada grants emergency-use authorization to Eli Lilly's COVID-19 antibody treatment. <https://www.ctvnews.ca/health/coronavirus/health-canada-grants-emergency-use-authorization-to-eli-lilly-s-covid-19-antibody-treatment-1.5199999> (accessed 11.03.21).

Ng, R., 2015. Drugs: From Discovery to Approval: From Discovery to Approval. John Wiley & Sons, Incorporated, New Jersey.

Pacifici, E., Bain, S. (Eds.), 2018. An Overview of FDA Regulated Products: From Drugs and Cosmetics to Food and Tobacco. Elsevier Science & Technology, California.

Patrick, W., Harrison-Woolrych, M., 2017. An Introduction to Pharmacovigilance. John Wiley & Sons, Incorporated, West Sussex.

Pharma Manufacturing, Pharma manufacturing essential reference guide. <https://www.pharmamanufacturing.com/fundamentals/pharma-manufacturing-essential-reference-guide/> (accessed 19.01.21).

Rosier, J.A., Martens, M.A., Thomas, J.R., 2014. Global New Drug Development: An Introduction. John Wiley & Sons, Ltd, West Sussex, UK.

Salminen, W.F., et al., 2013. Nonclinical Study Contracting and Monitoring: A Practical Guide. Elsevier Science & Technology, Massachusetts.

Shukla, J., 2017. Physicochemical parameters of preformulation study [PowerPoint slides]. <https://www.researchgate.net/publication/319980566_PREFORMULATION_STUDIES>.

Singla, B.D., Sakhuja, N., 2012. Stability testing of pharmaceutical products. J. Appl. Pharm. Sci. 02 (03), 129–138.

SPharm, The drug approval process in canada an e-guide. <https://spharm-inc.com/the-drug-review-and-approval-process-in-canada-an-eguide/> (accessed 15.03.21).

Tamimi, N.A., Ellis, P., 2009. Drug development: from concept to marketing!. Nephron Clin. Practice. 113 (3), 125_1231. <https://pubmed.ncbi.nlm.nih.gov/19729922/>.

TDR, 2009. Good laboratory practice (GLC) handbook, 2nd Edition. <https://www.who.int/tdr/publications/training-guideline-publications/good-laboratory-practice-handbook/en/>.

The European Parliament And The Council Of The European Union, 2014. Regulation (Eu) No 536/2014 of the European Parliament and of the council. <https://ec.europa.eu/health/sites/health/files/files/eudralex/vol-1/reg_2014_536/reg_2014_536_en.pdf> (accessed 02.03.21).

Thomas, D. (Ed.), 2019. Clinical Pharmacy Education, Practice and Research: Clinical Pharmacy, Drug Information, Pharmacovigilance, Pharmacoeconomics and Clinical Research. Elsevier, Massachusetts.

Thomas, F., 2020. Stability testing: the crucial development step. Pharm. Technol. 44 (3), 40–43. 03-02-2020. <https://www.pharmtech.com/view/stability-testing-crucial-development-step>.

U.S. Dept. of Health and Human Services, 2013. Guidance for industry. Labeling for human prescription drug and biological products—implementing the PLR content and format requirements. <https://www.fda.gov/media/71836/download> (accessed 11.03.21).

US Food & Drug Administration, 2003. Guidance for industry Q1A(R2) stability testing of new drug substances and products. <https://www.fda.gov/regulatory-information/search-fda-guidance-documents/q1ar2-stability-testing-new-drug-substances-and-products> (accessed 12.03.21).

US Food & Drug Administration, 2010. M3(R2) nonclinical safety studies for the conduct of human clinical trials and marketing authorization for pharmaceuticals. <https://www.fda.gov/regulatory-information/search-fda-guidance-documents/m3r2-nonclinical-safety-studies-conduct-human-clinical-trials-and-marketing-authorization>.

US Food & Drug Administration, 2012. Kefauver-Harris amendments revolutionized drug development. <https://www.fda.gov/consumers/consumer-updates/kefauver-harris-amendments-revolutionized-drug-development> (accessed 22.03.21).

US Food & Drug Administration, 2014. Expiration dating and stability testing for human drug products. <https://www.fda.gov/inspections-compliance-enforcement-and-criminal-investigations/inspection-technical-guides/expiration-dating-and-stability-testing-human-drug-products> (accessed 12.02.21).

US Food & Drug Administration, 2018. Milestones in U.S. food and drug law history. <https://www.fda.gov/about-fda/fdas-evolving-regulatory-powers/milestones-us-food-and-drug-law-history> (accessed 11.03.21).

US Food & Drug Administration, 2019. New drug application (NDA). <https://www.fda.gov/drugs/types-applications/new-drug-application-nda> (accessed 11.03.21).

US Food & Drug Administration,. 2021. FDA regulations: good clinical practice and clinical trials. <https://www.fda.gov/science-research/clinical-trials-and-human-subject-protection/regulations-good-clinical-practice-and-clinical-trials> (accessed 18.03.21).

US Food & Drug Administration, 2021. Advancing health through innovation: new drug approvals 2020. <https://www.fda.gov/media/144982/download>.

US Food & Drug Administration, 2021. Emergency use authorization. <https://www.fda.gov/emergency-preparedness-and-response/mcm-legal-regulatory-and-policy-framework/emergency-use-authorization> (accessed 11.03.21).

US Food & Drug Administration, Guidance for industry: M3(R2) nonclinical safety studies for the conduct of human clinical trials and marketing authorization for pharmaceuticals. <https://www.fda.gov/media/71542/download>(accessed 14.01.21).

US Food & Drug Administration, IND applications for clinical investigations: pharmacology and toxicology (PT) information. <https://www.fda.gov/drugs/investigational-new-drug-ind-application/ind-applications-clinical-investigations-pharmacology-and-toxicology-pt-information> (accessed 15.01.21).

US Food & Drug Administration, Inside clinical trials: testing medical products in people. <https://www.fda.gov/drugs/information-consumers-and-patients-drugs/inside-clinical-trials-testing-medical-products-people> (accessed 20.01.21).

US Food & Drug Administration, New Drugs at FDA: CDER's new molecular entities and new therapeutic biological products. <https://www.fda.gov/drugs/development-approval-process-drugs/new-drugs-fda-cders-new-molecular-entities-and-new-therapeutic-biological-products> (accessed 14.01.21).

US Food & Drug Administration, The drug development process. <https://www.fda.gov/patients/learn-about-drug-and-device-approvals/drug-development-process> (accessed 14.03.21).

Warwick. Good Lab Practice (GLP), <https://warwick.ac.uk/services/ris/research_integrity/code_of_practice_and_policies/research_code_of_practice/legal_regulatory_funding/glp/#:~:text=GOOD%20LABORATORY%20PRACTICE%20%28GLP%29%20In%20the%20European%20Union,The%20Good%20Laboratory%20Practice%20%28Codification%2C%20amendments%20etc%20> (accessed 17.03.21).

WHO, 2002. WHO handbook for good clinical practice. <https://www.who.int/medicines/areas/quality_safety/safety_efficacy/gcp1.pdf>.

World Health Organization, 2006. Stability testing of active substances and pharmaceutical products, Working document QAS/06.179. <https://www.who.int/medicines/services/expertcommittees/pharmprep/QAS06_179_StabilityGuidelineSept06.pdf> (accessed 23.03.21).

World Medical Association, 2018. WMA declaration of Helsinki — ethical principles for medical research involving human subjects. <https://www.wma.net/policies-post/wma-declaration-of-helsinki-ethical-principles-for-medical-research-involving-human-subjects/> (accessed 18.03.21).

CHAPTER 2

Good manufacturing practice

2.1 Introduction

As mentioned in Chapter 1, one of the primary responsibilities of regulatory agencies around the world is to ensure the quality and safety of all healthcare products that are marketed in their respective countries. To facilitate these responsibilities, "good practices," sometimes referred to as GxPs, and quality systems were developed. This chapter will focus on the good manufacturing practice (GMP) component of GxP. GMP refers to guidelines that encompass all the requirements to which manufacturers must comply to ensure the safe and effective manufacture of pharmaceutical products. GMP covers manufacturing, testing, and quality assurance (QA). GMP cannot be considered "best practices," rather, the GMP systems should establish the threshold standards that must be satisfied for a pharmaceutical manufacturing operation to be compliant. GMP is a very wide-ranging concept that is also recognized in other industries, in particular the food industry. GMP requirements work in parallel with quality systems. GMP establishes the element of QA that ensures products are consistently produced and controlled to the quality standards appropriate for their intended use as required by government regulations and product specifications. Chapter 3 will discuss how these systems work together to ensure the quality and safety of pharmaceutical products.

In Europe and many other parts of the world, good manufacturing practice is generally abbreviated as GMP; however, the United States has expanded the requirements of GMP with current GMP (CGMP) guidelines. This topic will be explored further in Section 2.2.1.

This chapter presents a review of the definition of GMP and a history of its development in different parts of the world. Additionally, comparisons are made between the various versions of GMP codes and guidelines in existence today. This is followed by a review of the basic requirements of GMP and how they are applied in pharmaceutical factories around the world. The chapter closes with a discussion of why there are often no "right answers" in questions of GMP and the need for interpretation of guidelines by individual practitioners.

2.2 Definition of good manufacturing practice

The WHO defines GMP as "that part of QA, which ensures that products are consistently produced and controlled to the quality standards appropriate to their

Quality
DOI: https://doi.org/10.1016/B978-0-323-90815-3.00009-8

intended use and as required by the marketing authorization" (https://gmpua.com/World/WHO/Annex4/trs908-4.pdf).

From this definition, there are a number of points that should be emphasized:

- GMP is part of QA. In other words, it is a preventive operation that is designed to make sure things happen in the correct manner. This means that, unlike quality control, the quality of any operation can be affected by the GMP measures that are put in place.
- There is a requirement for consistency. It is unacceptable for a company to produce a batch of products correctly one day if there is no guarantee that the same result can be obtained every day.
- GMP relates specifically to the manufacturing aspects of a product pipeline. This is defined as the point from which starting materials are purchased from approved suppliers to the point where the finished product leaves the factory. Indeed, there is also a responsibility to ensure the quality of the product during distribution, even though at this point it is often outside the control of the manufacturer.
- Quality standards should be appropriate for the intended use of the product. Hence the requirements to be fulfilled for the manufacture of an aseptically filled injection will be far more stringent than those for the manufacture of a multivitamin tablet, for example.
- The standards are previously defined in the application for marketing authorization. Hence there is a clearly defined process by which each product must be manufactured.

In a more simplistic definition, GMP can be described as the process of preventing cross-contamination and mix-ups. The difference between these two is as follows:

- Cross-contamination is where different materials or products become mixed, either in large quantities or as trace amounts. The latter will occur particularly if cleaning procedures or separation systems are not effective.
- Mix-ups are where printed packaging materials, particularly labels, are mixed together.

There is one final consideration when looking at the definition of GMP. The term is used in two different ways. First, and most correctly, it is used as the part of QA relating to manufacturing. As such, there are detailed lists of requirements to be fulfilled, as described later in this chapter. Second, it is used in the generic sense to describe everything relating to the quality of pharmaceuticals. Hence, various GMP guidelines, refer to Section 2.3, include sections on quality management and QA.

2.2.1 Current good manufacturing practice

As noted earlier current GMP (CGMP) is an extension of GMP that was developed in the United States. The US Food and Drug Administration (FDA) is responsible for ensuring the quality of drug products in the United States, and it carefully monitors drug manufacturers' compliance with CGMP regulations. The detailed CGMP requirements can be found in Title 21 of the FDA's Code of Federal Regulations (CFR), specifically, parts 210 and 211 (https://www.fda.gov/drugs/pharmaceutical-quality-resources/current-good-manufacturing-practice-CGMP-regulations).

There is a little difference between GMP and CGMP. CGMPs are minimal requirements that do not significantly affect most pharmaceutical companies because many companies already implement comprehensive, modern quality systems, and risk management methods that exceed these minimum standards. The "C" was added to certify that in addition to the GMP requirements, every step in the process of producing a product was completed in the most current manner available using up-to-date systems and technology. Even so, the FDA intentionally wrote the requirements so they would be flexible, as noted by the statement "…flexible in order to allow each manufacturer to decide individually how to best implement the necessary controls by using scientifically sound design, processing methods, and testing procedures." The flexibility in the requirements allows each manufacturer to individually decide how to best implement the necessary controls by using scientifically sound design, processing methods, and testing procedures. This flexibility allows companies to utilize continuous improvement along with innovative approaches and modern technologies to achieve higher quality, prevent contamination, mix-ups, and errors. Adherence to CGMP regulations ensures the identity, strength, quality, and purity of drug products by requiring manufacturers to adequately control their manufacturing operations. The control mechanisms should include establishing a strong quality management system, obtaining quality raw materials, establishing robust operating procedures, detecting and investigating deviations in product quality, and maintaining reliable testing laboratories. If a drug manufacturer does not comply with CGMP regulations, any drug it makes is considered adulterated. This does not mean that there is something wrong with the drug, but that the conditions under which it was made did not comply with CGMP. The product could be perfectly safe for use, but the US Federal Food, Drug, and Cosmetic (FD&C) Act establishes that drugs that are not manufactured according to CGMP requirements are adulterated.

2.3 Different versions of good manufacturing practice

There are many different versions of GMP in use around the world. As more and more countries improve the quality standards for their pharmaceutical industries, additional guidelines are developed. Some of these variants are described in this section. It should be noted that the wording of the various versions of GMP may differ slightly; however, the goal of what is to be achieved is practically identical. The degree of implementation and the interpretation may lead to minor differences between manufacturers.

2.3.1 Pharmaceutical Inspection Co-operation Scheme guide to good manufacturing practice

The Pharmaceutical Inspection Convention and Pharmaceutical Inspection Co-operation Scheme (jointly known as PIC/S) developed international standards between countries and pharmaceutical inspection authorities to provide a harmonized and constructive cooperation in the field of GMP. The original guide, published in 1972, was entitled "PIC Basic Standards." The most recent version, published July 1, 2018, aims to "facilitate the removal of barriers to trade in medicinal products, to promote uniformity in licensing decisions and to ensure the maintaining of high standards of QA in the development, manufacture and control of medicinal products."

In addition to the introduction document, the guide is divided into two parts and a host of annexes which are common to both parts. Part I covers GMP principles for the manufacture of medicinal products, Part II covers GMP for active substances used as starting materials, and the annexes provide detail on specific areas of activity, that is, sterile medicinal products, radiopharmaceuticals, biological medicinal products, medicinal gases, etc.

Since this book focuses on the manufacture of medicinal products, Part I is of primary interest. The chapters of Part I are listed in Table 2.1.

The following sections show a clearly defined parallel with GMP guidelines for different countries.

2.3.2 Good manufacturing practice and the WHO

The WHO is a United Nations agency with responsibility for international health matters and public health. The approach of the WHO to GMP is that there is a need for a "comprehensive approach to QA, which, while retaining adequate rigor, had to

Table 2.1 PIC/S GMP chapters.

Chapter	Title
1	Pharmaceutical quality system
2	Personnel
3	Premises and equipment
4	Documentation
5	Production
6	Quality control
7	Outsourced activities
8	Complaints and product recall
9	Self-inspection

be adaptable to the needs and economic circumstances of developing countries" (WHO Expert Committee on Specifications for Pharmaceutical Preparations. Thirty-second Report, 1992).

The first version of the WHO GMP arose from the WHO Health Assembly in 1967. It was published in 1968. Several revisions have been drafted since the original document with the most current version published as WHO Technical Report Series, No. 986, 2014 entitled "Annex 2 WHO good manufacturing practices for pharmaceutical products: main principles."

The chapters of the WHO guidelines are similar to the PIC/S and EU guidelines; however, where the topics of some chapters are combined in the latter guidelines, they are treated as standalone chapters in the WHO guidelines (e.g., Premises and equipment and Complaints and recalls). Additionally, the WHO guidelines includes several chapters that are not covered in the other guidelines. The chapters for the WHO guidelines are shown in Table 2.2.

It should be noted that the current WHO guideline has been significantly expanded when compared to the earlier versions. A chapter on validation was added, a section on "Product quality review" was added to Chapter 1, the concept of risk management was added, the concept of a "quality unit" was introduced, and the term "drugs" was replaced by the term "medicines."

Table 2.2 WHO GMP chapters.

Chapter	Title
1	Pharmaceutical quality system
2	Good manufacturing practices for pharmaceutical products
3	Sanitation and hygiene
4	Qualification and validation
5	Complaints
6	Product recalls
7	Contract production, analysis and other activities
8	Self-inspection, quality audits and suppliers' audits and approval
9	Personnel
10	Training
11	Personal hygiene
12	Premises
13	Equipment
14	Materials
15	Documentation
16	Good practices in production
17	Good practices in quality control

2.3.3 Good manufacturing practice in the United Kingdom

The first GMP guide produced in the United Kingdom was published in 1971. It was subsequently updated in 1977 [when the concept of good distribution practice (GDP) for wholesalers was introduced] and again in 1983. The United Kingdom became part of the European Union in 1975. For a number of years, there were different GMP standards for the manufacture of pharmaceuticals/drugs across Europe, that is, British GMP, German GMP, French GMP, etc. As a result, pharmaceutical manufacturing sites would be inspected by their own national regulatory authority as well as the neighboring countries' authorities. In the mid-1980s, work began to harmonize the versions of GMP. One outcome of this was the European Union GMP (EU GMP), published in 1991. From this point forward, individual GMP guidelines for each member state became obsolete and were replaced by a single EU GMP that was adopted across all the European Union. From this agreement, member states were no longer inspected by regulatory authorities from other EU countries but by their own regulatory authority on behalf of the whole of Europe. Currently, this is the largest mutual agreement for GMP across the world, with all the EU regulatory authorities working together to get consistent inspections.

In Europe, directives are issued by the European Union, and these directives must then be incorporated in national law by each member state of the European Union. Two GMP directives were issued in 1991, one for human medicinal products (91/356/EEC) and one for animal medical products (91/412/EEC). This section focuses on the directive for human medicinal products. This directive was updated in 2003 due to the additional requirements for clinical trial materials. Directive 2003/94/EC was issued on October 8, 2003, to replace Directive 91/356/EEC.

The familiar volume, known in the United Kingdom and many other parts of the world as "The Orange Guide" after the color of the cover, continues to be published in the United Kingdom. Its correct title is "Rules and Guidance for Pharmaceutical Manufacturers and Distributors." The latest edition, issued in 2017, has been updated to incorporate changes and additions made to the European Commission guidelines on GMP, including Annexes 15 and 16.

The United Kingdom left the European Union in 2020. However, the trade deal agreed in January 2021 includes an annex on medicinal products that provides for mutual recognition of GMP inspections and certifications, meaning that manufacturing facilities do not need to undergo separate UK and EU inspections.

2.3.4 Good manufacturing practice in the European Union

As noted earlier, the principles of GMP within the European Union are detailed in Directive 91/356/EEC. Upon approval of this directive, all member states were required to comply by January 1, 1992. The directive covers all medicinal products sold in the European Union, including products imported from elsewhere and products manufactured in the European Union for sale elsewhere. Until 2001, the application of the guidelines to the manufacture of clinical trials material depended on national legislation. However, as described in Chapter 1, the introduction of the Clinical Trials Directive 2001/20/EC has changed this situation.

The European Union legislation for the pharmaceutical sector is compiled in the EudraLex. EudraLex Volume 4 (GMP guidelines) "contains guidance for the interpretation of the principles and guidelines of good manufacturing practices for medicinal products for human and veterinary use laid down in Commission Directives 91/356/EEC, as amended by Directive 2003/94/EC, and 91/412/EEC respectively" (https://ec.europa.eu/health/documents/eudralex/vol-4_en). Additionally, this volume is used for assessing applications for manufacturing authorizations and as a foundation for inspection of manufacturers of medicinal products. The volume is organized into three parts and supplemented by 19 annexes. Part I details GMP principles for the manufacture of medicinal products, Part II details GMP for active substances used as starting materials, and Part III covers GMP related documents that clarify regulatory expectations. The chapters of Part I, which focus on the "basic requirements," are based on principles as defined in Directives 2003/94/EC and 91/412/EEC.

Part I contains nine chapters, each of which focuses on a specific principle. Each chapter details the principles for following the quality management objectives of that chapter and provides details for implementing the principles. The chapters are summarized as follows:

1. *Pharmaceutical quality system*: The manufacturer shall establish, implement, and maintain an effective QA system involving active participation of management and personnel of the different departments.
2. *Personnel*: Requires sufficient personnel with appropriate qualifications and experience to carry out the duties that they have been assigned. It also covers the topics of training and personal hygiene.
3. *Premises and equipment*: Manufacturers must ensure the premises and manufacturing equipment are: located, designed, constructed, adapted, and maintained to suit the intended operations; laid out, designed and operated in such a way as to minimize the risk of error and to permit effective cleaning and maintenance; shall be subjected to appropriate qualification and validation, which are critical to the quality of the products.
4. *Documentation*: There are a variety of documents that are mandatory for companies to have in place when carrying out pharmaceutical manufacturing. These include specifications for all starting materials, packaging materials, bulk product, intermediates and finished products. Specifications are the documents defining the material and describing analytical tests, test parameters and acceptance criteria. Also required are the manufacturing formulae and packaging instructions which are the

master documents from which individual batch documents are derived; batch processing records which must be completed during the manufacture and packaging respectively of each individual batch of product; standard operating procedures which describe all activities that are not product-specific (such as operation of a piece of machinery or sanitation programmes for the various parts of a factory). This section also deals with the management of electronic data. When electronic, photographic, or other data processing systems are used instead of written documents, the manufacturer shall be required to first validate the systems by showing that the data will be appropriately stored, properly protected, backed up, and readily available in legible form upon the request of authorities.

5. *Production*: Different production operations shall be carried out in accordance with preestablished instructions and procedures following GMP. There must be adequate and sufficient resources available for in-process control. Appropriate technical organizational measures should be taken to avoid cross contamination and mix-ups. Any new or modified processes and critical phases of manufacturing shall be regularly validated or revalidated.

6. *Quality control*: The manufacturer shall establish and maintain a quality control system under the authority of a person who has requisite qualifications and is independent of production. That person shall have access to, or at his disposal, one or more appropriately staffed and equipped quality control laboratories that can be used to conduct necessary examination and testing of starting materials, packaging materials, and intermediate and finished products.

7. *Outsourced activities*: Any manufacturing operation which is carried out under contract shall have a written contract. The contract shall clearly define the responsibilities of each party and define the observance of GMP to be followed by the contract-acceptor and how the qualified person responsible for certifying each batch is to discharge their responsibilities. The contract-acceptor shall not subcontract any of the work entrusted to the manufacturer without written authorization from the contract-giver.

8. *Complaints and Product Recall*: The manufacturer shall implement a system for recording and reviewing complaints along with an effective system for promptly recalling products in the distribution network. The manufacturer shall record and investigate any defect complaint. The manufacturer shall inform the authorities of any defect that could result in a recall or abnormal restriction in supply and if possible, indicate the destination countries. A procedure for rapid unblinding of blinded products shall be implemented where there is a necessity for a prompt recall.

9. *Self-inspection*: Manufacturers shall conduct repeated self-inspection as part of QA to monitor the implementation of GMP and to propose necessary corrective measures. Records of such self-inspections and corrective action shall be maintained.

2.3.5 Good manufacturing practice in the United States

As noted in Section 2.2.1 CGMP, GMP in the United States is termed CGMP. The detailed CGMP requirements are found in Title 21 of the US FDA CFR. Guidelines for drugs are addressed in Parts 210 and 211 (https://www.fda.gov/drugs/pharmaceutical-quality-resources/current-good-manufacturing-practice-CGMP-regulations). Part 210 (Current Good Manufacturing Practice in Manufacturing Processing, Packing, or Holding of Drugs) discusses the status of CGMP regulations, their applicability, and definitions. Part 211 (Current Good Manufacturing Practice for Finished Pharmaceuticals) covers a wide range of topics under several subparts, each of which is broken down into several sections. The subparts and a summary of their contents are shown in Table 2.3.

2.3.6 Good manufacturing practice in Australia

In Australia GMP falls under the guidelines of Section 36 of the Therapeutic Goods Act 1989. The Minister for Health determines manufacturing practices that will be applied in the manufacture of therapeutic goods. The current Therapeutic Goods (Manufacturing Principles) Determination 2020 specifies that medicinal products supplied in Australia must meet the PIC/S Guide to GMP, except for Annexes 4, 5, and 14.

Table 2.3 Summary of US FDA title 21 CFR Part 211 contents.

Subpart	Title	Summary of contents
A	General provisions	Scope and definitions
B	Organization and personnel	Details roles and responsibilities
C	Buildings and facilities	Details design, construction and maintenance of buildings and facilities
D	Equipment	Details equipment requirements and other specific topic, that is, automatic equipment and filters
E	Control of components and drug product containers and closures	Reviews their handling throughout the manufacturing process, from receipt to use. Emphasizes primary packaging components should be treated no differently from other starting materials
F	Production and process controls	Reviews reconciliation, in-process controls, and testing.
G	Packaging and labeling controls	Details the requirements for the issue and use of labels and other packaging materials
H	Holding and distribution	Covers the aspects of manufacturing that relate to holding (storage) and distribution.
I	Laboratory controls	Details requirements for laboratory controls
J	Record and reports	Covers all aspects of records and reports
K	Returned and salvaged products	Covers returned and salvaged drug products

2.3.7 Good manufacturing practice in Brazil

Brazil is an emerging market in pharmaceutical products. Drug registration and the licensing of pharmaceutical companies fall under its National Health Surveillance Agency, Agência Nacional de Vigilância Sanitária (ANVISA). In April 2010, ANVISA revised the previous GMP guidelines to include standards set by the WHO, that is, quality, sanitation and hygiene, qualification and validation, and products and contracts. The current standards apply to pharmaceutical products negotiated within Mercosur, which includes Argentina, Brazil, Paraguay, Uruguay, and Venezuela. Countries with associate member status are Bolivia, Chile, Colombia, Ecuador, and Peru.

In addition to drug registration and licensing, ANVISA establishes regulations for clinical trials and drug pricing. The agency works with states and municipalities in the inspection of factories, monitoring of drug quality, postmarketing surveillance, pharmacovigilance actions, and the regulation of drug promotion and marketing. ANVISA also works along with the National Industrial Property Institute in analyzing patent requests related to pharmaceutical processes and products.

2.3.8 Good manufacturing practice in Canada

In Canada, the production of drug products is controlled by the Canadian Food and Drugs Act. Their GMP guidelines, entitled "Good manufacturing practices guide for drug products (GUI-0001)," were developed by Health Canada in consultation with stakeholders. GUI-0001 interprets the requirements for GMP as stated in Part C, Division 2 of the Food and Drug Regulations, which is part of the Food and Drugs Act. The scope of the GUI-0001 guide is broad and applies to pharmaceutical, radiopharmaceutical, biological, and veterinary drugs. The document states that the guideline was written with a view to harmonizing the GMP standards with the WHO, PIC/S, International Council for Harmonization (ICH), Veterinary International Conference on Harmonization (VICH), and other regulatory agencies in other countries.

The GMP guideline is divided into five chapters and three appendices with the GMP regulations, and their applications presented in Chapter 5. This chapter is subdivided into 16 subchapters that cover the specific requirements and their applications. The requirements are summarized in Table 2.4.

As the table shows, the sections of this guide are similar to the previously mentioned guidelines.

2.3.9 Good manufacturing practice in China

In China, the regulation of medicinal products falls under the Drug Administration Law of the People's Republic of China. Its "GMP for Drugs" was first proclaimed in 1988 and was revised in 1992 and 1998. The latest revision, 2010, released by the Ministry of Health, has been effective since March 1, 2011. This new version of GMP

Table 2.4 Chapters of Canadian GOP (GUI-0001) guidelines.

Chapter	Title
C.02.002	Regulations
C.02.003	Sale
C.02.003.3	Use in fabrication
C.02.004	Premises
C.02.005	Equipment
C.02.006	Personnel
C.02.007 and 0.008	Sanitation
C.02.009 and 0.010	Raw material testing
C.02.011 and 0.012	Manufacturing control
C.02.013, 0.014 and 0.015	Quality control department
C.02.016 and 0.017	Packaging material testing
C.02.018 and 0.019	Finished product testing
C.02.020, 0.021, 0.022, 0.023, 0.024, and 0.024.1	Records
C.02.025 and 0.026	Samples
C.02.027 and 0.028	Stability
C.02.029	Sterile products
C.02.030	Medical gases

consists of 14 chapters and 313 articles and aligns with WHO GMP relative to the concepts of quality risk management and tighter process control of drug manufacturing. Overseas manufacturers of drug products supplied to China must provide evidence that the products are manufactured to GMP standards that are equivalent to the standards expected of Chinese manufacturers of the same goods.

2.3.10 Good manufacturing practice in Japan

In Japan, the legal framework for GMP is set by the Pharmaceutical Affairs Law (PAL); whereas it is regulated and inspected by the Ministry of Health, Labor and Welfare (MHLW). Over the years, the MHLW has issued three Ministerial Ordinances that cover the legal requirements for Japanese GMP. In addition to medicines, these Ordinances cover requirements for cosmetics and medical devices. Ministerial Ordinance No. 2 was developed in 1961 and covers the basic requirements for suitable facilities. Because of its age and its ambiguity, it is rarely referenced anymore. Ministerial Ordinance No. 179, developed in 2004, covers standards for Manufacturing Control and the Quality Control of Drug Products and is more widely used and referred to. The Quality Control standards include the requirements for controlling production, avoiding cross-contamination, validation, change control, and control of deviations. Another widely used guidance is Ministerial Ordinance No. 136, developed in 2004. It covers the requirements for "good quality practices" (GQP) rather than GMP. In Japan, GQP is the nearest equivalent to GMP. Within this Ordinance are the requirements for the general manager (site head), personnel, documentation and records, storage, QA, internal audits, batch release, and recall. Collectively, these three ministerial ordinances hold the requirements for GMP in Japan. As a member of the ICH, Japan adopted the ICH guidance document Q7, "GMP Guide for Active Pharmaceutical Ingredients" and published it as Pharmaceutical and Food Safety Bureau (PFSB) Director—General Notification No. 1200, 2001 "Guidelines on GMP for Drug Substances." This guideline states the requirements for the manufacture of APIs.

2.3.11 Good manufacturing practice in India

In India, GMP is covered under Schedule M of the Drugs and Cosmetics Rules, 1945. The rules, last amended in December 2016, govern the production of drugs in India. For GMP, the rules state that the licensee shall comply with the GMPs laid down in Schedule M, last amended in June 2005. Schedule M is divided into eight parts: I, IA, IB, IC, ID, IE, IF, and II. The general requirements for GMP are covered in Part I (Good Manufacturing Practices for Premises and Materials). Part I is further divided into 29 chapters, as shown in Table 2.5.

2.3.12 Good manufacturing practice in South Africa

In South Africa (SA), the Medicines and Related Substances Control Act (Act 101 of 1965) controls the production of drug products. South Africa's GMP guidelines are housed under the "SA Guide to Good Manufacturing Practice for Medicines." This guide was implemented in 1997 and was last revised in July 2019. The guide states that "GMP describes a set of principles and procedures that, when followed, ensure that medicines and related substances are of high quality, safety and efficacy." The guide was published by the South African Health Products Regulatory Authority (SAHPRA) who is a participating authority with PIC/S. The guide requires that manufacturers, importers and exporters of medicines and related substances in South Africa meet the standards laid out in the PIC/S Guide to Good Manufacturing Practice (GMP). As such, SAHPRA has adopted the PIC/S Guide to GMP, and all prospective adaptations as prescribed by the PIC/S. Annex 16 of the PIC/S guide to GMP pertains to country specific requirements and should be replaced with the SA specific Annex 16 as detailed in Section 2.4 of this guideline. The SA GMP consists of five sections and several annexes. As stated above, the specific GMP guidelines are captured in Section 2.4 (Annex 16—South African Specific Requirements: Organization and Personnel). The subsections are shown in Table 2.6.

2.4 Comparisons of different good manufacturing practice guidelines

As witnessed in the previous sections, different guidelines present the GMP topics in differing degrees of depth, in different orders, and in different topic combinations. It is

Table 2.5 Chapters of India's schedule M Part I (Good Manufacturing Practices for Premises and Materials).

Chapter	Title
1	General requirements
2	Warehousing area
3	Production area
4	Ancillary areas
5	Quality control area
6	Personnel
7	Health, clothing and sanitation of workers
8	Manufacturing operations and controls
9	Sanitation in the manufacturing premises
10	Raw materials
11	Equipment
12	Documentation and records
13	Labels and other printed materials
14	Quality assurance
15	Self-inspection and quality audit
16	Quality control system
17	Specification
18	Master formula records
19	Packaging records
20	Batch packaging records
21	Batch processing records
22	Standard operating procedures (SOPs) and records
23	Reference samples
24	Reprocessing and recoveries
25	Distribution records
26	Validation and process validation
27	Product recalls
28	Complaints and adverse reactions
29	Site master file

often useful to consult several source documents to clarify specific aspects for the country in which the manufacturing company is located. There will always be one main reference document in use which should be a part of a company's quality system documentation.

2.5 Rules versus guidelines

The requirements of GMP are generally set out as guidelines, rather than rules. In fact, many of the reference documents have the word guidelines in their titles. GMP guidelines tell a company what is required. They rarely tell the company how that

Table 2.6 Section of 4 (Annex 16) of South African GMP contents.

Subsection	Title
4.1	Principles
4.2	Responsibilities of key personnel
4.3	Legal aspects
4.4	Qualifications
4.5	Training
4.6	Hygiene

requirement is to be achieved. In other words, in the world of GMP, there are no right answers but only interpretations.

There are often preferred solutions, which have developed through custom and practice within the industry. However, if a company chooses to adopt a different solution for a particular requirement, they are at liberty to do so. As a result, the company must prove to their government inspector, or other auditing body, that the approach they have taken is appropriate and scientifically proven to achieve the required result.

This reliance on personal interpretation of guidelines, rather than adherence to rigid rules, is an approach that is particularly difficult for some countries to adjust to—particularly companies in traditionally highly-regulated countries. For example, the Soviet Union (formerly the USSR) had a wide range of standards in place that laid down the rules for construction of factories and manufacturing of products. Many of these standards are still in place, and on occasion, can conflict with the accepted custom and practice of GMP around the world. On the other hand, the lack of clear statements on what is allowed can result in confusion both among companies and licensing authorities.

2.6 Application of good manufacturing practice

Earlier parts of this chapter reviewed the guidelines produced in different countries to assist their respective companies achieve GMP compliance. Specific sections of GMP are also covered in greater detail in other chapters in this book. This section discusses the applied approach to the implementation of the GMP concepts. This applied approach is sometimes called the "10 Commandments of GMP" or "10 Principles of GMP." The principles, which parallel the EU, WHO, and PIC/S guidelines, are summarized as follows:

1. *Clearly defined processes*: All manufacturing processes should be clearly defined during development and reviewed on an on-going basis to ensure that they are appropriate and capable of consistently producing the required result. Additionally, this principle applies to the external and internal environment. The external environment should be such that the manufacturing facility is in a location that is not subjected to the

potential for water damage, infestation, or contamination of any type. The building should be well-designed and constructed such that the air, water, lighting, ventilation, temperature, and humidity within (internal environment) the facility does not impact product quality. The equipment should be designed, located, and maintained to suit its intended use. The equipment should be in a logical and well-planned layout that will suit the sequence of operations, reduce the chances of cross contamination, and to avoid mix-ups and errors.

2. *Validated processes*: All critical steps within a manufacturing process should be validated when the product/process is first introduced and whenever there are any substantive changes made to that process. Validation means that there is documented evidence that provides a high degree of assurance that a specific process will consistently deliver product that meets its predetermined specifications and quality attributes. This ensures that the process not only performs consistently but also can be proved, with documented evidence, to do so.

3. *Necessary resources*: All necessary resources should be provided. The resources include: trained, qualified personnel; sufficient, suitable premises; appropriate equipment and services; materials, correctly labeled in appropriate containers; approved standard operating procedures; and appropriate arrangements for storage and transport.

4. *Clear documentation*: Manufacturing instructions and standard operating procedures should be clearly written in a manner that will be understood by the personnel for whom they are intended. They must be tailored to the specific facility in question. It is a GMP requirement that the written documents are followed.

5. *Trained operators*: Even with defined processes and clear documentation, manufacturing will not be carried out satisfactorily unless the operators are properly trained, and the procedures are carried out correctly.

6. *Appropriate records*: All activities taking place during manufacturing must be adequately recorded to demonstrate that defined procedures and instructions were followed and that the quantity and quality of product are as expected. The general approach is: if it is not written down, it didn't happen. The documentation may be completed manually or by electronic recording devices. There must be an effective control system for obtaining and maintaining these records. All process deviations must also be recorded and fully investigated before a batch can be released.

7. *Batch traceability*: It is important that all manufacturing and distribution records are maintained in a suitable format so that full traceability is available. This particularly includes distribution records, which are critical in the case of a batch recall.

8. *Quality maintained during distribution*: The responsibility for maintenance of quality does not end at the factory gate. It is important that throughout the distribution chain, appropriate controls and storage conditions are maintained. This is

reasonably easy when the manufacturer controls the distribution channel. However, even when the products are distributed by other entities (such as wholesalers), there is still a responsibility to ensure that the product is properly stored and distributed to minimize risk to the quality of the product.

9. *Recall system*: No company wants to deal with a recall situation, but it is necessary for all of them to be prepared for this potential incidence. A procedure must be in place to recall any batch of product from sale or supply.

10. *Complaints system*: All complaints must be investigated to determine whether they are justified. If they are justified, it is necessary to determine the cause of the quality defects. Actions must be taken to rectify any immediate problems and prevent any recurrence.

2.7 Good manufacturing practice and manufacture of clinical trial material

It is generally accepted that wherever possible, the manufacture of clinical trials material should be subject to the same GMP requirements as licensed products.

2.7.1 European Union requirements

In the European Union, Annex 13 of the EU Guidance on Good Manufacturing Practice applies. Each section refers back to the relevant chapter in the main text.

2.7.1.1 Quality management

This section highlights the requirement for a pharmaceutical quality system while acknowledging that processes may be variable from batch to batch. Requirements for the product specification file are detailed.

2.7.1.2 Personnel

The section on personnel acknowledges there are likely to be only a small number of personnel involved but emphasizes the importance of maintaining the independence of QC from production. It also outlines the responsibilities of the qualified person.

2.7.1.3 Premises and equipment

The section on premises and equipment recognizes that manufacturing of clinical trials material can differ from the production of licensed materials in the same way as the manufacturing of "specials." The batch size is small, and it is likely that different products could be in progress in different parts of the same facility at the same time. This has implications for product security systems and for cleaning procedures to ensure that no cross-contamination occurs.

There is an additional consideration in relation to the manufacture of highly sensitizing or biological products. Under GMP requirements, such products would normally be produced in separate facilities. However, at the stage of clinical trials, this is not practical. An acceptable alternative would be the use of campaign manufacture, but particular care needs to be taken with cleaning and product security systems.

Finally, the small batch sizes involved cause problems in the validation of sterile manufacturing processes. The required number of units will often be equivalent to a full batch. The fact that many operations could be manual will increase the need for environmental monitoring.

A quality risk management approach must be taken to assess and control the risks of cross contamination presented by the manufacture of clinical trails material.

2.7.1.4 Documentation

The section on documentation deals with the fact that the process may change during the time of the trial and hence it is important to have a good change control procedure to ensure full traceability of all the changes. In these circumstances, it is not essential to develop formal master formulation or processing instructions, as it would be for licensed products. There are detailed instructions for: specifications and instructions; orders; manufacturing formulae and processing instructions; packaging instructions; and batch records. Document retention periods are also specified.

2.7.1.5 Production

The section on production begins with a comment on the implications of possible variations in packaging materials. It then continues with a discussion on manufacturing operations. Due to lack of validation, there will tend to be less information from which to determine critical process parameters. It may be necessary to deduce process parameters from information obtained on other systems. The need for reconciliation is emphasized, particularly in relation to labeling. Additionally, there is mention of the increased levels of QC checks that may be required in relation to biological contamination, cleaning procedures and unvalidated processes such as mixing.

There is a review of the considerations to be made in the manufacture of clinical trials material for comparator product studies. It is important that the integrity of the product is maintained and the significance of any changes is recognized. Changes to the primary packaging used may have an effect on the use-by date that can be applied.

There is also a mention of the aspects of randomization codes and blinding operations. It is important that identification of the "blinded" product is possible and that appropriate samples are kept.

2.7.1.6 Quality control

The section on QC emphasizes the increased importance of end-product testing in the absence of validated processes. There is acknowledgment of the need for compliance with the aspects of the specification that relate to efficacy. Retained samples of clinical trials material must be kept. These samples will generally be kept in the same primary packaging as the administered doses. If by exception, an alternative pack is used, the effect on the shelf life must be considered.

2.7.1.7 Release of batches

This section details the process by which the Qualified Person can release batches for use and acknowledges there will be variations in the process based on such factors as the product's country of origin; the manufacturer; whether the product already has a marketing authorization; and the phase of its development.

2.7.1.8 Outsourced operations

Any outsourced operations must be covered by a written contract between the contract giver and the contract acceptor.

2.7.1.9 Complaints

Any complaints must be investigated as per normal GMP requirements. Additionally, the impact on the trial and the need for reporting a serious breach must be assessed.

2.7.1.10 Returns and destruction

The final section of the annex deals with returns and destruction. Any materials that are returned should be handled under carefully controlled conditions and should be stored in a segregated area. Destruction of materials should be carried out by or at least under the instructions of the sponsor.

2.7.2 Current good manufacturing practice requirements

CGMP helps to ensure the safety of human subjects when an investigational new drug is introduced to human subjects during the Phase I trials; however, 21 CFR Part 210.2(c) states that "An investigational drug for use in a Phase 1 study... is exempt from compliance with the regulations in part 211." As noted in Section 2.3.5 of this book, Part 211 specifies the CGMP regulations.

2.7.3 Pharmaceutical Inspection Co-operation Scheme requirements

The PIC/S approach to GMP during clinical trials relates to protecting human subjects and is detailed in an Aide Memoire document developed in 2002 by a team of PIC/S inspectors. The document entitled "GMP Particularities in The Manufacture of Medicinal Products to Be Used in Clinical Trials on Human Subjects" became active in January 2006. The guide states that the guidelines are "to be applied in addition to the applicable GMPs." Additionally, the guide states "The application of GMPs to the manufacture of investigational medicinal products (IMP) is intended to ensure that trial subjects are not placed at risk and that the results of clinical trials are unaffected by inadequate safety, quality, or efficacy arising from unsatisfactory manufacture." The guidance continues with guidelines relating to packaging of the IMP, training of personnel; added assurance with respect to safety, quality, and efficacy; and inspections. Also, the document states that its purpose is "to provide guidance for GMP inspectors in the evaluation of sites that manufacture, package and label IMPs."

2.7.4 Requirements of the WHO

Annex 2 of the WHO good manufacturing practices for pharmaceutical products states that the guide is also applicable to "operations for the manufacture of medicines in their finished dosage forms, including large-scale processes in hospitals and the preparation of supplies for use in clinical trials." Therefore the guidelines for clinical trial products fall under the same standards as the production of finished products.

2.8 Chapter summary

- GMP is the abbreviation for Good Manufacturing Practice.
- CGMP is the United States' expanded requirement for GMP where "C" refers to "current."
- The simplistic definition of GMP is the process of preventing cross-contamination and mix-ups.
- Cross-contamination is where different materials or products become mixed, either in large quantities or as trace amounts.
- Mix-ups are where printed packaging materials, particularly labels, are mixed together.
- The PIC/S and the WHO published international GMP guidelines.
- Many countries have published their own versions of GMP.
- The requirements of GMP are generally set out as guidelines, rather than rules.
- The GMP guidelines describe what should be achieved, rather than how it should be done and the "how" is often a question of interpretation and is the responsibility of the individual companies.
- The "10 Commandments of GMP" or "10 Principles of GMP" refer to the applied approach to the implementation of the GMP concepts.
- Nationally and internationally, the specific GMP requirements for clinical trials material may differ slightly from the requirements for the finished product.

2.9 Questions/problems

1. How does CGMP differ from GMP?
2. How is the PIC/S GMP different from the WHO GMP?
3. What are the two international GMP guides?
4. What is implied by the "10 Commandments of GMP" or "10 Principles of GMP"? How do they differ from other GMP guidelines?
5. How are the GMP requirements for the manufacture of finished products different for GMP for clinical trials material? Which guidelines state distinct differences in the requirements?

Further reading

Australian Government Department of Health, 2021. Manufacturing principles for medicinal products. https://www.tga.gov.au/publication/manufacturing-principles-medicinal-products (accessed 20.04.21).

Australian Government, 2021. Therapeutic Goods Act 1989. https://www.legislation.gov.au/Details/C2021C00142 (accessed 06.04.21).

Avanti Polar Lipids, 2020. CGMP and GMP: what's the difference? https://avantilipids.com/news/CGMP-and-gmp-whats-the-difference (accessed 06.04.21).

Bunn, G.P., 2019. Good Manufacturing Practices for Pharmaceuticals, seventh ed. CRC Press, Florida.

European Commission, 2021. EudraLex - EU Legislation. https://ec.europa.eu/health/documents/eudralex_en (accessed 22.04.21).

Government of India, 2016. The Drugs and Cosmetics Act and Rules, The Drugs and Cosmetics Act, 1940 and The Drugs and Cosmetics Rules, 1945.

Health Canada, 2020. Good manufacturing practices guide for drug products (GUI-0001). https://www.canada.ca/content/dam/hc-sc/documents/services/drugs-health-products/compliance-enforcement/good-manufacturing-practices/guidance-documents/gmp-guidelines-0001/gui-0001-eng.pdf (accessed 20.04.21).

Medicines and Healthcare products Regulatory Agency, 2017. Guidance for Pharmaceutical Manufacturers and Distributors 2017 (The Orange Guide). Pharmaceutical Press, London.

Ministry of Health and Family Welfare, 2005. Schedule M good manufacturing practices and requirements of premises, plant and equipment for pharmaceutical products. http://rajswasthya.nic.in/drug%20website%2021.01.11/revised%20schedule%20%20m%204.pdf (accessed 26.04.21).

National Institute of Health Sciences, http://www.nihs.go.jp (accessed 26.04.21).

Official Journal of the European Union, 2014. Regulation (Eu) No 536/2014 of the european parliament clinical trials on medicinal products for human use. Retrieved 4/29/2021 from https://ec.europa.eu/health/sites/health/files/files/eudralex/vol-1/reg_2014_536/reg_2014_536_en.pdf (accessed 29.04.21).

Official Journal of the European Union, 2017. Commission directive (EU) 2017/1572. September 16, 2017.

Pharmaceutical Inspection Convention Pharmaceutical Inspection Co-Operation Scheme (Pic/S), 2018. PIC/S guide to good manufacturing practice for medicinal products.

Pharmaceutical Inspection Convention Pharmaceutical Inspection Co-Operation Scheme (Pic/S), 2018. PIC/S guide to good manufacturing practice for medicinal products part I.

Pharmaceutical Inspection Convention Pharmaceutical Inspection Co-Operation Scheme (Pic/S), 2018. PIC/S guide to good manufacturing practice for medicinal products part II.

Pharmaceutical Inspection Convention Pharmaceutical Inspection Co-Operation Scheme (PIC/S), 2007. GMP particularities in the manufacture of medicinal products to be used in clinical trials on human subjects.

Pharmaceutical Press, 2017. Guidance for pharmaceutical manufacturers and distributors 2017 (The Orange Guide). https://www.pharmpress.com/product.asp?productid = 9780857112859&affiliateid = (accessed 13.04.21).

PharmOut, 2017. White paper: 10 golden rules of GMP. February 2016.

Rodríguez-Pérez, J., 2014. The FDA and Worldwide Current Good Manufacturing Practices and Quality System Requirements Guidebook for Finished Pharmaceuticals. Milwaukee, Wisconsin; American Society for Quality, Quality Press.

South African Health Products Regulatory Authority, 2017. 4.01_SA Guide to good manufacturing practice for medicines.

The Commission of the European Communities, 2003. Commission directive 2003/94/EC.

US FDA, 2008. Guidance for industry CGMP for phase 1 investigational drugs. https://www.fda.gov/media/70975/download (accessed 06.04.21).

US FDA, 2020. CFR — code of federal regulations title 21, part 211 current good manufacturing practice for finished pharmaceuticals, Retrieved 4/6/2021 from https://www.accessdata.fda.gov/scripts/cdrh/cfdocs/cfcfr/CFRSearch.cfm?CFRPart = 211 (accessed 06.04.21).

World Health Organization, 2003. Good manufacturing practices for pharmaceutical products: Main principles. https://gmpua.com/World/WHO/Annex4/trs908-4.pdf (accessed 06.04.21).

Zheng, X., 2012. Regulation of medicines in China. WHO drug information (Vol. 26, Issue 1). https://go.gale.com/ps/i.do?p = HRCA&u = ncliveecu&id = GALE%7CA291895144&v = 2.1&it = r&sid = summon (accessed 24.04.21).

CHAPTER 3

Elements of quality management

3.1 Introduction

Within the pharmaceutical manufacturing environment, various functions related to quality management are critical. This chapter discusses two of the three main functions, quality assurance (QA) and quality control (QC). The third element, good manufacturing practice (GMP) has been covered separately in Chapter 2.

For a complete understanding of quality management, it is important to understand the terminology and the difference between quality management, QA, and QC. Therefore the chapter begins with an overview of the concept of quality management systems and continues with a review of the interrelationship between the three concepts. It then follows a review of the definitions of each function and the differences between them before introducing sections covering the responsibilities of QA and QC in detail. The chapter concludes with a summary and suggested questions and problems for further consideration.

3.2 The quality management system

The topic of quality management systems in the formal sense of the word will be fully covered in Chapter 4 in the discussion on the ISO 9000 series of standards. There are a few examples of such registrations within the pharmaceutical industry itself, but more in the case of suppliers to the industry and medical device manufacturers.

There is a Pharmaceutical Inspection Convention/Pharmaceutical Inspection Co-operation Scheme (PIC/S) document that reviews the topic of quality systems, and while it is written primarily for pharmaceutical inspectorates, it provides a useful reference for companies as well. PI 002-3 *Recommendation on Quality System Requirements for Pharmaceutical Inspectorates* defines a quality system as

> *The sum of all that is necessary to implement an organization's quality policy and meet quality objectives. It includes organization structure, responsibilities, procedures, systems, processes and resources. Typically these features will be addressed in different kinds of documents as the quality manual and documented procedures, modus operandi, etc.*

The principal documentation of a quality system is contained in a quality manual and quality procedures. The quality manual is the document that describes how the

Quality
DOI: https://doi.org/10.1016/B978-0-323-90815-3.00002-5

organization addresses the various clauses within the quality standard. It will include reference to the quality procedures that describe the activities of the organization and how the quality system is to be maintained. PI 002-3 contains sections on organizational structure, documentation, and change control plus other quality system requirements such as records, procedures, internal audit, and corrective/preventive action.

3.3 Relationship between quality management, quality assurance, good manufacturing practice, and quality control

The relationship between quality management, QA, GMP, and QC can be viewed as a cascade arrangement as shown in Fig. 3.1.

Quality management, containing the overall policy of the organization toward quality, is over everything else. Next comes QA, which is the unit ensuring the policy is achieved. GMP is a part of QA. It builds quality into the product by addressing potential problems in advance and avoiding them. QC is the part of GMP that focuses on testing the environment and facilities, as well as testing the materials, components, and products under the standards.

While the previous paragraph is written in the context of the pharmaceutical company manufacturing the product, quality management is a much wider concept and should be applied across the entire organization. It also involves a structured approach to documentation.

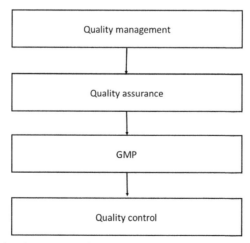

Figure 3.1 The relationship between quality management, quality assurance, good manufacturing practice, and quality control.

3.4 Documentation cascade

The analogy of a champagne fountain can be used to explain the documentation cascade. At the top of the cascade are the international and national policies, codes of practice, and standards, which govern everything in the pharmaceutical industry.

At the second level are the statements of goals, mission statement, and values to which the company wishes to adhere. These should be designed to meet all the national and international codes that apply. They set the overall framework within which the company will operate. This should include references to public health and the environment.

At the third level is the company quality manual which includes the policy statement stemming from the mission statement. The quality manual will be designed to deliver the mission statement, goals, and values the company has set for itself.

At the fourth level is the company quality system developed to provide details for the policy statement. The quality system is designed to ensure the quality policy is achieved in reality and is not just words.

At the fifth level are the major departments' strategies involving research and development (R&D), manufacturing, and QA. The documents explain how each department will achieve its contribution to the quality system, using the major policies to be implemented.

At the sixth level are the procedures and standards (including standard operating procedures (SOPs) and standard operating setpoints) developed in each department to implement the strategies. By this point, quality should be embedded into the work of each department.

At the base of the cascade are the individual job instructions and performance of the work to meet the standards and procedures, including the critical records of each part of the manufacturing process.

This arrangement forms all the elements of the documentation system into a closely linked cascade. Each level provides a reference for the level below. All the activities are closely aligned with one another and eventually to the achievement of the national and relevant international standards.

Having set the various functions within the overall context, the remainder of the chapter returns to the individual organization with specific reference to quality management, QA, and QC.

3.5 International guidelines

In the context of the pharmaceutical industry, the International Council for Harmonization (ICH) of Technical Requirements for Pharmaceuticals for Human Use guidelines are a major source of international guidance documents. The full database of such documents can be found at https://www.ich.org/page/search-index-ich-guidelines. The guidelines are divided into four categories:

- Efficacy
- Multidisciplinary
- Quality
- Safety

With quality management, it is only necessary to consider those in the third category, quality; and more specifically, guidelines Q7 to Q10.

3.5.1 Guideline for active pharmaceutical ingredients

ICH Q7 *Good manufacturing practice for active pharmaceutical ingredients* relates to the manufacturing of active pharmaceutical ingredients (APIs) and the quality management system required to ensure the APIs have the required level of quality and purity.

3.5.2 Guideline on pharmaceutical development

ICH Q8 (R2) *Pharmaceutical development* relates to the presentation of the development and manufacturing process knowledge, obtained through applying scientific approaches and quality risk management.

3.5.3 Guideline on quality risk management

ICH Q9 *Quality risk management* relates to the principles and tools for the application of quality risk management throughout all phases of the lifecycle of a pharmaceutical drug substance or a pharmaceutical drug product.

3.5.4 Guideline on pharmaceutical quality system

ICH Q10 *Pharmaceutical quality system* relates to the system required to manage the quality of pharmaceutical drug substances and products throughout the entire product lifecycle.

3.6 ICH Q10 expanded

Since quality management is the topic of this chapter, it is appropriate to explore this guideline in more detail than the others referenced in Section 3.5.

3.6.1 Relationship to other regulations and guidelines

ICH Q10 complements ICH Q8 and ICH Q9 and builds on the foundations provided by ICH Q7 and regional GMP requirements. Where the elements of ICH Q10 exceed the GMP requirements, they are optional rather than mandatory. The purpose is to facilitate the use of a science and risk-based approach to the pharmaceutical lifecycle.

3.6.2 Objectives of ICH Q10

There are three main objectives identified for the pharmaceutical quality system outlined in this guideline:

- *Product realization*: A system should be in place which ensures the appropriate quality attributes are obtained.
- *State of control*: Control and monitoring should be in place to ensure processes are both suitable and capable.
- *Continual improvement*: Programs should be in place to derive ongoing improvements in product quality, processes and the quality management system itself.

3.6.3 Enablers

There are two enablers identified within the guideline which facilitate its implementation:

- *Knowledge management*: A scientific approach at all stages of the product life cycle which comprises acquisition, analysis, storage, and dissemination of information on products, processes and components.
- *Quality risk management*: The identification, evaluation, and control of potential risks to quality, enabling process and product quality improvements.

3.6.4 Design and content of the quality management system

ICH Q10 lists seven aspects to be considered when designing a pharmaceutical quality system:

- A clear structure that can be easily communicated, understood, and applied.
- Appropriate and proportionate application at each of the different life cycle stages.
- The complexity of the company will dictate whether aspects of the system are applied at the company level or site level, although effectiveness should always be assessed at the site level.
- The system should extend to QA for outsourced activities and purchased materials.
- Management responsibilities are a key element.
- Process performance and product quality monitoring, corrective and preventive action (CAPA), change management, and management review are also key elements.
- Performance indicators are used to monitor the effectiveness of the pharmaceutical quality system.

3.6.5 Quality manual

Implementation of a pharmaceutical quality system, as outlined in ICH Q10, requires the establishment of a quality manual that includes the company's quality policy, the scope of the system, process descriptions, and management responsibilities.

3.6.6 Management responsibility

It is clearly stated in ICH Q10 that responsibility for the establishment and implementation of the pharmaceutical quality system rests squarely with senior management. The role encompasses the following activities:

- Establishment of an effective system.
- Support for implementation of the system.
- Communication and escalation of quality issues to appropriate management levels.
- Definition of roles, authorities, and responsibilities.
- Review of the ongoing effectiveness of the system.
- Support for continual improvement.
- Provision of appropriate resources.

Senior management must ensure the quality policy is established, communicated, and reviewed for effectiveness. They should be involved in the definition of quality objectives and manage the resourcing to ensure the objectives can be achieved. Their responsibilities extend to control of outsourced activities and purchased materials; and continue throughout the technology transfer associated with any change in product ownership.

3.6.7 Continual improvement of process performance and product quality

The objectives of ICH Q10 cover four stages of a pharmaceutical product: development; technology transfer; commercial manufacturing; and product discontinuation. This lifecycle approach requires four elements of the pharmaceutical quality system:

- *Process performance and product quality monitoring*: QC testing to ensure the finished product and the processes by which it is produced comply with all standards and specifications.
- *CAPA*: Investigation of all complaints and nonconformities to ensure problems are put right (corrective action) and prevented from reoccurring (preventive action).
- *Change management*: Management of changes to procedures or specifications to ensure the quality of the product is not adversely impacted in any way.
- *Management review*: Senior management must regularly review results of regulatory inspections, internal audits, and periodic reviews and ensure appropriate follow-up actions are put in place to protect the quality of the product and processes by which it is produced.

The document provides examples of how each element might be applied during the different stages of the product lifecycle.

3.6.8 Continual improvement of the pharmaceutical quality system

In the true spirit of quality management, there is a formal requirement to continually improve not only the processes and the product quality but also the quality system itself. The requirements are split into three elements:

- *Management review*: Senior management must regularly review all aspects of the quality system to ensure its successful operation.
- *Monitoring of internal and external factors*: Senior management must review factors such as regulatory issues; changes in the business environment; opportunities for enhancement of the quality system; and changes in product ownership to determine what effect these factors might have on the operation of the quality system.
- Actions arising from the previous two elements.

3.7 Definitions of quality management

Irrespective of whether a company adopts the requirements of ICH Q10 or not, there is an absolute requirement for a quality management system to ensure the quality and efficacy of the product.

The first chapter of the European Union (EU) GMP guidelines defines quality management as: "a wide-ranging concept, which covers all matters, which individually or collectively influence the quality of a product. It is the sum total of the organized arrangements made with the objective of ensuring that medicinal products are of the quality required for their intended use." (EU Guidelines for Good Manufacturing Practice for Medicinal Products for Human and Veterinary Use.)

The manufacturer is obliged to assume responsibility for the quality of the pharmaceutical products to ensure they are fit for their intended use, comply with the requirements of the marketing authorization, and do not place the patient at risk because of inadequate safety, quality, or efficacy.

The pharmaceutical product quality parameters are stated in individual product specifications. These specifications ensure the product fulfills the basic requirements of identity, purity, strength, and bioavailability. They are described in detail in the marketing authorization or product licence.

- *Identity*: The product must comply with the information given on the product label.
- *Strength/Potency*: The product contains the quantity of each ingredient claimed on its label, within the applicable limits of the specification for release and shelf life. This may be determined by chemical testing for strength or by reference to a biological standard of potency.

- *Purity*: Purity is defined as the extent to which raw material or a drug in the dosage form is free from undesirable or adulterating chemical, biological, or physical entities as defined by the specification.
- *Bioavailability/Biopharmaceutical properties*: Upon administration, the product must provide the active ingredient for the intended therapeutic/biological availability. Bioavailability is the rate and extent of absorption of a drug from a dosage form as determined by its concentration/time curve in the systematic circulation, or by its excretion in urine.

The commitment of the company to the general quality philosophy should be detailed in a document signed by management. This quality policy is a formal corporate statement by the senior managers of the company of its overall intentions and direction relating to quality. The senior managers of a company comprise the board of directors or the general manager of the company, the plant or factory managers together with the senior managers responsible for production and QC.

There are two basic elements to the function of quality management: quality system infrastructure and systematic actions.

3.7.1 Quality system infrastructure

There must be an infrastructure in place that covers the organizational structure for quality management, sets up the necessary procedures and processes, and ensures appropriate resources are available to carry out those procedures and processes. A company needs to have a plan to develop all these items and a statement of its intent to implement that plan. Once all the elements of this plan have been established, there is a system of quality management in place.

Any company or organization making pharmaceuticals should show there is a structure an organization dedicated to making the products correctly. This structure must have the backing of the most senior management of the company to ensure that it will succeed. This topic will be covered in more detail in Chapter 5.

3.7.2 Systematic actions

Once the infrastructure is in place, it results in systematic actions, which bring the quality policy to life. It is these actions that make up the function of QA.

3.8 Definition of quality assurance

Within the EU the term pharmaceutical QA system is considered interchangeable with the term pharmaceutical quality system. Hence, the definition in Section 3.7

applies here as well: "a wide-ranging concept, which covers all matters, which individually or collectively influence the quality of a product."

Inside an organization, QA is the tool by which senior management ensures the processes are operating successfully and the product is in full compliance. In contractual situations, QA provides confidence for the customer (whether that is a pharmacist, doctor, or patient) in the quality of the drug being supplied.

An important part of the systematic actions is the availability of a complete system of SOPs. They describe all the actions to be taken in a standardized way. This means everyone involved in pharmaceutical manufacturing has a book of procedures that guides them in how to perform their jobs. The SOP provides a standardized way of working.

Hence, although there is a specific department within the company called Quality Assurance, the achievement of QA is not the duty of this organizational unit alone but is the responsibility of all staff members who in any way can influence product quality.

One specific aspect of QA is encompassed in the term "quality assurance." It is the process that gives assurance that quality will be achieved. It puts procedures in place in advance so that everything goes according to plan and there are no problems with the quality of the final product. QA focuses on preventive measures. The topic of preventive rather than appraisal activities is discussed in more detail in Chapter 7, Quality Improvement Programs under the section on the cost of quality.

3.9 Responsibilities of quality assurance

Each of the various guidelines and codes of practice referred to in this textbook and listed in the references cover QA in a similar way, although the specific details tend to vary slightly. This section commences with a review of the approach taken with the EU guidelines and within the PIC/S guidelines. The same requirements are detailed in the WHO text. Specific differences within the US Food and Drug Administration (FDA) documents are discussed later.

3.9.1 Quality assurance requirements within EU, PIC/S, and WHO

3.9.1.1 Product realization

It is important to ensure products are formulated and developed in accordance with QA principles. If all the development work is carried out with a commitment to QA, it becomes easier to achieve QA in the rest of manufacturing. Compliance is not only with GMP but also with good laboratory practice (GLP) requirements. See Chapter 1 for a detailed discussion of quality requirements in the stages before manufacturing.

3.9.1.2 Specification for production and control

Written specifications are essential for all aspects of manufacturing and supply. These specifications should state what must be achieved and how. They will cover all starting materials, intermediates, and finished products, together with process specifications and analytical methodology.

3.9.1.3 Managerial responsibilities

There need to be a defined organizational structure and clear job descriptions for all personnel, particularly those in managerial positions. Organizational structure and job descriptions ensure there are sufficient qualified and experienced people available who have the correct training to perform their responsibilities. The topic of managerial responsibilities is covered in more detail in Chapter 5.

3.9.1.4 Control of starting and packaging materials

This requirement relates to the management of purchasing, receipt, sampling, and testing of raw materials and packaging materials, and demonstrates how quality is the responsibility of all functions within the organization. Purchasing personnel may not necessarily believe they can affect product quality. They may see themselves as more aligned with the finance department. Indeed they may report to finance. However, it is important they only purchase materials from approved suppliers and according to approved specifications. Their purchasing decisions should under no circumstances be based purely on purchasing at the lowest cost.

3.9.1.5 Control of outsourced activities

In a global industry such as pharmaceutical manufacturing, it has become common for some activities to be outsourced. For example, a tablet sold around the world might be manufactured in bulk in one or two key locations, while packaging in territory-specific packs might be outsourced to facilities all around the world. There must be systems in place to ensure the processes in these outsourced facilities have the same degree of QA as the main company.

3.9.1.6 Control of intermediate materials

There is a requirement to ensure all intermediate materials are controlled appropriately and all in-process checks are set up and made.

3.9.1.7 Control of finished products

Similarly, this requirement ensures all necessary measures are in place for the manufacture and testing of the finished product.

3.9.1.8 Continual improvement and change management

This requirement states systems must be in place to ensure processes are improved as the degree of knowledge of the product and the process grows. All changes must be planned, implemented, and evaluated in a controlled manner.

3.9.1.9 Investigation of deviations and CAPA

Following the principles of quality risk management, all deviations must be fully investigated and appropriate CAPA actions identified as a result.

3.9.1.10 Batch release

The batch release can only be authorized after all checks have been completed to ensure the product has been produced and controlled by the established specifications and the registered product details or other appropriate regulations. The registered product details will state what standards the product must meet.

3.9.1.11 Control of storage and distribution

During product development, stability testing will be completed. The outcome of this stability testing is a set of specified conditions under which the product should be stored. Normally this specification will include temperature and humidity requirements. Additionally, there may be a specification for exposure to light and/or other parameters. Arrangements should be in place throughout the storage and distribution chain so the product will not be exposed to conditions that could adversely affect its quality or efficacy. This means all aspects of the distribution chain from the factory through the wholesaler to the hospital, pharmacy or drug store need to be included. Since, in many cases, ownership of the product moves to another company once the product leaves the factory gates, this implies an influencing and educational role for the manufacturing company.

3.9.1.12 Self-inspection program

A key part of the management of the manufacturing operations is the auditing of the operations for compliance with all quality requirements. The auditing is done at several levels within the company, as discussed in Chapter 6. Self-inspection is the internal audit function existing within the individual departments.

Once all the above requirements have been addressed, a company can be said to be working within QA principles.

3.9.2 Quality assurance requirements within FDA

There is no reference to QA as a function within the FDA's Code of Federal Regulations (CFR) Title 21 Parts 210–211. However, various requirements listed in

Section 3.9.1 are covered within 21 CFR Part 211, except for product design and development and self-inspection programs.

3.10 Definition of quality control

Quality control is defined in the EU GMP guidelines Chapter 1 as:

that part of Good Manufacturing Practice which is concerned with sampling, specifications and testing, and with the organisation, documentation and release procedures which ensure that the necessary and relevant tests are actually carried out and that materials are not released for use, nor products released for sale or supply, until their quality has been judged to be satisfactory.

In the FDA's 21 CFR Subchapter C Part 210.3, quality control is defined as: "any person or organizational element designated by the firm to be responsible for the duties relating to QC." While this is a somewhat circular definition, it does not contradict the fuller definition from the EU.

In the strictest sense of the words, QC is an historical process that proves the appropriate level of quality has been achieved. QC cannot affect the quality of the product. It is merely a process for measuring quality.

The QC process is therefore primarily confined to laboratory operations, testing and/or inspecting samples of raw materials, packaging materials, in-process materials, and finished products. QC staff will also monitor aspects of the environment that affect product quality.

However, in many companies, the QC department also has responsibility for some of the areas relating to QA. For a fuller discussion of this, see Chapter 5, The Management of Quality.

3.11 Responsibilities of quality control

In the EU guidelines, QC has its section within the introductory paragraphs, outlining the requirements to be achieved in a satisfactory QC function. In addition, there is further material in a later chapter, which covers the requirements in more detail. A different approach is adopted in the FDA requirements, although in general the sentiments expressed are the same.

This section again begins with a review of the EU (and hence the PIC/S) documentation and then makes a comparison with the FDA.

3.11.1 Quality control requirements within EU and PIC/S
3.11.1.1 Adequate resources
The QC department must have adequate resources to fulfill its responsibilities: suitable laboratory facilities, either inhouse or by the use of government or contract

laboratories; qualified, trained, and experienced personnel; and approved documented procedures covering all operational duties of the department.

The operational tasks of the QC department are sampling; inspecting; analytical testing; monitoring of all materials and environmental conditions in the factory; releasing or rejecting materials for production use, and finished products.

The objects of these activities can be: starting materials (both APIs and excipients); packaging materials (both primary and secondary materials); intermediates; bulk products; finished products; and environmental conditions.

Hence, for a full audit of the level of QC resources within a company, it is possible to adopt a matrix approach, as shown in Table 3.1. By combining any one of the resources in the first column with any one of the tasks in the second column and any one of the objects in the third column, a checklist can be developed against which a gap analysis is performed.

3.11.1.2 Sampling

Sampling should be conducted according to methods approved by the QC department and only by approved personnel. It is not a requirement that all sampling be completed by QA or QC personnel. A sampling of incoming materials is generally, but not always, done by QC at the request of the warehouse personnel. In many companies, most in-process samples are taken by the production operatives. In some situations, such as in sterile areas or high-toxicity areas, where access is restricted, sampling of finished products is also conducted by production personnel. The key point is not the department in which the samplers work, but that they have been trained in the appropriate methods by the QC staff.

All samplings should be representative of the batch and done in accordance with an SOP. Where necessary, QC personnel must have access to the factory to undertake sampling.

3.11.1.3 Validated or verified test methods

All test methods used within the laboratories and in-process control areas should be validated or verified. When a test method is taken from a recognized source, normally

Table 3.1 Summary of quality control requirements.

Resources	Tasks	Objects
Adequate facilities	Sampling	Starting materials
Trained personnel	Inspecting	Packaging materials
Approved procedures	Testing	Intermediates
	Monitoring	Bulk products
	Releasing/rejecting	Finished products
		Environmental conditions

the national pharmacopoeia, it is sufficient to verify if it can be duplicated under the conditions existing within the company. A pharmacopoeia is an official publication containing a list of medicinal drugs with their effects and directions for their use. However, if an analytical method has been developed in-house, it must be fully validated.

The topic of validation of test methods is fully covered in the ICH Guidelines Q2 (R1) and, within this textbook, in Chapter 10. The validation of test methods includes consideration of accuracy, precision, linearity, repeatability, robustness, and specificity. This means the test method should be challenged to demonstrate its ability to give an accurate result on a repeatable basis. The method must be capable of being applied with precision. The results obtained must be linear over a range of acceptable responses. Finally, the results must be repeatable over several identical tests.

The actual parameters that are validated depend on the type of test. Tests can be categorized as identification tests; impurity/degradation tests, which may be quantitative or limit tests; and active assay/dissolution tests.

3.11.1.4 Adequate records

Records must be kept of all sampling, inspection, and testing of materials, intermediates, bulk, and finished products. Essential records are kept of the work done by QC and during in-process testing. This is a key part of traceability, which must be achievable for all batches of products released onto the market.

As batches are produced, any deviations from the normal manufacturing procedure are recorded or documented and the resulting impact on product quality is assessed. Additional product testing may be required, including possible additional stability testing.

3.11.1.5 Correct active ingredients and correct labeled containers

QC must ensure all finished products contain APIs in compliance with the qualitative and quantitative composition of the finished product described in the product registration dossier. Materials used in manufacturing must comply with the details registered in the marketing authorization, since this is the basis on which the product was developed, and the stability testing is done. All clinical trials must also have been completed using materials of a consistent specification.

Ingredients must be shown to be of the required purity since without starting materials of the specified quality, the company is unable to ensure the rest of the process can be completed successfully. Although the requirement specifically refers to APIs, it should be considered maintaining a consistent specification for excipients is important for the quality of the final product.

The importance of using the proper containers must also be recognized. During the development of the product, tests will be conducted on the compatibility of the product with the container. Testing will also be completed to determine the effectiveness of the container in ensuring product stability. The use of noncompliant or nonapproved containers will mean the product shelf life cannot be guaranteed.

Labeling of the finished-product is especially important. In some countries, more than half of all product recalls are caused by incorrectly printed components. These failures can be due to mix-ups in the printed components during printing, or labeling, and packing, or text errors in the printing which were not identified. If QC is conducted correctly, all such problems should be identified before the product is released. In fact, with an effective QA system, they should be prevented from occurring.

3.11.1.6 Assessment of results
The results of inspection and testing of all materials must be assessed against the appropriate specification to confirm compliance. This assessment must cover a full review of the process and packaging documentation. Any deviations must be fully investigated to confirm they do not impact, in any way, the finished product.

3.11.1.7 Product release
Release of batches of the finished product should only occur after the authorized person has certified production and QC to have been completed according to the requirements of the registered product details.

3.11.1.8 Reference samples
Sufficient retained samples of the finished product in its final pack should be kept for 1 year past the expiry date. Additionally, retained samples of starting materials should be kept for at least 2 years after the date of release of the finished product, assuming the stability of the material can be maintained for this period. This is to allow for an evaluation, should there be a need, of the product after it has been distributed and sold to consumers. It will also allow ongoing stability trials to be run. The trials provide confidence that the quality of the product is not deteriorating at a greater rate than might be expected over time. Full requirements on reference and retention samples are outlined in Annex 19 of the EU Guidelines for Good Manufacturing Practice for Medicinal Products for Human and Veterinary Use.

3.11.2 Good control laboratory practice in EU and PIC/S
The organization, management, and key responsibilities of the QC department are covered in Chapter 5. At this point, it is sufficient to emphasize that under GMP requirements, the QC department must be independent of production to be able to perform its responsibilities effectively.

Within the EU Guidelines for Good Manufacturing Practice for Medicinal Products for Human and Veterinary Use, Chapter 6 is dedicated to QC and encompasses how the department should operate. This can be termed as Good Control Laboratory Practice (GCLP). It should not be confused with GLP which, as discussed in Chapter 1, relates to the conduct of preclinical studies.

3.11.2.1 Premises and equipment

There are no defined requirements for the premises in which QC laboratories are housed. It depends on what activities are to take place in a specific area. For example, the requirements for a microbiology laboratory responsible for sterility testing on finished products would be more stringent than for a laboratory carrying out microbiological analysis on raw materials for nonsterile products.

The laboratories should be large enough to suit the level of production monitored and to prevent cross-contamination between samples. Since samples are never returned to production after analysis, there is no issue of reverse cross-contamination back to the manufacturing process.

Laboratories should be located close to, but physically separated from, production areas. Particular care needs to be taken with laboratories used to analyze biological materials or antibiotics. It is also necessary to separate some types of analysis from each other. For examples the antibiotic testing room should not be located close to the microbiology laboratory.

In physical or chemical laboratories, it is usual to separate instrumentation, particularly equipment such as balances which need to be protected from vibrations, from wet chemistry areas.

In many countries, particularly in developing industries where investment in equipment is low, some or all QC activities are contracted out. This is permissible, providing the contract laboratory is audited and all GMP requirements of contracting are complied with. This topic has been covered in more detail in Chapter 2.

Even in companies with sufficient facilities for their own QC functions under normal circumstances, it is common to contract out abnormal QC loads. For example, during the validation of a new facility, the environmental monitoring needed for commissioning the building and the additional sampling and testing required during the commissioning of the water treatment system will put a huge, short-term load on the microbiology department which they might not be able to satisfy.

3.11.2.2 Documentation

In general terms, the treatment of documentation within the QC department is no different from that for the rest of the manufacturing environment. However, there are a number of specific points made in relation to QC documentation. Key documents necessary for QC activities to be achieved satisfactorily are:

- specifications defining the characteristics of raw materials, packaging materials, intermediates, and finished products;
- sampling procedures for raw materials, packaging materials, intermediates, and finished products;
- testing procedures and results of analysis of raw materials, intermediates, and finished products (including all raw data);
- procedures for the investigation of results that deviate from the specification;
- analytical reports and/or certificates of analysis produced as a result of the tests;
- raw data from environmental monitoring programs such as particle counts, settle plates and pressure differential readings;
- data for the validation or verification of analytical methods, as appropriate; and
- methods and results of calibration of laboratory instruments and other preventive maintenance activities.

Critical documentation, that is, anything relating to a specific batch of product, must be archived for shelf life plus 1 year, together with the original data, such as laboratory notebooks and instrument printouts. Since the results will often be used in annual product reviews, consideration should be given to expressing the data in a form that allows for trend analysis. Data will frequently be transcribed into a Laboratory Information Management System (LIMS) and these transcribed results can be used for the purposes of trend analysis.

3.11.2.3 Sampling

There must be a written procedure covering different aspects of sampling:

- *How the sample is taken*: From which part of the batch, using what equipment, how much is required, and whether it should be kept as a single sample or subdivided.
- *What the samples should be placed in*: Type of container and the information that needs to go on the label.
- *Any special precautions*: Both in terms of protecting the material being sampled and protecting the person taking the samples.
- *Storage conditions*: Both before analysis and afterwards if the sample is retained.
- *Maintenance of sampling equipment*: How it should be cleaned after use, where it should be stored and whether it needs to be cleaned again prior to use.

In addition to the paragraphs within Chapter 6, of the EU guidelines, there is an additional reference source specifically dedicated to sampling of starting (i.e., raw) materials and packaging materials. This is found in Annex 8.

The annex begins with a statement of the precautions to be taken about the training of personnel who will take samples. As previously stated, these may be personnel from QC, production or, in some cases, warehousing. The training should focus on:

- *The procedure for sampling*: Plans to determine how many samples should be taken, how and with what equipment those samples should be taken.

- *Cross-contamination issues*: Particularly with sterile or toxic material.
- *Visual inspection before sampling*: The state of containers, labeling details, etc., and the importance of recording unusual observation.

3.11.2.4 Sampling for identity testing

The sampling of starting materials is an issue which, in the experience of the author, can confuse in some companies. The sampling rule of $\sqrt{n + 1}$, where n is the number of containers, is often quoted during audits as the basis for a sampling plan for identity tests. However, according to Annex 8, all containers should be sampled and individually tested as a general rule, since this is the only true way to ensure every container has the correct contents.

It is permissible to adopt a reduced sampling program for identity testing provided: "a validated procedure has been established to ensure that no single container of starting material has been incorrectly labeled."

There are several areas to focus on in achieving such validation, including:

- the nature of the supplier and the validity of their QA program;
- the manufacturing conditions under which the material has been produced; and
- the nature of the material.

For example, it is possible to consider such reduced testing where the material is purchased directly from the manufacturer and where the company is known to have a good understanding of GMP requirements and to operate to this level of quality. As a prerequisite for reduced sampling, there is the expectation that the purchaser will have audited the supplier, including visiting the manufacturing site.

It is unlikely such reduced testing would be acceptable where the material is being purchased through a broker. In this case, the original supplier may not be known and may change from delivery to delivery. Hence, it would be impossible to gain sufficient assurance of the quality of manufacture to be certain all containers would hold what the label claimed. Reduced testing should not be considered for materials that will be used in the manufacture of parenterals. A parenteral is defined as a medicine administered by some means other than oral intake, particularly intravenously or by injection.

3.11.2.5 Sampling for other purposes

For analysis of a material to check its compliance with the specification, it is permissible to sample a representative number of containers, and in some cases, to combine samples together. The method of sampling and the sampling plan may be defined in the pharmacopeia or other national regulations. In any case, it should be the subject of a written procedure.

For packaging materials, it is also necessary to develop a sampling plan and to determine statistically how many samples should be taken. There will be many factors to be considered, including the source and nature of the material, together with the history of the supplier's performance and QA system.

3.11.2.6 Testing

All tests referred to in the marketing authorization should use the correct methodology, which must be validated or verified. All results should be checked to ensure they are correct. The implication of this is that calculations and other data within laboratory notebooks should be checked and countersigned.

There is a statement of the minimum amount of information to be recorded in the case of a set of test results.

Whether the testing is done in the laboratory by a QC analyst or in the in-process control laboratory within the manufacturing area, by a production operative, the correct methodology, approved by QC, must be used.

There should be a procedure for the preparation of such working materials as reagents, reference standards, and culture media. This should include reference to the method of preparation, the labeling requirements, expiry date, storage conditions, and records to be kept.

Where animals are used for testing purposes, there is a need for appropriate quarantine procedures, identification, and records.

3.11.2.7 Ongoing stability program

There must be a program for identifying stability issues throughout the shelf life of a finished pack and, where appropriate, for the bulk products or intermediates that are subject to prolonged storage periods. The program should comply with normal GMP requirements for documentation (EU GMP guidelines Chapter 4), premises and equipment (EU GMP guidelines Chapter 3), and validation and verification (EU GMP guidelines Annex 15). There is a list provided of the minimal parameters to be included.

Variation from the protocol for the initial long-term stability studies is permitted but must be justified. A minimum of one batch per year, per strength, and per primary packaging type must be studied. Significant changes or deviations within the process or packaging would require additional sampling and testing.

Results must be communicated to the qualified person(s) and available at the manufacturing site for review by the regulatory authority. All deviations must be investigated, and the implications reviewed for batches still in the marketplace, as per the requirements on complaints and product recall (EU GMP guidelines Chapter 8).

3.11.3 Quality control requirements within FDA

The first mention of QC within 21 CFR Part 211 is in subpart B, Organization and Personnel, where the role of the QC unit is outlined. Responsibilities include testing and release of all raw materials, packaging materials, intermediates, and finished products and reviewing of documentation associated with all aspects of manufacturing. These responsibilities cover not only in-house manufacture, but also product manufactured by contractors. There must be suitable facilities available for the unit to fulfill its responsibilities. The responsibility for approving all specifications and procedures also sits with this unit; thus there is a clear element of QA included here. The management of quality within the United States is covered in more detail in Chapter 5.

QC is a key factor throughout the FDA requirements. However, there are a number of subparts within 21 CFR 211 that relate specifically to QC activities.

3.11.3.1 Control of components and drug product containers and closures (subpart E)

This section deals with the need for written procedures covering all aspects of control. There is a reference to the need for visual inspection on receipt and quarantining of deliveries pending testing and release. The sampling procedure is covered in some detail, as are the testing requirements. There are also references to stock rotation, retesting requirements, and the handling of rejected materials.

Finally, there is a section relating specifically to drug product containers and closures, which are described elsewhere in this chapter as primary packaging components. This section covers such topics as compatibility of the materials with the drug, the integrity of closure systems, and cleanliness requirements including those for sterile products.

3.11.3.2 Production and process controls (subpart F)

This section deals with controls within manufacturing. It covers writing and approval of procedures; how to control the charge-in of components; responsibilities relating to yield calculation; equipment identification; sampling and testing of in-process materials and drug products; limitations on processing times; control of microbiological contamination; and reprocessing control. Specific responsibilities sitting with the QC unit are highlighted throughout.

3.11.3.3 Laboratory controls (subpart I)

There are seven different sections under this subpart of 21 CFR 211.
*   General requirements make reference to the writing and approval of control mechanisms such as specifications, sampling plans, and test procedures, and a review of which controls need to be in place.
*   Testing and release for distribution covers the criteria to be achieved before a batch can be released and the circumstances under which an exception can be made. Testing should include microbiological analysis if appropriate. The need for a

written procedure for both sampling and testing is emphasized. The action to be taken with product that fails to meet acceptance criteria is also discussed.

- A stability-testing program must be established and described in writing. The circumstances under which accelerated stability studies may be used are reviewed. Requirements with homeopathic drugs are also covered.
- Special testing requirements covers drugs that are sterile or pyrogen-free, to demonstrate the absence of microorganisms or pyrogens; ophthalmic ointments, to demonstrate the absence of foreign particles or harsh or abrasive substances; and controlled-release dosage forms, to demonstrate the rate of release of the API.
- Reserve samples are defined separately for APIs and finished products. Under general conditions, both active materials and finished product samples must be kept for 1 year past the expiry date of the finished product. However, there are special conditions quoted for radioactive materials, where the storage requirements are between three and six months after the expiry date of the product. For certain over-the-counter (OTC) products, which have no expiry date, and for the active ingredients contained in them, samples must be kept for 3 years after distribution of the batch.
- Laboratory animals require good control and records.
- Penicillin contamination, if detected in nonpenicillin drugs, will result in the release of the batch being prohibited.

3.11.3.4 Records and reports (subpart J)

Much of this subpart deals with the requirements for record-keeping during manufacturing. However, Section 211.194 covers the specific topic of laboratory records. Records must include details of the sample; test methodology; quantity of the sample used in each test; all raw data obtained during the tests; a record of the calculations performed; results of the test, and a comparison with the appropriate acceptance criteria; signatures of the analyst and the person who checked the records and the calculations. Records must also be kept of any changes to the established methodology; all standards and reagents; calibration of test equipment; and all stability tests performed.

3.12 Quality management in Japan

Since the 1950s, Japan has led the world in the development of quality management and QC practices. The Japanese Ministry of Health, Labor and Welfare (MHLW) in combination with the Japanese Pharmaceuticals and Medical Devices Agency (PMDA) was a founding member of ICH. Two representatives of the Japanese Pharmaceutical Manufacturers Association (JPMA) sit on the ICH Project Committee. Japan is a signatory to ICH Q10 and it was implemented February 1, 2010.

Regulation of pharmaceutical manufacturing in Japan comes under the Pharmaceuticals and Medical Devices Act (PMD Act), also known as the Act on

Securing Quality, Efficacy, and Safety of Pharmaceuticals, Medical Devices, Regenerative and Cellular Therapy Products, Gene Therapy Products, and Cosmetics. There is a requirement for all manufacturers to comply with GMP, and within that, to have effective QC systems. QA is not a term commonly used.

3.13 Quality management in Canada

In Canada, regulation of pharmaceutical manufacturing is overseen by the Therapeutic Products Directorate (TPD), within the legal framework of Part 2, Division C of the Food and Drug Regulations. The main guidance document is Good manufacturing practices guide for drug products (GUI-0001).

GUI-0001describes the need for a quality management system that incorporates GMP and quality risk management. The system must be fully documented and monitored to demonstrate effectiveness. Reference is made to ICH Q10.

The relationship between QA, GMP, and QC is the same as in the EU. The requirements to be fulfilled by QC cover all aspects outlined in Section 3.11.1.

3.14 Chapter summary

- The quality management system is the sum of all that is necessary to implement an organization's quality policy and meet quality objectives.
- The quality management system incorporates QA. QA incorporates GMP. GMP incorporates QC.
- Documentation for pharmaceutical manufacturing can be described as a cascade and begins with the national or international regulations and guidelines. From these, the company develops its goals, mission statement, and values. The quality manual contains the policy by which the goals, mission statement, and values will be achieved. The details of the policy are enshrined within the quality management system and individual functions within the company will develop strategies for their approach to the policy. Specifics will be presented in procedures and standards, from which are derived work instructions and records of activities.
- The International Council for Harmonization of Technical Requirements for Pharmaceuticals for Human Use (ICH) guidelines are a major source of international guidance documents.
- Key documents of relevance to this textbook include ICH Q7 (APIs); ICH Q8 (pharmaceutical development); ICH Q9 (quality risk management); ICH Q10 (pharmaceutical quality system). ICH Q10 builds on ICH Q7 and complements ICH Q8 and Q9. The purpose is to facilitate the use of a science and risk-based approach to the pharmaceutical lifecycle.

- The three main objectives for the pharmaceutical quality system outlined in ICH Q10 are product realization, state of control, and continual improvement.
- There are two enablers identified within ICH Q10 that facilitate its implementation: knowledge management and quality risk management.
- The seven key elements identified for an effective pharmaceutical quality system are clear structure; appropriate and proportionate application at each of the different life cycle stages; company or site level applications, depending on the complexity of the company; extension to outsourced activities and purchased materials; management responsibilities; the importance of process performance, product quality monitoring, CAPA, change management, and management review; and the use of performance indicators to monitor the effectiveness of the pharmaceutical quality system.
- The key responsibilities of senior management include the establishment of, support for, and communication about an effective system; definition of roles and responsibilities, plus adequate resourcing; continual monitoring and improvement of the effectiveness of the system.
- Continual improvement applies both to process performance and product quality, and to the quality system itself.
- While implementation of ICH Q10 is voluntary, the requirement for a quality management system is mandatory in many countries and is mentioned in regulatory and guidance documents.
- Within the WU, the terms pharmaceutical quality system and QA are used synonymously. In other major markets, such as the United States and Japan, the term QA is not used.
- The EU, WHO, and PIC/S guidelines outline the responsibilities of QA in terms of product realization; specifications for production and control; managerial responsibilities; control of materials at all stages in the production cycle from starting materials through to the finished product, and outsourced activities; continual improvement, change management and CAPA; batch release; control of storage and distribution; and self-inspection.
- QC is a term used in all regulatory systems. While the wording is different between, for example, the EU and the United States, the intention is the same and the key elements include resources; sampling; test methods; records; correct materials and packaging; results assessment; product release and reference samples.
- Within the EU and PIC/S guidance, there is a GCLP, which relates to control of manufacturing and should not be confused with Good Laboratory Practice, which relates to preclinical studies. It discusses premises and equipment; documentation; sampling; testing; and stability programs.
- A brief review of quality management requirements in Japan and Canada confirms that although the wording may be different in some cases, the need for a quality management system is now a major element of pharmaceutical manufacturing in all major markets.

3.15 Questions/problems

1. You have taken a post as QA Manager in a small tablet manufacturing facility in the United Kingdom. What documents would you expect to find within the quality management system?

2. What is the relevance of ICH Q7—Q10 in a company in the United States producing OTC cough mixture for children?

3. What does ICH Q10 describe as the three main purposes of a pharmaceutical quality management system and what are the two main enablers?

4. You are the QC Manager for a print company producing secondary packaging for a large multinational parenterals manufacturer. Describe your QC systems.

5. You are the Purchasing Manager for a tablet manufacturing and packaging company in the United States. You receive a report from the QC department about the delivery of packaging materials that do not comply with the specification. What would you do?

6. Compare and contrast the QC requirements as outlined in the EU GMP guidelines and US 21 CFR 211.

Further reading

European Commission, 2013. Health and Consumers Directorate-General. The Rules Governing Medicinal Products in the European Union. Volume 4. EU guidelines for good manufacturing practice for medicinal products for human and veterinary use. Chapter 1Pharmaceutical quality system. <https://ec.europa.eu/health/sites/health/files/files/eudralex/vol-4/vol4-chap1_2013-01_en.pdf> (accessed 04.09.21).

European Commission, 2014. Health and Consumers Directorate-General. The Rules Governing Medicinal Products in the European Union. Volume 4. EU guidelines for good manufacturing practice for medicinal products for human and veterinary use. Chapter 6 Quality control. <https://ec.europa.eu/health/sites/health/files/files/eudralex/vol-4/2014-11_vol4_chapter_6.pdf> (accessed 04.12.21).

European Commission, n.d. Health and Consumers Directorate-General. The Rules Governing Medicinal Products in the European Union. Volume 4. EU guidelines for good manufacturing practice for medicinal products for human and veterinary use. Annex 8 sampling of starting and packaging materials. <https://ec.europa.eu/health/sites/health/files/files/eudralex/vol-4/pdfs-en/anx08_en.pdf> (accessed 04.12.21).

European Commission, 2005. Health and Consumers Directorate-General. The Rules Governing Medicinal Products in the European Union. Volume 4. EU guidelines for good manufacturing practice for medicinal products for human and veterinary use. Annex 19 Reference and retention samples. <https://ec.europa.eu/health/sites/health/files/files/eudralex/vol-4/pdfs-en/2005_12_14_annex19_en.pdf> (accessed 04.12.21).

Health Canada, 2020. Good Manufacturing Practices Guide for Drug Products (GUI-0001). <https://www.canada.ca/en/health-canada/services/drugs-health-products/compliance-enforcement/good-manufacturing-practices/guidance-documents/gmp-guidelines-0001/document.html> (accessed 05.01.21).

International Conference on Harmonisation of Technical Requirements for Registration of Pharmaceuticals for Human Use, 2005. ICH Harmonised Tripartite Guideline. Validation of analytical procedures: Text and methodology Q2(R1). <https://database.ich.org/sites/default/files/Q2%28R1%29%20Guideline.pdf> (accessed 04.12.21).

International Conference on Harmonisation of Technical Requirements for Registration of Pharmaceuticals for Human Use, 2000. ICH Tripartite Guideline. Good manufacturing practice guide for active pharmaceutical ingredients Q7. <https://database.ich.org/sites/default/files/Q7%20Guideline.pdf> (accessed 04.08.21).

International Conference on Harmonisation of Technical Requirements for Registration of Pharmaceuticals for Human Use, 2009. Ich Harmonised Tripartite Guideline Pharmaceutical Development Q8(R2). <https://database.ich.org/sites/default/files/Q8%28R2%29%20Guideline.pdf> (accessed 04.08.21).

International Conference on Harmonisation of Technical Requirements for Registration of Pharmaceuticals for Human Use, 2005. ICH Harmonised Tripartite Guideline. Quality risk management Q9. <https://database.ich.org/sites/default/files/Q9%20Guideline.pdf> (accessed 04.08.21).

International Conference on Harmonisation of Technical Requirements for Registration of Pharmaceuticals for Human Use, 2008. ICH Harmonised Tripartite Guideline. Pharmaceutical quality system. Q10. <https://database.ich.org/sites/default/files/Q10%20Guideline.pdf> (accessed 04.08.21).

Pharmaceutical Inspection Convention/Pharmaceutical Inspection Co-operation Scheme, (2007). Pi002−3 Recommendation on Quality System Requirement for Pharmaceutical Inspectorates. <https://picscheme.org/docview/3462> (accessed 04.06.21).

US Food and Drug Administration, 2021. Electronic Code of Federal Regulations Title 21, Chapter 1, Sub-chapter C, Part 210: Current good manufacturing practice in manufacturing, processing, packing, or holding of drugs; general. <https://www.ecfr.gov/cgi-bin/text-idx?SID = 8a82b9e207fb272a6476ed0ce1df1766&mc = true&node = pt21.4.210&rgn = div5> (accessed 04.12.21).

US Food and Drug Administration, 2021. Electronic Code of Federal Regulations Title 21, Chapter 1, Sub-chapter C, Part 211: Current good manufacturing practice for finished pharmaceuticals. <https://www.ecfr.gov/cgi-bin/text-idx?SID = 4e633f7767685e679f3e535a2a92f0a0&mc = true&node = se21.4.211_13&rgn = div8> (accessed 04.12.21).

CHAPTER 4

Quality systems and international standards

4.1 Introduction

This chapter deals with the subject of quality systems from the point of view of internationally recognized standards. One major standard, ISO 9000, is reviewed in detail here. ISO 9000 is the series related to satisfaction of customer requirements. Another standard, ISO 14000, is also discussed briefly. ISO 14000 is the series related to the management of the environment.

For ISO 9000, a review of the makeup of the standard is presented, including a brief overview of its development history. This is followed by a discussion on how each of the standards can be applied within the pharmaceutical industry.

4.2 International Organization for Standardization

The International Organization for Standardization (ISO) is an independent, non-governmental international agency comprising the national standards bodies of 165 countries or territories. With a central secretariat based in Switzerland, it coordinates the sharing of knowledge and development of voluntary, consensus-based international standards supporting innovation and providing solutions to global challenges.

The standards discussed in this chapter fall under the remit of the ISO Technical Committee (TC) 176, which was established in 1979. Its responsibilities are: "Standardization in the field of quality management (generic quality management systems and supporting technologies), as well as quality management standardization in specific sectors at the request of the affected sector and the ISO Technical Management Board."

4.3 History of ISO 9000 series

The purpose of this series of standards is to guarantee a company has a system and processes which ensure the delivery of a product or service in conformance with customer and regulatory requirements, recognize and effect opportunities to enhance the customer satisfaction, address risks, and demonstrate compliance.

Quality
DOI: https://doi.org/10.1016/B978-0-323-90815-3.00003-7

The ISO 9000 series of quality standards was first published in 1987 and revised in 1994, 2000, 2008, and 2015. While the purpose and principles of the standards have not changed significantly, there has been a major shift in emphasis and in presentation of those principles, as the concept of QMSs has developed over the years. A brief overview of these changes now follows.

4.3.1 ISO 9000: 1987 and 1994 series

Originally, there were different standards available for different types of organizations:

- ISO 9001: *Quality systems—Model for quality assurance in design, development, production, installation, and servicing* was appropriate for a supplier who provided all aspects of a business. This would include the original design of the product/service through manufacturing and supply to servicing according to contractual agreements. In this context, servicing related to an agreement to periodically provide a service, rather than one-off activities relating to repairs. For example, an instrument manufacturer that designs the equipment, manufactures, and sells the units and offers an annual recalibration service.

- ISO 9002: *Quality systems—Model for quality assurance in production, installation and servicing* was appropriate for a supplier who was involved in all aspects other than the original design of the product/service. For example, a company producing pharmaceuticals under licence, which sold the products and dealt with any customer complaints.

- ISO 9003: *Quality systems—Model for quality assurance in final inspection and test* was appropriate for a supplier who made or supplied items from materials provided by a third party, carried out an inspection process and then delivered and serviced a product/service, but was not involved in the original design or production. For example, a contract medical device company that assembled the finished articles from components supplied by the patent holder, tested the finished product and had a contractual agreement to provide servicing to the patient.

In addition to these main standards, there were a number of supplementary standards that provided help in application. Of particular note were ISO 8402, which dealt with terminology, and ISO 9000 parts 1—3, which provided guidelines on how to apply the standards in practice.

4.3.2 ISO 9000: 2000 and 2008 series

Publication of the ISO 9000: 2000 series of standards represented a significant revamp and a fundamental shift in emphasis. To start with, the language in which it was written was more straightforward. The layout of the document, with a full-page column of text, rather than the previous double column, made for easier reading.

The terminology used for the three members of the supply chain was amended to bring it into line with that used more commonly in organizations. The company providing materials, product or subcontracting services was called "the supplier" rather than "the subcontractor." The company to which the standard was being applied was called "the organization" rather than "the supplier." The term and definition of customer remained unchanged, being the company to which the product or service was being supplied.

At this point, the revised series consisted of three standards in total:

- ISO 9000: 2000 *Quality Management Systems—Fundamentals and vocabulary* replaced ISO 8402:1994 and ISO 9000-1: 1994. It presented a comprehensive glossary and described the background to the development of a quality system.
- ISO 9001: 2000 *Quality Management Systems—Requirements* replaced ISO 9001−9003 (1994 series) and presented in detail the requirements that a company had to comply with in order to obtain certification to the standard.
- ISO 9004: 2000 *Quality Management Systems—Guidelines for performance improvements* replaced ISO 9004 parts 1−4, published between 1991 and 1994. It dealt with continuous improvement in quality and was not intended as a standard to which companies would become accredited.

The ISO 9001: 2008 revision was a minor one, providing clarification on issues raised following the previous major revision.

4.3.3 ISO 9000: 2015 series

The latest version of the series, dating from 2015 and 2018, incorporates another major revision and as of September 2018, any company accredited to ISO 9001: 2008 was expected to have completed their transition to the new standard. The standard now takes a process approach to quality systems, using the Plan-Do-Check-Act (PDCA) cycle and a risk-based approach. This will be discussed in more detail in Section 4.6.1.

The latest versions of the three standards are:

- ISO 9000: 2015 *Quality Management Systems—Fundamentals and vocabulary*
- ISO 9001: 2015 *Quality Management Systems—Requirements*
- ISO 9004: 2018 *Quality management—Quality of an organization—Guidance to achieve sustained success*

4.4 Quality management principles

The topic of quality management has been fully covered in Chapter 3. However, it is worth briefly revisiting the topic before looking at the current standard in more detail. The current ISO 9000 series outlines seven principles of quality management:

- *Customer focus:* Since organizations can only continue to exist if they have satisfied customers, there is a requirement to recognize customer requirements and to ensure that these requirements are at least met, if not exceeded.

- *Leadership:* This recognizes the importance of the leaders of the organization in identifying objectives, communicating those objectives throughout the company and providing appropriate resources and environment to ensure that the objectives are achieved.
- *Engagement of people:* Just as the leaders are important to the success of the organization, so are the remainder of the team. This requires provision of appropriate training and development, coupled with involvement and empowerment.
- *Process approach:* A process is defined as a system of activities that uses resources to transform inputs into outputs. The focus on processes requires the activities of the organization to be considered as a series of interconnected processes which can be managed together. It also implies more effective management of an organization by viewing it as a series of interrelated horizontal processes, rather than a set of discrete vertical functions—often described as functional silos—as in the past.
- *Improvement:* This is seen as an ongoing objective of the organization. It is the point at which ISO 9000 and Total Quality Management (TQM) really come together. See Chapters 7 and 8, for a full discussion of TQM and other quality techniques.
- *Evidence-based decision making:* This recognizes the need for data to be analyzed and information taken into account when making decisions.
- *Relationship management:* It is important for companies to develop a win–win situation in their dealings with suppliers since a partnership approach is beneficial for both parties.

4.5 Quality system documentation

There are four main elements to a quality system, and they can be equated to the documentation required for an effective system: the quality manual, the quality plans, the quality procedures, and the quality records.

4.5.1 Quality manual

The quality manual is the key document which describes the company's quality system in detail. It contains the statement of quality objectives, which should be signed by the managing director. It also describes how the company addresses each of the clauses within the standard and identifies any that are not applicable. It refers to the quality procedures that relate to each aspect of the operation of the quality system.

This is a controlled document, which means it has an approval signature, issue number, and date. All changes are recorded in a change control register, and only the latest version of the document should be in circulation.

4.5.2 Quality plans

Quality plans are the documents which describe how a company's quality system is applied to a specific contract or project. They are operational by nature and as such are controlled documents, usually according to project requirements.

4.5.3 Quality procedures

Quality procedures describe how various activities take place. They cover what has to be done, who is responsible, the frequency and, if appropriate, the location of the activities. Quality procedures cover both the operation of the quality system and the operational aspects of the company's business. Each procedure should cross-reference to the quality instructions for and the quality records produced as a result of each activity. Once again, these are controlled documents, with the same requirements as those described for the quality manual above.

4.5.4 Quality records

Quality records are produced during the operation of the company. They cover both the operation of the quality system, such as minutes of management review meetings and reports of internal quality audits, and the normal activities of the company. The operational documents are not controlled in the same way as per the manual or the procedures, although their design will be subject to control.

4.6 ISO 9001: 2015

ISO 9001: 2015 comprises 10 clauses, two annexes, and a bibliography. The key clauses outlining the requirements to be achieved to comply with the standard are Clauses 4—10. These clauses are discussed individually in Sections 4.6.2—4.6.8. There is also an introductory section, dealing with the theory behind the process approach to quality systems.

4.6.1 Process approach to quality systems

The process approach to quality systems incorporates the PDCA cycle and risk-based thinking.

The PDCA cycle ensures processes are planned, resourced, managed, and improved effectively. Clauses 4—10 of the standard can each be applied to an aspect of the PDCA as shown in Fig. 4.1.

The risk-based approach requires identification of factors potentially impacting on the operation of the processes, then taking measures to prevent adverse effects while maximizing opportunities. While this may be a new term within the standard,

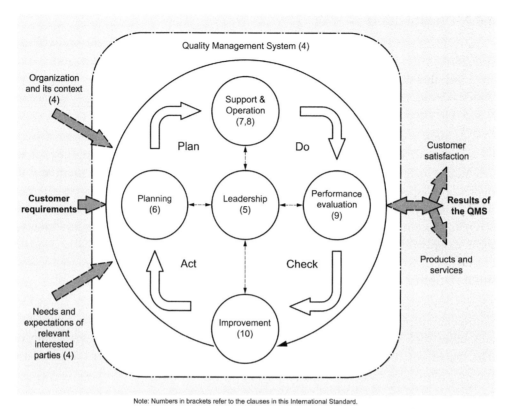

Note: Numbers in brackets refer to the clauses in this International Standard.

Figure 4.1 PDCA cycle. *Source*: Permission to reproduce extracts from ISO 9001: 2015 is granted by BSI.

elements such as corrective and preventive actions (CAPA) have been in previous versions, and therefore the concept is not a completely new one.

4.6.2 Context of the organization (Clause 4)

It is a requirement of the standard that the organization identify issues, either internal or external, which may impact on the purpose of the QMS. It should also consider the impact of any interested parties. The boundaries and applicability of the QMS must be defined; and the processes set up to achieve the QMS.

4.6.3 Leadership (Clause 5)

Senior management within the organization must demonstrate both leadership and commitment to the QMS and ensure a customer focus is maintained. A quality policy must be established and communicated both across the organization and to all interested parties. Appropriate roles, responsibility and authority must be allocated, communicated, and understood.

4.6.4 Planning (Clause 6)

Planning for the QMS requires the organization to identify any risks or opportunities that need to be addressed. Quality objectives must be established, together with plans for how they will be achieved. Additionally, any changes to the QMS must be undertaken in a controlled manner.

4.6.5 Support (Clause 7)

The organization must identify all resources required for operation of the QMS, and ensure they are available. These resources will include people; infrastructure elements such as buildings, equipment, and technology; the appropriate environment, both tangible and intangible; monitoring and measurement systems; and the organization's knowledge base. There is a requirement to ensure all personnel have the right level of training and competency. They must also be aware of the details of the QMS and the need for compliance. Suitable communication channels must be established. There must be a system for creation and control of documentation.

4.6.6 Operation (Clause 8)

The processes required to deliver the product or service must be planned, implemented, and controlled. This starts with identification of customer requirements, plus any regulatory requirements. Planning, implementation, and control must be applied to design and development of the product or service (if applicable); to processes, products or services that are sourced externally to the organization; to in-house production activities; and to release to the customer. Any nonconforming outputs from processes must be controlled to ensure they are not used or delivered to the customer.

4.6.7 Performance evaluation (Clause 9)

There needs to be systems in place for all necessary monitoring, measurement, analysis, and evaluation. This should cover both the processes for delivery of product or service and the operation of the QMS. Customer satisfaction should also be monitored. All results must be documented. An internal audit system must be established to ensure the QMS is operating effectively. And finally, senior management must review the QMS regularly.

4.6.8 Improvement (Clause 10)

The organization must identify and put into practice opportunities to improve customer satisfaction. All nonconformities must be investigated, and corrective actions applied and documented. There must also be a system for continually monitoring the QMS for improvement opportunities.

4.6.9 Annexes

Annex A provides clarification on the revised structure of the standard, its terminology, and concepts. Annex B lists an additional 16 standards developed by ISO/TC 176 as supplementary guidance for organizations working toward ISO 9001: 2015. They are informative only and do no amend the requirements of the main standard.

4.7 Application of ISO 9000 standards to the pharmaceutical industry

The ISO 9000 standards are generic ones that can be applied to any industry. In the past, many companies, particularly those in regions such as Eastern Europe and the Former Soviet Union, where the industry was just emerging, used to consider using this route to achieve compliance to international pharmaceutical standards. The author was frequently asked what is the difference between ISO 9001 and guidelines for Good Manufacturing Practice (GMP), and on occasion, companies stated they had no need to work toward GMP because they were working toward ISO 9001 instead.

It is certainly true there is a degree of similarity in the approach taken toward the two—and in fact, the latest version of GMP guidelines such as the EU and WHO guides both refer to an ISO 9001—type quality system. However, the two are not completely equivalent. It is probably fair to say any company which had in place all the systems required to comply with GMP would have little difficulty in obtaining ISO 9001 accreditation, at least in relation to its manufacturing operation. However, GMP has little to say about the areas of sales and marketing. On the other hand, it is not necessarily the case that a company with ISO 9001 accreditation would automatically be able to demonstrate compliance to GMP.

One aspect that particularly stands out as a difference between the two is validation. This is illustrated by reviewing Clause 8.5.1.f of ISO 9001: 2015, which calls for: "the validation and periodic revalidation, of the ability to achieve planned results of the processes for production and service provision, where the resulting output cannot be verified by subsequent monitoring or measurement." This implies inspection and testing is the preferred route to assurance of quality. However, in the pharmaceutical industry, this would be considered as quality control; and the concept of quality assurance being of greater importance than quality control has long been established. Hence, for a pharmaceutical company, validation is a critical element.

Another example of differences could be the approach to product release. Clause 8.6 of ISO 9001: 2015 on release of products and services states: "The release of products and services to the customer shall not proceed until the planned arrangements have been satisfactorily completed, unless otherwise approved by a relevant authority and, as applicable, by the customer." In the pharmaceutical industry, this should never happen. It is a requirement of GMP that all batches of finished product are approved by the appropriate person before they can be released into the marketplace.

There have been no guides written to date that discuss how to apply ISO 9000 standards in the pharmaceutical industry. There are guides available for suppliers to the pharmaceutical industry. For example, in the United Kingdom, the Pharmaceutical Quality Group developed the PS 9000 standard on requirements and guidance for GMP relating to the manufacture of packaging materials for medicinal products, including orally inhaled and nasal drug products. The latest version, PS 9000: 2016 is in accordance with ISO 9001: 2015. There are also many similarities between ISO quality standards and the regulations for the manufacture of medical devices.

4.8 ISO 14000 series

The ISO 14000 series of standards deal with environmental management policy. ISO 14001 was first issued in 1996, revised in 2004 and again in 2015. ISO 14001: 2015 is therefore the current version. It requires a company to demonstrate that they have an environmental management system, including environmental policy; assessment of the impacts of products or services and other activities on the environment; setting up environmental objectives with quantifiable targets; activities to achieve these objectives; systems for corrective action; and management review. Once again, the system must be documented and must have appropriate monitoring and control programs. Unlike ISO 9000, which is essentially a confidential system (apart from the relationship between the organization and its assessors), the environmental policy produced by a company accredited to ISO 14001 must be available to the public.

When the first edition of this book was published in 2002, environmental management was a relatively new topic. However, it was pointed out that the pharmaceutical industry uses large quantities of chemicals both in the primary synthesis of its actives and in the formulation of its finished products; and the amount of waste material at these stages can be high. Additionally, the amount of waste materials produced during packaging can also be high, particularly in a blistering operation. On this basis, the pharmaceutical industry was a prime candidate for ISO 14001.

Nearly 20 years later, as we write this second edition, the situation has become much more critical and environmental management is no longer an additional public relations tool, but a regulatory requirement in most countries. Companies are required to have policies and systems in place; and many of them make these public on their websites. This is a far larger topic than it was previously and outside the scope of this book.

4.9 Chapter summary

• The International Organization for Standardization (ISO) is an independent, nongovernmental international agency comprising the national standards bodies of 165 countries or territories.

- The responsibilities of ISO Technical Committee (TC) 176 are: "Standardization in the field of quality management (generic quality management systems and supporting technologies), as well as quality management standardization in specific sectors at the request of the affected sector and the ISO Technical Management Board."
- The ISO 9000 series of quality standards was first published in 1987 and revised in 1994, 2000, 2008, and 2015.
- The current revision comprises three main standards. Only ISO 9001: 2015 offers accreditation for companies.
- There are 16 supplementary standards, providing guidance for companies working toward accreditation. They are advisory rather than mandatory.
- ISO 9001: 2015 outlines seven principles of quality management: customer focus; leadership; engagement of people; process approach; improvement; evidence-based decision making; and relationship management.
- The four main elements of a QMS's documentation are the quality manual, quality policies, quality procedures, and quality records.
- The process approach to quality systems incorporates the PDCA cycle and risk-based thinking.
- The PDCA cycle ensures processes are planned, resourced, managed, and improved effectively.
- The risk-based approach requires identification of factors potentially impacting the operation of the processes, then taking measures to prevent adverse effects while maximizing opportunities.
- The key clauses of ISO 9001: 2015 which must be addressed in establishing and controlling the QMS are context of the organization, leadership, planning, support, operation, performance evaluation, and improvement.
- There is considerable overlap between ISO 9001: 2015 and GMP, but the two are not completely interchangeable.
- While environmental management is a key element of management and control for the pharmaceutical industry, it has grown in criticality in the past 20 years and is no longer within the scope of this book.

4.10 Questions/problems

1. What are the seven principles of a QMS, as described in ISO 9001: 2015. How might they be applied to a pharmaceutical manufacturing company?
2. Describe the PDCA cycle for a company producing packaging materials for a pharmaceutical tablet manufacturer.
3. How would risk-based thinking impact on the supplier of active pharmaceutical ingredients to a sterile products manufacturing company?

4. Choose three of the clauses of ISO 9001: 2015 and describe the quality plans required for a liquids and creams manufacturer who wishes to achieve accreditation.

5. Identify five examples within a pharmaceutical development and manufacturing company where compliance to ISO 9001: 2015 would not necessarily ensure compliance to GMP.

6. Identify five examples within a pharmaceutical development and manufacturing company where compliance to GMP would not necessarily ensure compliance to ISO 9001: 2015.

Further reading

International Organization for Standardization. (2015a). *Environmental management* (ISO Standard No. 14001:2015).

International Organization for Standardization. (2015b). Quality management systems - Fundamentals and vocabulary (ISO Standard No. 9000:2015).

International Organization for Standardization. (2015c). Quality management systems — Requirements (ISO Standard No 9001:2015).

International Organization for Standardization. (2018). Quality management — Quality of an organization — Guidance to achieve sustained success (ISO Standard No 9004:2018).

CHAPTER 5

The management of quality

5.1 Introduction

This chapter discusses the management of the quality function. The chapter begins with the evolution of quality within the organization from a subordinated laboratory service to a fully integrated and independent area of responsibility. The discussion addresses the position of the quality function within the organizational structure and the technical and business responsibilities of the senior personnel. This is followed by a detailed review of the responsibility for batch release, contrasting the qualified person (QP) within Europe and the authorized person (AP) in other parts of the world.

Each holder of a manufacturing licence must have a quality control (QC) function. In other words, there must be people clearly responsible for all QC activities, with access to sufficient numbers of trained and experienced staff, and an appropriately designed laboratory, suitably equipped to enable all QC functions to be carried out in accordance with specifications. The independence of QC from production is fundamental. The QC manager should not report to the production manager. Conversely, the production manager should not report to the QC manager. Legislation in different countries deals with this issue in different ways. Ideally, the head of the QC function reports directly to the president of the company. This ensures there is no interference from manufacturing staff in key decisions on product quality. An alternative to this, which might in some circumstances be preferable, is that the quality controller reports to a professionally qualified technical director, who would also be responsible for production activities. The advantage of this approach is a scientific and professional review of product quality against standards and the product's use. This scientific evaluation of the product may not be possible with a chief executive who has no scientific background.

5.2 Evolution of the quality function

The development of the quality function within a company has tended to be an evolutionary process. For companies in the United States and much of Europe, this is a process which started in the 1970s or even earlier and is now in the late stages of maturity. However, there are still companies in some parts of the world that are in the early stages. A brief overview of the evolutionary steps might be useful at this point.

Quality
DOI: https://doi.org/10.1016/B978-0-323-90815-3.00014-1

5.2.1 Laboratory function

In the first stage, there is only a laboratory function. All countries, no matter what the stage of maturity their industry has reached, have a registration process for pharmaceuticals which issues licences before a product is launched onto the marketplace. This implies a requirement for analysis of raw materials, intermediates, and finished products. The position of the laboratory within the company at this point tends to be as a service to production. Often, it reports to the production manager. In some cases, there is no laboratory within the company itself and the process is subcontracted out, either to a government organization or a private company.

Within the company hierarchy, the laboratory personnel do not have the same status as the production personnel. The concept of independence of QC from production does not exist. Responsibility for releasing the product remains with production.

5.2.2 Subordinated quality control function

The next stage tends to be the widening of the role of the laboratory to cover other testing requirements such as environmental monitoring. At this point, the company may be said to have a QC function. The responsibility for product release tends to move at this point to the QC manager. There are still occasions, however, where this function is subordinated to production.

The process of document audit however does not yet form part of the release process. Process records exist but were often in logbooks at the point of production, rather than gathered together into a batch dossier. In the author's experience, the view of both production and QC personnel at this point is "QC is responsible for physical testing only. The documentation belongs to, and is the business of, production."

5.2.3 Independent quality control function

At the next stage, there is a recognition of the need to separate the responsibilities of QC and production. The QC function no longer reports to the production manager, although where it becomes located within the organization varies from company to company. In some companies, QC reports to the development department, if such a function exists. In other companies, QC reports to a technical director, along with, but not necessarily at the same level as, the production department(s). The process of document audit might be added to the QC responsibilities, but this is not necessarily the case.

At some point, the importance of QC relative to production is recognized and the production manager and the QC manager reach a point of equilibrium within the organizational hierarchy.

5.2.4 Introduction of quality assurance

The next stage is where the function of quality assurance (QA) first appears within an organization. This is often the point where a company makes huge steps forward towards achievement of good manufacturing practice (GMP) compliance. QA tends to begin with responsibility for such topics as validation, document audit and GMP training. Often, responsibility is given to a single person to set up the function and their main problem is determining how to cover such a huge range of responsibilities on their own.

During GMP audits, one of the questions many companies at this stage in their development ask is "where should QA be located in the organization?" At this point, there is often no direct relationship between QA and QC. The latter, wherever it is situated in the organization chart, is still seen as providing a service to production. On the other hand, QA is seen as a staff function. Frequently, it reports to the General Manager or senior technical person within the organization.

5.3 Alternative models for management of quality

As the organization matures, the role of QA grows and the number of personnel working within the department increases. However, there are a number of different organizational models that are adopted by companies.

In some, QA evolves into quality management and QC becomes absorbed as one of the departments. At this point, the laboratory function may remain as part of QC or it may revert to being a pure service center for production.

Conversely, there are companies in which QA becomes one of the departments of QC, alongside the laboratories.

In other companies, QC and QA remain as distinct functions with a complete separation of responsibilities. Document audit may at this point be the responsibility of either department. The QP or AP with responsibility for batch release does not have a fixed position and their location within the organizational structure is variable.

5.4 Management of quality in a multinational company

The models described above can be seen both in companies with single sites and in much larger organizations. However, there is a further aspect which is seen within a multinational company (MNC), that of the corporate quality function.

The MNC has a number of factories around the world, producing products to corporate specifications and standards. Some factories will be wholly owned subsidiaries, some will be joint ventures with local companies, and some will be contract manufacturers or licensees. Each factory will have its own quality management system, covering QC and QA. However, there is frequently a corporate function as well, which operates from the head office. This department covers such functions as development of company-wide quality standards and procedures, auditing of individual factories, and approval of contractors.

5.5 The role of the quality manager

Chapter 3, covers the requirements to be fulfilled to ensure a company has an effective quality management system. These requirements will be the same in all companies. But the personnel responsible for carrying out the various activities will vary from company to company. This chapter looks at the topic from a different angle and discusses the role of the quality manager within a company. The role can be looked at from two viewpoints: technical, and business.

5.5.1 Technical responsibilities of the quality manager

The quality manager is firstly responsible for the approval or rejection of all starting and packaging materials and all intermediate, bulk, and finished products. This is a critical area where independence is paramount.

Secondly, the quality manager is responsible for the evaluation of batch records coming from production. This should be done as part of the product release process. The purpose is to ensure everything has been produced in accordance with the agreed process and meets specifications. If there have been any deviations from the agreed process, these must be authorized by responsible persons (RPs).

The quality manager is also responsible for ensuring all required testing is completed in accordance with specifications, and for approving all the instructions required for the organization and implementation of testing. However, the development of all these instructions, policies, and procedures may well be done in cooperation with production and development personnel, as discussed in Section 5.5.2.

The quality manager is responsible not only for in-house analysis but also for testing carried out under contract by third parties. There must be certainty that the contract acceptor can conduct the testing to the required standard, has all the necessary personnel and equipment to conduct the testing, and has a written contract specifying the responsibilities of all parties to the agreement.

The quality manager is responsible for ensuring proper maintenance of all facilities and equipment under their control. Validation of analytical methods and calibration of laboratory equipment must be done. This validation ensures the results achieved by following the validated processes can be relied upon to indicate the correct result. Some aspects of validation will almost inevitably be shared with production and engineering, as discussed in Section 5.5.2.

Finally, the quality manager must ensure the people who carry out all this work are well trained and motivated at the commencement of their work and receive regular training and retraining.

5.5.2 Shared technical responsibilities of the quality manager

As mentioned in Section 5.5.1, there are a number of responsibilities the quality manager will share with the equivalent persons within other functions of the organization. In order to ensure nothing is missed and there is no duplication, all organizational positions must have clear written job descriptions, showing where the responsibilities are shared.

Approval of all procedures and documents used in manufacturing is a shared responsibility. There is also a requirement to ensure an effective change control system is established. As documents are updated, all users must be given the latest version.

Monitoring of the manufacturing environment is shared between QA/QC, production, and engineering. They should conduct the monitoring and testing as appropriate, with the results available to all who need to know them.

Both quality and production have a role to play in the development and maintenance of an appropriate factory sanitation and hygiene management system. Similarly, both have a major contribution to make in the validation of processes and the calibration of equipment.

Just as a comprehensive organization chart is required for a factory, a comprehensive training program is also required for all its personnel. Both production and QC have a role to play in the development of that training program and shared responsibility for its implementation.

Approval of all suppliers and contract manufacturers is also an area of shared responsibility, with each function contributing their own particular expertise. The specification and monitoring of storage conditions will also be shared, but with the additional involvement of the development function.

Since both quality and production functions are responsible for the generation of records relevant to batches, the arrangements for the storage of those records may be a shared responsibility. Alternatively, a separate department may have responsibility for all aspects of documentation and batch records. The practicalities of document management and storage are often decided by such peripheral issues as where adequate space is available.

Monitoring of compliance with GMP is very much a shared responsibility, emphasizing the understanding that the achievement of GMP is everyone's responsibility.

Some aspects of sampling may be conducted by people other than QC personnel. If this is the case, there must be a clear definition of who is taking what sort of sample and when, to provide confidence that what is being done is appropriate. Sampling should only be done by persons trained in the methods to be used.

5.5.3 Business role of the quality manager

The quality manager may be independent of production in terms of the technical functions of the position. However, they are also part of the management team running the organization, and as such have a responsibility to ensure the business is not adversely affected by any of the activities of quality management. Aspects of the business which may be impacted by quality management include cost, regulatory aspects, quality, staff motivation, and operational viability/flexibility. If any of these elements is negatively affected, the quality manager is not operating effectively.

It is therefore important for the quality manager to work cooperatively with people at many different departments within the organization, including not only technical colleagues in production, development, engineering, and warehousing but also others such as purchasing and marketing.

5.6 Responsibility for batch release

Any company responsible for supplying pharmaceuticals needs to appoint one or more person(s) whose responsibility is to release batches of product onto the marketplace. However, this person's job title varies across countries and regions.

The term "qualified person" is universally recognized in Europe and has a particular legal basis within the European Union (EU). In other parts of the world, other terms, such as "authorized person" or "responsible person" are more frequently used. However, whatever the precise terminology, the role of such a person is to ensure the final user of any drug, the patient, can be sure that drug meets all requirements of safety, quality, and efficacy. It is the final act of quality assurance by the company.

It is not only the terminology that varies around the world. The degree of development of the system for appointing and controlling such people is also variable. The system within the EU has been developing over the past 40 + years and is evolving still. Yet, even here, there are significant differences in interpretation and approach.

5.6.1 The qualified person in the European Union and the United Kingdom

Any company that manufactures pharmaceuticals in, or imports pharmaceuticals into, the EU, or is authorized to produce materials for clinical trials, must appoint a QP, who will be named on the appropriate documentation. The licensing authority has the right to accept or reject the nominated individual.

The United Kingdom ceased to be a member state of the EU in January 2021. However she was a member state throughout the period when the role of the QP was being developed and there is still a legal requirement for pharmaceutical companies within the United Kingdom to operate a QP system.

5.6.1.1 The European Union directive

The requirement for a company to appoint a QP first appeared in the 1975 EU Directive 75/319/EEC, which was amended in 1985 and 1993 before being superseded in 2001 by directive 2001/83/EC, the consolidated version of which was approved in July 2019. The section of the directive dealing with QPs is Articles 48 to 52 relating, respectively, to:

- the requirement to appoint a QP;
- qualifications and experience required to become a QP;
- transitional arrangements, the so-called grandfather clause;
- responsibilities of a QP; and
- and the code of conduct.

As a result of this directive, the requirements are then included in the national legislation of each member state. In some cases, additional literature is then issued by the national licensing authority or accreditation bodies to describe the required procedures. For example, in the United Kingdom, the joint accreditation bodies are the Royal Pharmaceutical Society, the Royal Society of Biology, and the Royal Society of Chemistry. They jointly produced a Code of Conduct for QPs operating within the United Kingdom, as discussed in Section 5.6.1.3.

5.6.1.2 Qualified person eligibility

The EU Directive states that to be a QP, a person must have appropriate knowledge and industrial experience. The original discipline of that person may be pharmacy, medicine, veterinary medicine, chemistry, pharmaceutical chemistry, and technology, or biology. However, the application of this rule varies within the member states.

Within the United Kingdom, the Republic of Ireland, and the Scandinavian countries, all disciplines listed in the directive are accepted. This wide interpretation may be in part a reflection of the fact that the number of industrial pharmacists is relatively low in these countries. A similar situation also exists in Spain. However, in France, for example, there is an absolute requirement for the QP to be a pharmacist (the *Pharmacien Responsible*).

5.6.1.3 Qualified person disciplinary action

The EU directive requires the performance of the duties of a QP to be subject to some manner of control. One option is to operate according to a code of practice. As mentioned in Section 5.6.1.1, such a code was developed and originally published in 1993 by three professional bodies in the United Kingdom, in discussion with the Medicines Control Authority (the forerunner of the Medicines and Healthcare products Regulatory Agency). The document has been updated and reissued a number of times and the latest version was published in 2015. The text of this Code of Practice can be downloaded from the websites of any of the three professional bodies (Qualified Persons in the Pharmaceutical Industry Code of Practice.)

Since the EU directive is binding on all member states, there was a need for other countries to adopt a code of practice or a suitable alternative. From 1996 onward, a similar code was adopted by the European Industrial Pharmacists Group (EIPG). This code can be obtained from the EIPG website (Code of Practice for Qualified Persons).

In most of the EU member states, disciplinary matters are dealt with by the regulatory authorities. This approach contrasts with the United Kingdom, where discipline is a joint responsibility of the regulatory authority and the appropriate professional body. It is generally assumed, although not always the case, that a QP is a member of an appropriate professional body and will thus be bound by the rules and guidelines of that body. If a QP fails to carry out their duties in an appropriate manner, they can be considered to be guilty of professional misconduct and can have their professional status removed. Failure to adhere to the QP code of practice would be considered as such a case of misconduct.

The codes of practice emphasize QPs have a responsibility not only to the companies employing them but also to the licensing authority and the inspectorate. QPs have a duty to highlight any aspects of the quality system not complying with requirements. Should an aspect of the situation in which they are being asked to operate be outside their sphere of knowledge and experience, the QPs have a duty to refuse to act in this context. For example, a QP whose only experience is in the manufacture of dry products would not automatically be competent to act as a QP if the company moved into the manufacture of sterile products.

5.6.1.4 Qualified person registration

There are two categories of person defined in the directive who can be registered as eligible to serve as a QP: permanent and transitional provisions. Under the permanent provisions, a specific course of study is defined and must be undertaken together with an appropriate period of work experience before a person can be nominated for the role of QP.

However, at the time the role of QP was being formalized across the EU, there were a large number of people who were already carrying out such a function within their companies. These people had experience in the role but had not studied for the formal qualification. Under the transitional provisions, these people were permitted to apply for QP status on the basis of experience alone.

One issue currently being faced within Europe is the QPs who were registered under the transitional provisions are coming to the end of their careers. This means more people are leaving the register than joining it. Due to the major investment in time (by the candidate and their employer) and money (usually by the employer) to achieve registration, there is a slowdown in people eligible for the role.

5.6.1.5 Qualified person training
The knowledge required by someone working toward eligibility via the permanent transitions (the only way now open to potential QPs in Europe) is very detailed and covers 12 major subject areas. Once again, there are differences in approach. Much of the knowledge required by the QP is covered by the pharmacy degree, although the amount of industrial pharmacy content covered by these university courses is not always in-depth. Graduates of other disciplines are unlikely to have covered all the required topics and will need to take additional training courses. Training is generally modular and can be carried out in any order. Depending on the previous experience and qualifications of an individual, either the whole course or just some sections will be studied.

5.6.1.6 Role of the qualified person
The role of the QP can be specifically described as ensuring:
- Each batch of product is manufactured in compliance with both the manufacturing authorization and the specific marketing authorization.
- Each batch of product imported from outside the EU has been fully tested to prove it complies with all requirements of the marketing authorization.
- Each batch of product imported from a country outside the EU, where the EU has an agreement that products are manufactured to at least the same standard as that in the EU, can be accepted without carrying out additional testing.
- Each approved batch of product is entered in an appropriate register as soon as possible after manufacture or importation.

5.6.1.7 Routine duties of the qualified person
In the process of approving a batch of products for release onto the marketplace, there are a number of checks a QP must make to ensure all requirements have been achieved as follows:
- The batch must comply with the requirements of the product licence and the manufacturing authorization.
- All aspects of GMP guidelines have been fulfilled.
- Critical processes have been validated.
- All QC checks have been carried out satisfactorily and a review of manufacturing and packaging records has been completed.
- Any process deviations have been recorded and investigated to determine the effect on product quality. (In some cases, depending on the nature of the deviation, this would imply notification to the national regulatory authority.)

- If required as a result of a process deviation, all extra QC checks have been carried out satisfactorily.
- The documentation review has been carried out and signed off by appropriately qualified personnel.
- Self-inspections and other regular audits have been carried out.
- All other aspects, such as calibration and environmental monitoring, are satisfactory.
- All legal aspects relating to products imported from outside the EU are covered as required.

Depending on the size of the company, the QP may carry out some or all of these checks personally. However, in larger organizations, it is acceptable, and indeed necessary, for the QP to rely on other people to carry out individual checks on a day-to-day basis. In this case, the principal responsibility of the QP is to ensure the appropriate elements of the quality system are in place and there are sufficient controls within the system to prevent problems being missed. Hence the QP relies on the activities of other people and has to have good interpersonal skills to maintain good relationships with those people.

The QP will also be involved in routine dealings with the regulatory authorities. In some member states, this will be as part of a team. However, in France, the regulatory authority will only deal with the *Pharmacien Responsable*.

5.6.1.8 Requirements for number and location of qualified persons

According to the directives and guidelines, companies are only required to nominate a single person to serve as a QP. However, going down the route of a single nomination means there is no cover for holidays and/or sickness absences. When there are a very small number of batches for approval, an absence is not likely to be a problem and the company would need to identify a suitable alternative person as a deputy.

In the situation where an organization is a large one, or one that operates on more than one manufacturing site, it is permissible for a number of people to be nominated on the manufacturing authorization.

5.6.1.9 The qualified person and quality control/quality assurance

There is no specific requirement that the QP and the head of QC be the same person. The EU guideline specifically states in GMP Chapter 2, paragraph 2.5: "Senior Management should appoint Key Management Personnel including the head of Production, the head of QC, and if at least one of these persons is not responsible for the duties described in Article 51 of Directive 2001/83/EC, an adequate number, but at least one, Qualified Person(s) designated for the purpose." (EU Guidelines for Good Manufacturing Practice for Medicinal Products for Human and Veterinary Use. Part 1. Chapter 2: Personnel).

In a small organization, it is quite likely the same person would be responsible for QA, QC and be the QP. However, in a larger organization, QC is often one of the departments within the QA function. The QPs in this situation could be the head of QA and/or some of their deputies.

5.6.1.10 Contracted qualified persons

It is not a requirement for the QP to be an employee of the company. It is acceptable for the QP to be working under contract to the company, in a self-employed status. This is particularly relevant for small companies, who may only have a few batches to be released each week and for whom the expense of employing a full-time QP would not be justified.

In such a situation, the responsibility of the QP in relation to the professional aspects of the role is exactly the same as if there were an employer–employee relationship. However, there should be a written contract between the two parties, detailing the expectations and responsibilities of both.

In addition to signing off batch releases, the QP would be expected to take part in training, auditing and other activities and be in attendance during regulatory inspections.

5.6.1.11 Contract manufacture

In the situation where one company (the contract acceptor) is manufacturing a product under contract for a second company (the contract giver), there is no clear rule as to where the QP shall be located. The contract giver would normally hold the marketing authorization and the contract acceptor would hold the manufacturing authorization. The QP may be located in either company but must have full access to all appropriate information from both parties. The arrangement must be clearly stated in the contract.

5.6.1.12 Continuing professional development

Many professional bodies nowadays require their members to carry out an element of continuing professional development (CPD) as a prerequisite to maintaining their membership. The three professional bodies involved in the drafting of the QP Code of Practice in United Kingdom are no exception to this rule. Their positions are spelled out in paragraph 12 of the code and expanded in Appendix 1.

However, a QP, whether or not they are a member of a professional body, also has a responsibility to keep their knowledge and experience up to date, as emphasized in the Code of Conduct from the EIPG. There is a requirement for the QP to keep a written record of this CPD.

5.7 The equivalent role in the United States

There is no defined role of qualified or authorized person in the United States. Responsibility for batch release sits with the QC unit (Electronic Code of Federal Regulations Title 21, Chapter 1, Subchapter C, Part 211 Subpart B—Organization and Personnel Sec. 211.22 Responsibilities of QC unit). By reviewing the various clauses of Title 21CFR211, all the requirements outlined as the routine duties of the QP can be seen to be covered by the Food and Drug Administration (FDA) rules. However, there is no link between the person signing the batch release certificate and a professional membership that can be withdrawn in the case of misconduct. In the United States, the primary emphasis is on setting up the systems and validating those systems. Thereafter, the responsibility for batch release may be delegated to a technician in the QC unit.

5.8 Other parts of the world

Just as there are variations in the approach taken within different member states of the EU, so there are differences in other parts of the world. Some countries have no such official position in place. Many others will only accept pharmacists in the role. In all cases, the situation is a matter of national regulation.

5.8.1 Batch release and Pharmaceutical Inspection Co-operation Scheme

The Pharmaceutical Inspection Co-operation Scheme (PIC/S) guide to GMP uses the term "Authorized Person" in place of QP. In the glossary to this guide, the term is defined as: "Person recognized by the authority as having the necessary basic scientific and technical background and experience." Clause 1.4 xv of the same guide states the requirement for certification by an authorized person: "that each production batch has been produced and controlled in accordance with the requirements of the Marketing Authorization and any other regulations relevant to the production, control and release of medicinal products" (PE 009-15 GMP Guide).

5.8.2 Release for supply of medicines in Australia

As an example of how the PIC/S guidance is being implemented, The Therapeutic Goods Administration (TGA) in Australia issued its latest guidance on release for supply (RFS) in 2019. (Release for supply of medicines Technical guidance on the interpretation of the PIC/S Guide to GMP.) It makes specific reference to the PIC/S guidance and requires the appointment of an authorized person to release every batch. While there is no formal accreditation scheme as seen for QPs in Europe, there is a requirement for appropriate knowledge, experience and background. The TGA guidance states: "The person nominated to have control of QC under section 37(1) (e), Therapeutic Goods Act 1989 would be an obvious choice to be an authorized person, but other arrangements can be considered, including delegation." The company must nominate the AP(s) and they must be listed in the quality management system.

5.9 Chapter summary

- Every holder of a manufacturing licence must have a quality function. This function must operate independently from production.
- The quality function must have access to the appropriate levels of trained and experienced staff; suitable equipment; and validated methodology to test all materials, products, and systems.
- There is an evolutionary process from a simple laboratory reporting to production to a fully developed, independent quality function comprising both QC and QA. This evolution is completed in many regions but still operates in some countries where the industry and regulation are less well developed.
- There are no fixed organizational structures for the quality function and a number of alternative models exist.
- In a multinational company with multiple manufacturing sites, an additional level of quality management exists, based at the head office, with responsibility for corporate quality affairs.
- The quality manager has a significant technical role within the organization. Some responsibilities are theirs alone. Others are shared with the managers of other technical departments.
- The quality manager also has a business role as a member of the company's senior management team.
- Any company responsible for supplying pharmaceuticals must appoint one or more persons with responsibility for releasing batches onto the marketplace.
- The batch release should only take place if there is assurance that the product meets all requirements of safety, quality, and efficacy.
- Within the EU and the United Kingdom, there is a formal role as qualified person, whose education, training, and experience are specified within the Directive. While all member states must at least comply with the directive, in some countries, the eligibility requirements are even stricter.
- The QP has a responsibility not only to their company but also to the regulatory authority The QP is bound by a code of conduct and can have their registration removed in the case of misconduct.
- There is a detailed description of the role of the QP, and a definition of their routine duties.

- The number of QPs nominated by a company may vary depending on the size of the role. Not all companies need to employ a QP; the use of a contractor on a part-time basis is also permitted.
- QPs must engage in Continuing Professional Development.
- There is no equivalent role to QP in the United States. However, all the duties of a QP are specified as being the responsibility of the QC unit.
- The Pharmaceutical Inspection Co-operation Scheme uses the term "Authorised Person." This role is implemented in many of the PIC/S member countries. For example, an AP is required as part of the process of Release for Supply in Australia.

5.10 Questions/problems

1. What stages does a company go through in moving from a laboratory reporting to production to a fully independent quality function?
2. Outline three different models for the organizational structure of the quality function. What are the pros and cons of each model?
3. Develop the job description for the quality manager of a small manufacturing company in the United States. Indicate which responsibilities would be theirs alone, and which would be shared with other managers within the organization?
4. Develop the person specification for a QP to be recruited for a manufacturing company just outside Paris producing a range of tablets, capsules and infusion products.
5. How would the role of a QP differ in a large multiproduct manufacturing site of a MNC in Ireland from that of a small unit producing clinical trials materials in Scotland?
6. A company in Ukraine is hoping to obtain a license to manufacture the products of a MNC based in the United States. What provisions would it need to make to demonstrate an effective QC unit?

Further reading

Australian Government Department of Health. Therapeutic goods administration. Release for supply of medicines technical guidance on the interpretation of the PIC/S guide to GMP. Available at: https://www.tga.gov.au/sites/default/files/release-supply-medicines.pdf (accessed 18.05.21).

Electronic Code of Federal Regulations. Title 21, Chapter 1, Sub-chapter C, Part 211 Subpart B—organization and personnel Sec. 211.22 responsibilities of quality control unit. Available at: https://www.accessdata.fda.gov/scripts/cdrh/cfdocs/cfcfr/cfrsearch.cfm?fr = 211.22 (accessed 18.05.21).

EudreLex. The rules governing medicinal products in the european union. Volume 4. EU guidelines for good manufacturing practice for medicinal products for human and veterinary use. Chapter 2 personnel. Available at: https://ec.europa.eu/health/sites/default/files/files/eudralex/vol-4/2014-03_chapter_2.pdf (accessed 18.05.21).

European Industrial Pharmacists Group, 2004. Code of practice for qualified persons. Available at: https://eipg.eu/wp-content/uploads/2013/07/eipg-qp-code-of-practice.pdf (accessed 18.05.21).

Royal Pharmaceutical Society, Royal Society of Biology & Royal Society of Chemistry, 2015. Qualified persons in the pharmaceutical industry code of practice. Available at: https://www.rsb.org.uk/images/QP_Code_of_Practice_2015v1.pdf (accessed 17.05.21).

The European Parliament & The Council of the European Union, 2001. Directive 2001/83/EC of the European Parliament and of the council of the European Union on the community code relating to medicinal products for human use. Available at: https://eur-ex.europa.eu/eli/dir/2001/83/2019-07-26 (accessed 17.05.21).

The Pharmaceutical Inspection Co-operation Scheme (PIC/S), 2015. PE 009-15 GMP guide. Available at https://picscheme.org/en/publications?tri = gmp#zone (accessed 28.05.21).

CHAPTER 6

Inspections and auditing

6.1 Introduction

A major facet of the pharmaceutical industry is the process of inspections or auditing of facilities and quality systems to ensure they comply with the requirements of relevant standards and that all necessary processes are in place.

In many cases, the words inspection and audit are used interchangeably. However, there is a difference between the two processes. An inspection is a one-way process in which a review is carried out and compliance (or otherwise) is confirmed. There is no discussion on how improvements can be made. This process is generally used in the regulatory context. An audit, on the other hand, is a two-way process in which compliance (or otherwise) is reviewed and discussion takes place on how improvements can be achieved. This approach is more appropriate in the context of internal audits and consultancy situations. To prevent confusion, the term "inspection" will be used throughout this chapter, apart from the section dealing with auditing suppliers. However, in all but the regulatory situations, it can be assumed an inspection will also include an element of auditing as well.

The chapter starts with a review of the different types of inspections that companies are subjected to. There are internal ones, primarily the self-inspection program, but also, on occasion, independent quality assurance (QA) activities. From an external viewpoint, companies will receive inspections from regulatory authorities, from potential contract givers, and possibly from independent consultants. On the other hand, the same companies will carry out inspections on suppliers' premises.

In a global industry such as pharmaceutical manufacturing and supply, many companies enter export markets and hence become involved in inspection requirements from other countries. To reduce the cost and time resources required for these activities, there are several mutual recognition activities established around the world. The major ones are reviewed in this chapter.

Following this is a review of the particular skills required to prepare for and participate in inspections. These skills range from the technical aspects like knowledge of the standards and of the facility to the more people-oriented issues relating to communication.

Finally, there is a discussion of the issues faced by countries that are not yet in the mainstream of the pharmaceutical industry but with the need to demonstrate they can comply with current requirements to compete in the global marketplace.

Quality
DOI: https://doi.org/10.1016/B978-0-323-90815-3.00010-4

6.2 Types of inspections

Pharmaceutical manufacturing companies are accustomed to being inspected regularly and also need to be able to organize and run inspections themselves. This section deals with the different types of inspections a company will be involved with, either as the inspected or the inspector.

Inspections of manufacturing facilities tend to go through many stages, which together build towards a cohesive inspection program. At the first level, an informal self-inspection takes place everyday by operators and managers alike. If something is seen to be wrong, it is immediately fixed.

Next, there is a formal self-inspection process that takes place regularly and is a specified requirement of good manufacturing practice (GMP). The purpose of this is to take a step back from the day-to-day activities, review for compliance to GMP, and look for ways to improve the system. There may also be a need to conduct self-inspections as a result of a specific problem such as frequent complaints.

The next stage may or may not take place, depending on the size of the organization. It involves the use of QA staff as internal auditors to review the system for compliance. In a smaller company, this step and the previous one tend to blend into one another.

Finally, there is an external inspection. This will come from many sources. There will be national regulatory inspections related to manufacturing authorizations and marketing authorizations. If a company is planning to export its products, there may be inspections from overseas regulators. In addition, if a company is entering into a contract manufacturing relationship with one or more other companies, the inspectors from those companies will want to ensure there is no risk to their products. Some companies also use consultants to support them in GMP improvement projects. In such a case, a GMP inspection, against the appropriate national or international standards, would be the first step in the process.

6.2.1 Internal inspections

For most companies, the internal inspection will be in the form of a self-inspection program. This program should include a written procedure detailing what is to be inspected and at what frequency. It should be used to ensure a consistent approach is achieved.

The areas to be inspected would include, but would not necessarily be limited to are:

- the personnel working in the facility;
- production and ancillary facilities;
- maintenance of the factory and plant;
- warehousing of all materials;
- manufacturing and testing equipment;

- production and in-process controls;
- quality control procedures;
- documentation preparation, use, and compliance;
- sanitation and hygiene regimes;
- validation and monitoring programs;
- instrument calibration;
- recall procedures;
- handling of complaints;
- control of printed components;
- label control;
- purchasing; and
- a follow-up to previous self-inspections.

In other words, a complete review of all aspects of GMP.

The self-inspection team is appointed by the management of the company and is composed of a mixture of personnel, including experts in GMP and those familiar with the area in question. It is useful to have representation from production, quality control, and engineering on the team, as they will bring different perspectives to the inspection.

It can be a good training exercise to involve operators in the process, as well. It is also possible to involve people from other parts of the company, or even outside the company if it will add value to the process. It is important the team members are encouraged to be objective in their evaluation.

The team leader should be someone with access to the resources to produce a report at the end of the process, and with the authority and experience to organize and manage a team activity. Hence, it is usually, but not always, a manager or supervisor. The leader should be from a different department to take a more impartial viewpoint.

The frequency with which self-inspections are carried out will be dependent on the company. For a small company that can cover all its operations in one inspection, a quarterly or half-yearly review might be sufficient. However, for a larger company that needs to split the inspection into many sections, a program of monthly inspections, covering the whole factory in 3—6 months might be more appropriate.

All inspections need reports as an outcome; otherwise, there is no formal record of the findings and recommendations. This report should be issued as quickly as possible while things are fresh in people's minds. It does not need to be an elaborate, wordy document that no one will read. A simple list of findings with recommendations for corrective action is sufficient. However, it is important that responsibility for action and a time frame are agreed upon either during the inspection or soon after the report is issued.

An inspection on its own is unlikely to be particularly effective and it is important that the company management ensures follow-up actions are carried out to the agreed timetable.

Larger companies may have teams of auditors within the QA department, whose responsibilities would be to inspect the various parts of the factory. These auditors will take part in self-inspection programs but may also conduct their own inspections. These latter inspections are on occasion used as "dry-runs" in companies preparing for regulatory or other external inspections.

Whatever the objective of an internal inspection, it must be recognized as beneficial by all parties. See Section 6.6.1 Case study 1 for an example of a self-inspection program that went astray.

6.2.2 External inspections

As discussed previously, there are several different reasons why a company is inspected by an external body. However, the main reason, and the one common to all companies, is the inspection by the regulatory authority carried out as part of the process of licensing the factory and approving the products for sale.

Inspections by regulatory authorities take several different forms, depending on the purpose of the inspection, the length of time since the previous inspection, and the inspection history of the company.

6.2.2.1 Regulatory inspections—routine

A routine inspection is a full review of all aspects of GMP within a facility. Routine inspections may be announced or unannounced, depending on the history of the company, previous inspections, and the policy of the country.

It is appropriate under the following circumstances:

- when a new facility is opened;
- when a manufacturing authorization is due for renewal;
- if there have been significant changes such as new product lines, modification to processes, or changes in key personnel or premises;
- if the company has a history of noncompliance to GMP; or
- if an inspection has not been carried out within the past 3–5 years.

6.2.2.2 Regulatory inspections—concise

A concise inspection is the examination of limited aspects relating to GMP compliance within a facility. In some countries, they are known as abbreviated inspections. It also involves inspection of any significant changes that have taken place since the last inspection. Depending on the national practice, a company would normally be warned about a concise inspection.

A concise inspection is applicable under the following circumstances:

- where a company has a good history of GMP compliance through routine inspections in the past; or

- where a sample of aspects can be taken as a good indication of the overall level of GMP compliance.

However, if the concise inspection uncovers evidence suggesting the level of GMP compliance has fallen, it may be appropriate to carry out a full GMP inspection at some point in the near future.

6.2.2.3 Regulatory inspections—follow-up

A follow-up inspection is performed specifically to monitor the response to corrective actions arising from a previous inspection. The company would not necessarily know in advance about the follow-up inspection.

A follow-up inspection is not limited ONLY to subjects of corrective actions, but to monitor the result of corrective actions. They are limited to specific GMP requirements that have not been observed or that have been inadequately implemented.

Depending on the nature of the work required, they could be carried out between 6 weeks and 6 months after the original inspection has taken place.

6.2.2.4 Regulatory inspections—special

There are several circumstances in which special inspections may be necessary. The company may or may not be aware in advance of the inspection, depending on the reason for it.

- If there have been complaints about a specific product suggesting there may be defects, then a spot check can take place.
- If there has been a product recall, this can trigger an inspection.
- If there has been an adverse drug reaction, this can trigger an inspection.

In each of these three cases, the inspection would focus on the suspect product or aspect of production. It is unlikely the company would be warned in these cases.

- If the company has made an application for marketing authorization or an export license/authorization, this may also trigger an inspection.
- Finally, if a company has asked for advice on specific regulatory requirements, it may be necessary for the inspectors to visit before they can provide that advice.

6.2.2.5 Regulatory inspections—quality systems review

The purpose of a quality systems review is to inspect the quality management system. The quality manual is a document describing the quality system including the entire operational process, quality management and quality assurance approach of the company.

This type of review is similar to that carried out when a company is applying for accreditation to ISO 9000. It is an approach that has been used by the United States (US) Food and Drug Administration (FDA) in their medical devices inspections and in some of their medicinal products inspections. See Chapters 3 and 4, for a full discussion of quality management systems.

6.2.2.6 Regulatory inspections – timetable

Although there may be ideal timetables that should be achieved for inspections, in practice a number of factors influence the frequency:
- the type of inspection being undertaken;
- the number of inspectors available and their workload;
- the number of companies to be inspected;
- and the size of the company. For example, a large company with several major departments may be inspected in several stages covering the period of the manufacturing license.

An ideal timetable would be an annual visit. This gives the inspectors sufficient information to ensure the company is achieving GMP compliance. From the company's point of view, it is not too onerous in terms of preparation time.

In terms of the duration, this will again depend on a number of factors:
- the size of the company,
- the purpose of the visit, and
- the size of the inspectorate team.

6.2.2.7 Regulatory inspections – dealing with problems

The powers an inspectorate has to deal with unsatisfactory situations are controlled by national legislation. These powers often include:
- suspension or revoking of the marketing authorization;
- delay in the approval of licenses or marketing authorizations;
- delay in issue of a GMP certificate;
- closure of a facility (only used in an extreme case where the failure of a system or process has been identified which presents a significant risk to the patient); or
- the initiation of a product recall.

6.2.2.8 Differences between regulatory inspections in the European Union and the United States

Although the principles on inspection are the same for all regulatory bodies, there are some key differences between those carried out by European inspectors and those carried out by the US FDA. Both focus on the quality, safety, and efficacy of the product. However, while the European Union (EU) inspectors check for compliance to GMP guidelines, the FDA inspectors require compliance to the Code of Federal Regulations (CFRs). The EU approach focuses on future activities and the facility, while the FDA approach focuses on past activities, primarily in documentation. EU inspectors are experienced practitioners from industry, while FDA inspectors are trained for the role and may not have industry experience. Reports from EU inspections are confidential, while those in the United States are covered by the Freedom of Information Act and can be obtained on request.

6.2.3 Suppliers

The EU code of GMP requires materials to only be purchased from approved suppliers and all aspects of manufacture and distribution of materials to be reviewed with the supplier and with the manufacturer if they are not one and the same company. By implication, this means wherever possible, an audit of the suppliers' premises should be carried out as part of the approval process.

A supplier audit will involve more than one function within the company. The process will generally be led by the quality assurance department but will also concern the purchasing department, as well as production and possibly engineering departments, depending on the material being purchased. Not all these departments need to be represented during the audit, but all should be involved in the preparatory work and the decision on whether or not to approve the supplier.

Most companies have a long-established list of suppliers, many of whom may not have been audited in the past. If this were the case, then the first step in preparing for an audit would be to review the history of the relationship between the company and the supplier. What is their performance on deliveries, in terms of accuracy and timeliness? How does the material perform during processing; does it cause problems within production? What other information is already on file about the supplier?

For a potential new supplier, there is less information available, although analysis of a sample of material to ensure it complies with the purchase specification should be a first step.

In either case, it is useful to send the supplier a preaudit questionnaire, to be completed in advance of the visit. In the author's experience, it is better to keep this questionnaire to just a few pages and to provide it to the supplier at least 1 month before the date of the audit, to guarantee receipt of the completed form in good time.

When carrying out the audit, the team should focus on any major issues highlighted by the questionnaire, but also review the systems and premises against the requirements of GMP. This would also be an opportunity to review any problems experienced with previous deliveries, in the case of an existing supplier, and to confirm details of the purchase specification. It is worth remembering the suppliers are the experts with their materials and they might have constructive input into the development of the specifications.

Once a supplier has been approved, it will be necessary to monitor their performance over time and occasionally revisit the premises. However, it is unlikely to be necessary to carry out an annual visit, as would be expected for regulatory inspections of manufacturers' facilities.

6.2.4 Approaches to inspections

Irrespective of the purpose of the inspection, there are a number of approaches the inspectors might take. The end result will tend to be the same; it is the processes that differ.

6.2.4.1 Process inspections

This approach reviews the processes running through the factory, independent of specific products. It includes a review of documentation, how it is issued and controlled; measurement, methods, and calibration; manufacturing processes, planning, procedures, validation, deviations, and traceability; distribution systems; reject control; and corrective actions.

6.2.4.2 Product inspections

This is an inspection in which one or more products are examined in detail. It includes a review of design; development; change control; documentation; compliance; process control; quality control; complaints; packaging; stability; and validation.

6.2.4.3 Systems inspections

This is an inspection in which the quality systems of the company are reviewed to see whether they are appropriate and whether they are in compliance.

6.2.4.4 General themes

Whichever approach is used, there are several questions that can be addressed:

- What should be happening, that is, what is required?
- What is the described procedure, that is, what has been planned?
- What is taking place in practice, that is, what is happening?
- How does the plan compare with the requirement, that is, does the standard need to be amended?
- How does the actual compare with the plan, that is, does the performance need to be amended?

6.3 Mutual recognition of inspections

While all good pharmaceutical manufacturers recognize the importance of inspections as part of the continuing quality assurance program for the company, it is true to say the preparation for and participation in a full inspection is a time-consuming and resource-intensive activity. For companies operating as contract manufacturers for multiple principals (contract giving companies), it can become almost a full-time occupation for certain members of the team.

For companies exporting to many different countries, it would be disadvantageous to have to satisfy different sets of inspectors from each of the different countries. Fortunately, there are several mutual recognition agreements in place to make the situation more manageable. These agreements reduce the need for foreign inspectors from importing companies having to re-inspect facilities that have already been approved by their regulatory authorities. Additionally, it should reduce the requirement for full retesting of finished products once they have been imported into a country.

In addition to the benefits coming from mutual recognition in terms of inspections and analysis, harmonization of standards, in general, is also beneficial.

6.3.1 Pharmaceutical Inspection Convention and the Pharmaceutical Inspection Co-operation Scheme

PIC/S stands for the Pharmaceutical Inspection Convention and the Pharmaceutical Inspection Co-operation Scheme, a pair of international agreements that operate together.

6.3.1.1 Pharmaceutical Inspection Convention

PIC was set up in 1970 under the auspices of the European Free Trade Association (EFTA). Its full title was "The Convention for the Mutual Recognition of Inspections in Respect of the Manufacture of Pharmaceutical Products."

The purpose of PIC was:
- to establish mutual recognition of inspections between member countries;
- to bring about harmonization in GMP standards;
- to ensure equivalent inspection methodology was used in the member countries;
- to provide a mechanism for the training of inspectors;
- to set up a forum for the exchange of information between inspectors and inspectorates in the member countries; and
- to allow member countries to have mutual confidence in the results of inspections carried out by inspectors in other countries.

In other words, if a company was planning to export a product to another country within PIC, the inspectorate of the importing country would not necessarily have to inspect the exporter if a satisfactory inspection history by the national inspectorate was in existence.

PIC is a legally binding treaty between countries. The original signatories were: Austria, Denmark, Finland, Iceland, Liechtenstein, Norway, Portugal, Sweden, Switzerland, and the United Kingdom, these being the members of EFTA in 1970. Subsequently, Hungary, Ireland, Romania, Germany, Italy, Belgium, France, and Australia joined PIC between 1971 and 1993. At this point, it became clear there was a legal problem requiring a change of strategy.

6.3.1.2 Pharmaceutical Inspection Co-operation Scheme

Under EU law, it is not permissible for individual member states to sign treaties with countries outside the EU. Only the European Commission can sign such treaties. However, the European Commission was not a member of PIC. If the work of PIC was not to be lost, a compromise needed to be found.

The PIC Scheme was set up in 1995. It differs from PIC in that it is an informal agreement between regulatory authorities in member countries and is not legally binding. However, its goals are an extension of those of PIC, as shown on the PIC/S website:

- Developing and promoting harmonized GMP standards and guidance documents
- Training competent authorities, in particular Inspectors
- Assessing (and reassessing) Inspectorates
- Facilitating the cooperation and networking for competent authorities and international organizations (PIC/S\Strategic Development, n.d.).

PIC/S is open to the regulatory authorities from any country which has a comparable GMP inspection system. As of May 2021, 54 regulatory authorities are participating in PIC/S. An up-to-date list can be obtained at any time from the PIC/S website (PIC/S\Members, n.d.).

6.3.1.3 Principal activities of PIC/S

An annual training seminar is organized for inspectors from the member countries. Countries that are considering joining PIC/S and other interested parties may attend these seminars as observers. Each seminar takes a specific aspect of GMP as its theme. The outcome of the seminar will usually be the setting up of a working party to draft documentation on the theme, which will be published by PIC/S at a later date.

Training of inspectors within PIC/S is enhanced by the organization of joint visits where inspectors from three different countries observe inspections in each of the three countries. Apart from a useful training exercise, this is also a good way of highlighting any differences in inspection practices between members countries.

Many "Expert Circles" have been set up as special interest groups to facilitate the exchange of experiences and knowledge on particular topics. These circles meet at least annually and develop new documentation on the topic in question.

The publication of documentation is a major activity within PIC/S. These documents take a number of forms: guidelines, guidance documents, recommendations, explanatory notes, and *aide-memoir*. In addition, the proceedings of seminars are published.

To become a member of PIC/S, countries must demonstrate they have an effective licensing and inspection system at least comparable with the standard achieved by other PIC/S members. A detailed assessment is made by current members before an application is approved, including a review of the systems in place and observations of inspections being carried out in practice.

6.3.2 Mutual recognition between PIC/S and the European Union

In virtually all the member states of the EU, the regulatory authorities are either already participants in PIC/S or have applied for accession. However, there is also a history of cooperation between PIC/S and the EU itself. Both the European

Medicines Agency (EMA) and the European Directorate for the Quality of Medicines (EDQM) are associated partners of PIC/S. The EU and PIC/S GMP guides are equivalent. And formal, albeit nonbinding, agreements are in place to facilitate the exchange of information and sharing of inspection reports, particularly with nonPIC/S countries.

6.3.3 PIC/S and other international organizations

PIC/S has also established nonbinding partnerships with many international organizations to pursue its aims:

- *United Nations International Children's Emergency Fund (UNICEF)*: Cooperation in the areas of training of inspectors and sharing inspection planning.
- *World Health Organization (WHO)*: Cooperation in the areas of training of inspectors and sharing inspection planning. The first PIC/S GMP guide was based on the WHO GMP guide.
- *World Organization for Animal Health*: Cooperation in the areas of GMP and quality of veterinary medicines including vaccines.

6.3.4 International Council for Harmonization

The original title of International Council for Harmonization (ICH) was The International Conference on Harmonization of Technical Requirements for Registration of Pharmaceuticals for Human Use. In October 2015 it underwent a reorganization and a change of title. The new ICH or International Council for Harmonization was established as an international association and a legal entity under Swiss law.

While ICH is not primarily involved in the organization, monitoring, or operation of inspections, it is a major player in the move towards harmonization of standards and hence it is appropriate to briefly review its purpose and activities here.

ICH was set up in 1990 as a joint forum between regulatory authorities and the pharmaceutical industry, with a focus on testing procedures to monitor the safety, quality, and efficacy of medicines. The mission of ICH is:

> *to achieve greater harmonization worldwide to ensure that safe, effective, and high quality medicines are developed and registered in the most resource-efficient manner. Harmonization is achieved through the development of ICH Guidelines via a process of scientific consensus with regulatory and industry experts working side-by-side. Key to the success of this process is the commitment of the ICH regulators to implement the final Guidelines.*
>
> **(ICH\Home\About ICH\Mission, n.d.)**

6.3.4.1 Members of ICH

As of May 2021, there are 17 members and 32 observers of ICH. An up-to-date list can be found on the ICH website (ICH Home\Organisation\Members & Observers, n.d.).

The founder members of ICH were the regulatory authorities and the national industry bodies for each of three regions:

- The European Commission represents the regulatory authorities of the member states of the EU.
- The European Federation of Pharmaceutical Industries' Associations (EFPIA) represents national associations, leading pharmaceutical companies plus small and medium-sized enterprises across Europe.
- The Ministry of Health and Welfare, Japan (MHW) has the brief for public health, amongst other things, in Japan.
- Japan Pharmaceutical Manufacturers Association (JPMA) represents the manufacturing companies within the Japanese industry.
- The FDA is the regulatory authority for the United States.
- Pharmaceutical Research and Manufacturers of America (PhRMA) was formerly known as the Pharmaceutical Manufacturers Association (PMA). It represents the research-based section of the pharmaceutical industry in the United States.

In addition, there are members in the categories of Standing Regulatory Members, regulatory members, and industry members.

To ensure ICH maintains a link with countries outside its membership and other key organizations, there are a large number of observers to the process, including two Standing Observers:

- The WHO that deals primarily with countries in the developing nations or where the industry is just emerging.
- International Federation of Pharmaceutical Manufacturers Associations (IFPMA), which represents the global research industry.

Additional observers are drawn from legislative or administrative authorities, regional harmonization initiatives, international pharmaceutical industry organizations, and international organizations regulated or affected by ICH guidelines.

6.3.4.2 Activities of ICH

At the initial meeting of ICH in 1990, eleven topics were identified for harmonization work, divided into three main themes of quality, safety, and efficacy. Each topic became the subject of an Expert Working Group. Thirty years on, there are now four themes, with the addition of multidisciplinary guidelines and nearly 60 topics in total.

The formal process of harmonization involves five steps:

- *Step 1 Consensus building*: A draft guideline is prepared, and consensus sought between the members of the Expert Working Group.
- *Step 2 Confirmation of consensus and endorsement by regulatory members*: Once consensus has been confirmed at the biannual Assembly, the regulatory members will develop and endorse the draft guideline.

- *Step 3 Regulatory consultation*: Extensive consultation takes place between regulatory authorities both within and external to ICH.
- *Step 4 Adoption of an ICH harmonized guideline*: Once consensus is confirmed by the Assembly, the regulatory members adopt the document as a harmonized guideline.
- *Step 5 Implementation*: The document is implemented via the normal national/regional routes within each ICH region.

6.3.5 WHO certification scheme

There are many companies in countries not members of PIC/S who may wish to either export or import finished products. In the former case, they need to be able to convince the regulatory authorities in the importing country their products are safe, efficacious, and manufactured in compliance with all GMP requirements. In the latter case, they need assurance the product being brought into the country is satisfactory in the same way. However, the time and money required to arrange inspections are not always available.

The WHO certification scheme was set up to facilitate these situations. The full title of the scheme is "the WHO certification scheme on the quality of pharmaceutical products moving in international commerce." The scheme was originally proposed in 1969, at the same time as the requirements for "GMP as recommended by the WHO" were endorsed. These requirements are considered to be equivalent to those in operation in PIC/S countries.

The scheme is essentially an administrative tool available to any member state of the United Nations who wishes to register for it. All members can use the scheme to monitor the quality of imports. However, if a member state wishes to use the scheme to facilitate exports, they must be able to demonstrate compliance with several requirements:

- There must be a licensing framework in place that covers not only the authorization of products but also the manufacturers and distributors working within the industry.
- There must be a national GMP code in place, at least equivalent to the WHO requirements and it must be enforced across the country. (Adoption of appropriate international guidelines such as the EU guide would be an acceptable alternative.)
- There must be a system of quality control for finished products produced within the country, including an independent quality control laboratory.
- There must be a competent national inspectorate, which is part of the regulatory authority, and which has the knowledge, experience, resources, and authority to reinforce the GMP requirements across the industry.
- There must be resources available to administer the scheme within the country. This will involve issuing certificates and monitoring the scheme to ensure it is operating correctly and any quality problems are highlighted immediately.

The WHO scheme relates to specific products rather than to the whole operations of any one manufacturer. When an interested party from the importing country initiates an enquiry regarding a particular product, the regulatory authority of the exporting country issues a certificate to the following effect:

- The product has a marketing authorization within the country of export, or if not, the reasons why not.
- The manufacturing facility in which the product is produced is inspected regularly by the national regulatory inspectors and has been demonstrated to achieve GMP compliance.
- The product documentation, including labeling, is authorized in the exporting country.

6.4 Guidance on participating in inspections

Participating in an inspection, either as an inspector or inspectee, requires a certain level of knowledge and experience in a variety of different areas. Firstly, it is important to have a detailed understanding of the standards against which the facility is being inspected. Secondly, it is critical that the representative of the inspected entity knows the facility well and can answer the majority of the questions accurately. For the inspector, it is helpful and will increase the effectiveness of the inspection, if sufficient preparation has been carried out to ensure at least a basic knowledge of the facility.

Thirdly, inspections are communication exercises. The interaction between the various parties will affect how the inspection proceeds and will determine whether it is effective or not. Hence, there is an aspect of personal interaction which is very important but is often forgotten in the process of training inspectors.

Finally, there is the actual process of carrying out an inspection:
- how to prepare effectively,
- how to carry out the inspection effectively, and
- how to ensure effective follow-up.

Each of these aspects is addressed separately within this section. The section is written both from the viewpoint of the inspector and the inspectee, but inevitably, the emphasis will be on the former role. However, bearing in mind all companies need to carry out their internal inspections and supplier audits as a minimum, there are many instances where company personnel will carry out both the role of inspector and that of inspectee on different occasions and hence there should be something for everyone in the rest of this chapter.

6.4.1 Inspection guidelines

There are several sources of guidance for inspectors, regarding the first area of knowledge—the technical aspects. There are the source documents, the various

GMP guidelines, and regulatory publications. However, there are also some documents written specifically about the inspection process that might be useful, particularly for relatively new inspectors.

6.4.1.1 Pharmaceutical Inspection Convention and the Pharmaceutical Inspection Co-operation Scheme

As discussed previously in Section 6.3.1, PIC/S issues documents on a variety of topics. While these documents are primarily intended for the guidance of inspectorates, they are also useful documents for companies regarding questions of implementation. All these documents are listed on the PIC/S website, and many can be downloaded for free (PIC/S\Publications, n.d.).

6.4.1.2 Food and Drug Administration

The FDA has over the years published a series of guides to inspections. While primarily intended to support the activities of the FDA inspectors, they are freely available and can be downloaded from the FDA website (FDA\Home\Inspections, Compliance, Enforcement, and Criminal Investigations\Inspection References\Inspection Guides, n.d.). They are particularly useful in preparing for an FDA inspection, but can also be helpful for companies who are developing activities in a particular area, although it has to be said that many of the documents date from the 1980s and 1990s. The guides to inspections under the category of drugs include:

- High purity water systems
- Lyophilization of parenterals
- Microbiological pharmaceutical quality control laboratories
- Validation of cleaning processes
- Dosage form drug manufacturers—CGMPs
- Oral solid dosage forms pre/post approval issues
- Sterile drug substance manufacturers
- Topical drug products
- Oral solutions and suspensions

In addition, FDA publishes guides to inspections related to biotechnology, computer issues, devices, and inspection of foreign manufacturers. Also published and freely available are the FDA Investigations Operations Manual, and International Inspection Manual, and Travel Guide. These are a combination of technical and administrative items. All these reference documents can be downloaded from the FDA website. (FDA\Home \Inspections, Compliance, Enforcement, and Criminal Investigations\Inspection Reference, n.d.). However, once again, many of the documents were written years ago and hence their relevance must be reviewed in each individual case.

6.4.1.3 World Health Organization

In 1992, the WHO published a document entitled "Provisional guidelines on the inspection of pharmaceutical manufacturers," intending to harmonize the activities of inspectorates among the member states. The document was expanded and published in 2002 as Annex 7 Guidelines on preapproval inspections (WHO, 2002). While it is aimed primarily at regulatory inspectors, it is also useful for manufacturing companies, both as a preparation for an external inspection and as a reference text for the planning of internal inspection programs. The guidelines cover both the process of carrying out an inspection and the technical content thereof.

The guidelines are applicable mainly to the manufacture of secondary pharmaceuticals and to active pharmaceutical ingredients but may also be applied to the inspection of facilities for the production of other products, which may be covered by national legislation in some companies. Examples of these products would include biologicals, medical devices, diagnostics, or food.

Since the competent inspection of manufacturing facilities is a key element of the WHO certification scheme discussed above, this guideline should certainly be used by any country registered to export under that scheme. However, it may also be useful in planning and carrying out inspections of quality systems against ISO 9001, as discussed in Chapter 4, or for supplier audits.

6.4.2 Developing knowledge of the facility

Knowledge of the individual facility will be different in every inspection and can only be dealt with on a case-by-case basis, although some suggestions are made in this section.

From the point of view of the company being inspected, it would be easy to assume someone very familiar with the facility and its systems would be delegated to accompany the inspector throughout the visit. This person would not necessarily be able to answer all the questions themselves, but they would know whom to contact to get the answers. However, in the author's experience, this is not always the approach taken by companies, particularly those not familiar with the inspection process. See Section 6.6.2, Case study 2, for an example of how not to deal with a regulatory inspector.

From the point of view of inspectors, it is not likely they will know the facility very well, unless they have visited it many times. However, any information obtained during the preparation stage is likely to increase the effectiveness of the inspection process.

For an initial inspection, there are several potential sources of information about the company. If it is a regulatory inspection, then the application dossier will include information about the company, including a site master file. For a nonregulatory inspection, such as in a potential contract manufacturing situation, the company should be asked to complete a preinspection questionnaire and/or provide layout diagrams. Sufficient time should always be allowed for these documents to be provided. Requesting information or documentation at the last minute is almost guaranteed to reduce the effectiveness of the inspection since it will either involve significant extra work for the inspectee to comply with the request, or the information will fail to materialize in time.

Documentation such as manuals and procedures can also give an overview of the company for the inspector. This will depend on company policy—some companies treat all such documents as confidential and do not allow them to leave the site. However, in the case of ISO 9001 certification inspections, provision of the quality manual and procedures is a prerequisite to setting up the inspection in the first place.

The annual report, if the company is required to produce one, is a useful background document. While this rarely has any technical detail, it helps to provide a full overview of the company and its culture.

Where an inspection is not the first one to be carried out in a company, there will be a certain amount of information already available to the inspector, whether a representative of a regulatory body or someone carrying out an inspection on behalf of a private company.

There should be a company file, which will contain information obtained before or during other visits. However, it is important to be aware that this information is dated and may not be completely accurate. If the company produces a site master file, this will also be a useful document.

Specifically for regulatory inspections, information is also available from the site manufacturing license and from the registration dossiers submitted for the products being manufactured. A further source of information is monitoring data, not just of inspections, but also of any recalls, complaints, or product testing.

A visit to a company should always start with a review of progress against recommendations made during the last inspection. Hence, the inspector must be fully familiar with this material.

6.4.3 Inspections: an exercise in communications

Inspections are a snapshot in time. They are relatively short by nature—it is unlikely an inspection will last longer than 5 days, unless the manufacturing facility is very large. Hence, the time needs to be used effectively. From the point of view of the inspector, it is necessary to get as much information as possible, together with the evidence to back up that information. From the point of view of the inspectee, it is important to be able to communicate the point of view of the company, explain any problems, and justify any approaches that appear unusual to the inspector. Hence, this is an exercise in communications and two-way communications at that.

6.4.3.1 The role of the inspector

There are many different approaches an inspector can take, which will affect how the inspection is completed. The most appropriate one will depend on the nature of the inspection, the relationship between the inspector and the inspectee, and the history of previous inspections.

The primary role of an inspector must be as an observer of facts. It is a key responsibility to report factually on the standards being achieved within the factory. This can be termed as a policing role. It will be the main approach taken by a regulatory inspector and will also be appropriate in initial inspections by other external bodies. It would be less appropriate in the case of a self-inspection activity.

However, there are many occasions when an inspector takes the role of adviser or coach and uses the opportunity of the inspection to suggest ways of improving manufacture or control. The company may also see the inspection as an opportunity to seek support and guidance in particular areas where compliance is in question. This is particularly appropriate in situations where there is a business relationship between the inspector and the inspectee. See Section 6.6.3 Case study 3 for an example of this approach.

In the past, regulatory inspectors were reluctant to provide advice to companies on topics such as the design of new buildings, in case any such advice was taken as a tacit approval of one particular approach over another. However, this view has now changed, and inspectors are more willing to review plans while they are still on the drawing board, rather than waiting until the building is complete, and it is too late to make major changes. It must be stressed, however, that this approach must always be made within the context of national policy.

There are a few circumstances in which the inspector and the inspectee can take a partnership approach to the process of inspections. This is particularly appropriate in the case of supplier audits, where cooperation on the improvement of a specific process can produce a win-win situation between the two parties. This would also be the case where an independent consultant is working with a company to help them improve their GMP compliance.

6.4.3.2 The inspector as communicator

In order to communicate effectively, it is important to use the language most appropriate to the level of the organization being addressed. An inspector will meet and may have to communicate with many people within a company from members of the board to the shop floor operators, and good inspectors are able to both give and receive information on all occasions—and to recognize where it is most appropriate to ask particular questions. For example, a board member or senior manager would be able to answer questions about investments and company policies, but to determine the answers to technical questions such as "how is this process carried out in practice," the inspector would be more likely to talk to someone in the production area such as the supervisor or the operator.

It is important for both the inspector and the company representatives to be aware of their body language. If the inspector asks a question, particularly a difficult one, then it is important to be seen to be interested in the answer. Looking around or paying attention to something else would only increase the nervousness or the irritation of the person making the reply.

Both parties should try to keep their arms open, rather than crossed. This indicates receptiveness to the discussion in progress, rather than defensiveness or aggression.

An inspector must be aware of and sensitive to the company culture in relation to visitors. In general, it may be perfectly acceptable to talk directly to people encountered during the factory visit but in some companies, it is preferable that questions be addressed through the company representative.

In the case of a regulatory inspector, there is always the right to insist on talking to anyone and seeing anything. In the interest of establishing or maintaining a good relationship with the company, doing things the way they would prefer would tend to be the best approach. However, this would only be valid if it does not create a barrier to getting answers. It may be necessary to find ways around the company culture if this happens.

For inspectors working outside their own country, it is important to remember different countries have different cultures and social behaviors which need to be recognized and taken into account. On occasion, this can have a major impact on the effectiveness of communications.

Effective inspectors would always be aware of the potential or perceived impact of their actions, particularly in a situation where there are major noncompliance issues. It is the inspector's role independently to observe and report the facts. People in the company may have concerns about the outcome of the inspection that may be unjustified, but which could be caused by the inspector's behavior. This would affect communications and would reduce the likelihood of the company representatives being open in their answers.

One of the biggest barriers to effective communications is a misunderstanding over the purpose of those communications. A full understanding and agreement on the objectives, both in the planning stage and during the inspection, is critical.

6.4.3.3 Relieving the stress of an inspection

An inspection is a stressful situation for both parties. This will tend to affect the way people behave. A recognition of some typical behaviors and how to avoid the negative effects is a useful addition to the tool-bag of both inspectors and inspectee.

All discussions should be held on a factual basis. Inspectors should collect the evidence in all situations, and company representatives should be happy to provide it.

There should be no discussions that become personal and descend to blaming individuals. A calm, measured comment made after the event would be more effective than perceived critical comments made in the heat of the moment.

It is always important to remain polite, even if the other party becomes rude, and from the author's experience, this will happen on occasion, particularly if the company representative feels they are being accused of something.

The more professional an approach both parties make to an inspection, the more relaxed they will be and hence the more effective the whole process will be. This can only help to make the inspection go more successfully. The key to a professional approach is preparation. The inspector will have a full agenda prepared and be aware of the key issues to be reviewed. Equally, the company that puts lots of preparation into an inspection will be a company appearing more professional to the inspector.

An inspector must maintain a consistent approach to a company, both within a single inspection and from one inspection to another. Companies need to know where they stand on the various issues likely to arise.

Inspectors should ensure questions or requests are made clearly and check for understanding. The inspectee should ensure their responses and explanations are fully understood. Just because a speaker understands what they are saying, they should never assume everyone else will. Getting impatient with someone who misunderstands a question, or response will not help the situation. It will only make people more nervous.

This point is particularly critical for inspectors who are working overseas via an interpreter or with people whose first language is not the same as their own. It may be necessary to ask a question more than once, in different ways, to ensure it has been understood. From the author's experience, it is also necessary to check back on answers received, to ensure what has been said and translated is what was actually meant.

Integrity is a critical part of all communications, and particularly in a situation like a regulatory inspection. Decisions inspectors make can have a significant effect on the business performance of the companies being inspected, not to mention the health of the patient. Hence, it is important the inspector's reputation is above question.

Both parties should remain tactful and diplomatic at all times. An antagonistic attitude should not be allowed to cause provocation. In all cases, the objective is to collect evidence, not to have an argument about it.

As has been mentioned several times before, an inspection, while an essential part of running a pharmaceutical company, is also a resource-intensive activity, both before and during the inspection itself. It is important both parties, but particularly the inspector, contribute to the effectiveness of the process by being well prepared, clear and direct in questions and discussions.

6.4.3.4 Maintaining independence as an inspector

This section deals with the process of successful communications and their importance in carrying out an effective inspection. However, it is important to conclude by emphasizing the independence of the inspector. Above all, the inspectors have a responsibility to ensure the evidence assembled is true and accurate. It is necessary to be rigorous in investigations and not take the easy way out of only looking at the parts the company wants looked at. After all, it is unlikely a company will volunteer information about their problem areas, even in a situation where an excellent relationship exists between the inspector and the inspectee.

6.4.4 Preparing for and conducting an inspection

Apart from the technical aspects of an inspection, and the importance of developing effective relationships with the people involved, it is also important an inspector is equipped with the skills to handle the mechanics of an inspection; from the preparation, through the inspection itself to the report and follow-up actions. There are no regulations or guidelines for this, although the WHO guide mentioned above has some suggestions. The following suggestions are taken from the author's experiences of more than 20 years and hundreds of company inspections.

6.4.4.1 Preparing for an inspection

The first step in preparation is to define the purpose and scope of the inspection. There are several different types of inspections, as discussed earlier. However, it is also necessary to decide whether the inspection will cover the entire facility or just part of it. For example, if a company produces a range of dosage types such as liquids, tablets and sterile products, it may be preferable to take one area at a time, rather than covering everything in one go.

Once the purpose of the inspection and the depth have been decided upon, it is then necessary to decide how much time will be required to complete it. It is also appropriate at this point to decide when the inspection will take place. Whether this is done in conjunction with the company in question will depend on whether it is to be an announced or unannounced inspection. For regulatory inspections, this will depend on the objective of the inspection and the accepted practice within the inspectorate. For all other types of inspections, it is unlikely they would be unannounced.

Some inspections are carried out by one person, while others are completed by a team of inspectors. In the author's experience, a team approach is preferable if possible since it allows the workload to be split. For example, it is easier to ask questions and listen carefully to the answers if a second person is taking notes. A team approach also increases the range of knowledge and expertise of the inspectors and provides a "sounding board" for development of recommendations.

Once the timing of the inspection is finalized, there will be a number of people who need to be notified. These will include the company (in the case of an announced inspection), the members of the inspection team, and other interested parties such as administrators who organize travel.

In the case of a regulatory inspection, there may be other sections of the authority that have dealings with the company and may need to be informed. If such an inspection is to be undertaken in other countries, the regulatory authorities of those countries would be informed as a matter of courtesy.

6.4.4.2 Conducting the inspection

During the preparation stage, a draft program will have been prepared for the inspection. While every inspection will be different in the detail, there are some standard items that can be included in all of them:

- All inspections should start with an opening meeting to ensure everyone has been briefed on the purpose of the inspections and the objectives are understood.
- A request should have been made for any help needed by the inspectors, including the provision of technical officers to accompany them during their visit.
- It is useful to have an orientation tour of the plant, particularly if it is the first visit the inspectors have made. However, they should remember this is an initial walk-through only and not be pulled into detailed discussions at this point.

Once the introductions have been completed, it is time to begin the main activity of the inspection, the fact-finding to assess compliance to GMP. Periodically, it is necessary to review the program to see whether it needs to be revised in light of the information obtained thus far. That is why the original agenda is never more than a draft. In the author's experience, most inspections throw up surprises necessitating a change of emphasis. The inspection then continues using the revised plan. It is important to make the management of the company aware of any changes, so they can amend their plans accordingly.

There are three main approaches that can be used to carry out an inspection:

- To trace forward is to start at the receipt of goods and follow the system through the factory logically to the dispatch warehouse at the end. This will tend to be a hypothetical exercise concentrating on the physical systems.
- To trace backward is to take a pack of finished products off the shelf in the warehouse and review its entire history back through the system. This will be a fact-based exercise concentrating on documentation.
- The random approach is to start from points around the factory that appear to be significant and see where they lead. This approach is probably not a recommended one for an inexperienced inspector.

The choice of method will depend on the purpose of the inspection, the previous inspection history of the company, and the personal choice of the inspector.

In eliciting facts from people, it is important to ask questions in a way that will lead to an appropriate response. For this reason, closed questions, which lead to a "yes" or "no" answer are much less useful than open questions that require explanations. For example "is there a procedure for this operation?" will tend to bring out far less information than "can you talk me through the procedure for this operation?"

One of the key skills needed for a successful inspection is that of note-taking. There is no point in asking all the right questions if at the end of the inspection there is not an accurate record of the answers. As mentioned previously, this is one of the advantages of the team approach to inspections. While one person is talking, the other one can take notes. However, when the inspection is carried out by an individual, it is necessary both to ask the questions and record the responses.

There are a few key points to be remembered when taking notes:

- It is important to record all the relevant facts at the appropriate level of detail. Facts should always be verified, not taken on trust or based on assumptions.
- Records should be of specific information, not general impressions.
- Details should be recorded as they are seen, not as the company says they should be.
- Accuracy is paramount. There is nothing that undermines the credibility and authority of an inspector more than being proved wrong, particularly in front of senior management.
- The notes can be made in an open manner. The results of the inspection will be the subject of a report, so no secrets need to be hidden.

There are several specific ways in which records can be made. The chosen one will be a combination of what is most appropriate at the time and personal choice. Each method has advantages and disadvantages:

- Many inspectors take detailed but rough notes that can be reviewed and tidied up later. This allows them to concentrate on the discussion. However, it involves extra work outside the daily inspection program, since the notes need to be refined as soon as possible, while the memories are fresh.
- Checklists are a detailed but structured way of taking notes. They are a good way of ensuring all topics are covered, and hence may be useful in particular for inexperienced inspectors. However, they tend to be composed of closed questions and can stifle further discussion if not used flexibly.
- Flowcharts can be a good way for the inspectors to check their understanding of an operation and how it fits into the overall system.
- A tape recorder has been used by inspectors in the past. However, this may be problematic for the person being interviewed as it makes the inspector seem more remote.
- A video camera is useful for recording information about the plant and premises but will be of little use in getting information, as it will prevent people from relaxing and answering questions sensibly.

- A still camera may also be useful for recording information about the plant or premises. It should be noted that for both the camera and the video, permission might need to be obtained from the company before they can be used, unless, in the case of a regulatory inspection, national legislation provides the inspector with the authority to use such equipment.

Where the inspection has been completed by a team, there needs to be some time at the end of the visit for the inspectors to review their findings in advance of the closing meeting. This is particularly so when members of the team have been visiting different parts of the site at the same time.

The first step is to pool noncompliances so the whole team has the same set of information. The noncompliances are then categorized into critical, major, and minor or some similar system. Depending on the number of noncompliances identified, it may not be possible or advisable to cover all of them in the closing meeting. In this case, they can be ranked in order of priority so the key ones can be discussed.

It is important for the inspectors to anticipate what questions might be raised by the inspectees at the closing meeting and have answers ready. This is particularly true if there are likely to be any contentious issues.

The last activity at the company is the closing meeting with the management team, where the inspectors will give initial feedback of findings. This meeting has two main objectives:

- It is an opportunity for the management team to learn from the inspector. Companies often widen the audience for these meetings to more than the immediate technical team.
- It ensures there will be no surprises in the report. The bad news, or the good news, will be reviewed and clarified on the spot.

In the author's experience, there is sometimes a third objective, in the case of nonregulatory inspections. In a company, particularly a small one, where the technical management has had difficulty convincing the financial managers that significant investment in the factory is required to achieve GMP, the closing meeting is used to add weight to the argument, by adding the opinion of an independent, external authority.

6.4.4.3 Inspection reports

The final output of an inspection is a written report of the findings. For nonregulatory inspections, this will often include recommendations for improvements in levels of compliance. In the case of regulatory inspections, the nonconformance is highlighted, but it is generally left to the company to respond and say how they intend to overcome the problem. In all cases, there should be a timeframe for a required response from the inspectee.

The WHO guideline on inspections mentioned previously provides an example of the type of report that can be written after an inspection. The report is split into four parts:

- General information about the company can be taken directly from the information provided by the company itself, assuming it is annotated as such and has been verified during the inspection.
- The description of the inspection lists all the inspected parts of the factory.
- The next part is devoted to observations, either negative or positive, including any major changes that have taken place since the previous visit. Negative observations should differentiate between poor systems, and failure to comply with a good system.
- The final part consists of the inspectors' conclusions, including corrective actions required and recommendations on how to improve.

For some types of inspections, such as supplier audits, a much simpler style with a list of issues and required actions might be more appropriate. For regulatory inspections, there will tend to be a "house style" used by the whole inspectorate, to ensure consistency and to prevent confusion for companies when their inspector changes.

6.5 GMP certification in the developing world

While compliance to international standards of GMP is relatively well-established in the developed world, there are many companies in Eastern Europe, the Middle East, and Africa which are going through rapid change to catch up. In many cases, these countries are working with independent consultants, either funded privately or, more often, through EU-funded and similar programs. In all cases, one of the first questions asked of the consultant is "how can we get our factory certified to GMP." This is usually because they want to develop their export market or apply for international tenders.

The answer is not a straightforward one. The easiest solution is for the national regulatory authority to carry out inspections. However, in some countries, the infrastructure is only just being developed and there might not be a competent inspectorate in place. This immediately precludes the country from registering for the WHO certification scheme.

To get an inspector from an EU member state or from the FDA to visit the factory, it is necessary for a registration dossier to have been submitted. In many cases, it is far too early for the companies to think about this.

Hence, there is an impasse developing, which can only be solved by encouraging the companies to work towards GMP standards in parallel with the development of the national inspectorate. Since everyone is learning together, this can lead to an interesting culture of cooperation in areas where traditionally the divide between the regulatory authorities and industry has been much wider.

6.6 Case studies

6.6.1 Case study 1

A company in the Middle East employed a GMP consultant to help them improve their level of GMP compliance as an initial step towards exporting their products to Europe. During the initial GMP inspection, it became apparent the company did not have a self-inspection program in place. One of the recommendations was hence for such a program to be set up.

During the second visit to the company, the consultant was assured by the QA department everything was going very well, and many of the recommendations were already being implemented. The self-inspection program had been planned and the first round of inspections was in progress. However, the story from the production department was a little different. They were unhappy the QA personnel had set up "yet another policing mechanism" and saw the whole thing as a bad idea.

On reviewing the situation with both parties, it was discovered the QA manager had taken all the decisions and presented the production manager with a *fait accomplis*. Once the objectives of the program were fully reviewed, and the production department became involved in both the planning and the operation of the program, they realized self-inspection was about improvement rather than blame and became much more enthusiastic about it.

6.6.2 Case study 2

In the late 1970s, the UK pharmaceutical industry was getting used to the idea that increased legislation, GMP guidelines, and a regular program of inspections by regulatory authorities were the facts of life from now on.

A tiny, research-based company had been developing a small-scale manufacturing operation in their facility, which was primarily a laboratory and office building. They were told by the Department of Health and Social Security inspectors, who were the forerunners of the Medicines and Healthcare products Regulatory Agency (MHRA), they must build a purpose-built factory or cease production. They rented an old warehouse, refurbished it and moved the production equipment in. Slowly but surely, they were getting everything in place, but obviously, it would take time to reach full compliance.

A couple of months later, the first inspection of the facility was held. The Managing Director (MD) wanted to ensure everything went smoothly and decided to accompany the inspector himself. He did most of the talking during the visit and insisted on answering all the inspector's questions.

Anxious to put on a good performance but blissfully unaware of the full technical requirements of GMP, the MD proceeded to give all the answers he felt the inspector wanted to hear: of course, they had a suitable ventilation system; obviously, all the procedures were correctly written and in place; certainly, all the personnel was fully trained. The technical manager, who was a fairly recent graduate, listened to this discussion with a sinking heart. He knew sooner or later the inspector would ask for evidence of all these assertions, none of which was accurate—and also knew he would not be able to produce the evidence. This would reinforce the view of the inspector of a badly run and technically incompetent company, rather than a small technical team trying to deal as best it could with a rapidly changing environment.

While this case study is many years old, the same story is being repeated today in countries that are behind the developed world and are desperately running to try and catch up.

6.6.3 Case study 3

A major multinational pharmaceutical company with subsidiaries around the world had a program of inspections carried out in all their factories. The inspectors were drawn from corporate headquarters and had expertise in production, QA, development, and engineering. On average, the inspections took place on an annual basis.

When the inspections were first started in the mid-1980s, the role taken by the inspectors was primarily a policing one. It was an opportunity to check up on what the subsidiaries were doing and to make sure the quality of the product was consistent all around the world. The response from the subsidiaries was mixed, but in many cases, there was a feeling "those guys from head office turn up, criticize all the hard work we have done under difficult circumstances, and then go home, leaving us with a long list of things we have to do—and pay for!"

In the early 1990s, the pharmaceutical world was starting to change, and a much more commercially aware approach was required. The inspectors found they had to justify their expensive trips in financial terms. It was no longer good enough to say quality demanded these inspections. After all, each of the subsidiaries had its own QA systems, QC controls, and national regulatory bodies to satisfy.

The emphasis of the inspections changed, and the inspectors began to take the role of coaches, helping the subsidiaries to improve not only their quality standards but also the business performance of the factory. Benchmarking exercises were used to disseminate best practice from individual factories to the rest of the group. The entire process became much more positive, and the annual visits became a welcome part of the calendar for all the subsidiaries.

6.7 Chapter summary

- All pharmaceutical companies take part in different types of audits and inspections, either as the inspected company or as the inspector.
- An inspection tends to be a one-way process where inspectors check for compliance with GMP.

- An audit is a two-way process where auditors identify areas where compliance to GMP needs to be improved and then work with the auditee to determine ways to achieve that compliance.
- In this chapter, the term inspection is used throughout, but in all situations apart from the regulatory one, an element of auditing may be assumed to also take place.
- There are several levels of internal inspection from day-to-day informal review of processes, through the formal self-inspection program, to inspections by local or corporate QA teams, depending on the size of the organization.
- The most critical external inspection is that by the regulatory authority. There are a number of different types of such inspection, and the choice of which takes place depends on a range of circumstances.
- While all regulatory inspections are based on the same principle of compliance to GMP, there are some significant differences between inspections completed by EU inspectors and those from the FDA.
- Suppliers of raw materials and packaging materials should be approved by the manufacturing company and, wherever possible, this approval should be preceded by a supplier audit and site visit.
- There are several different approaches that can be taken for an inspection, focusing on processes, products, systems, or general themes. But in all cases, the inspection should consider whether requirements are appropriate and whether they are being achieved. In other words, how does practice compare with planning?
- Mutual recognition of inspections is a widely-developed process to reduce the resources, both time and money, spent by inspectors and inspectees in the duplication of efforts across the world.
- The PIC/S is a major player in the mutual recognition of inspections and more than 50 regulatory authorities are participating in the scheme.
- The ICH, while not primarily involved with inspections, is a major player in the harmonization of international standards which have a significant effect on GMP requirements and hence on inspections.
- The WHO operates a certification scheme on the quality of pharmaceutical products moving in international commerce, which is aimed at supporting companies in countries that are not yet members of PIC/S.
- To participate in an inspection, either as an inspector or as an inspectee, it is necessary to have a good knowledge and understanding both of the facility being inspected and the standards to which it is being inspected.
- In addition to the national and international guidelines relating to GMP requirements, there is a body of documentation available on how to participate in inspections. While primarily aimed at inspectors, the documents are freely available to companies as well, and can be very useful for preparation purposes.

- The process of participating in an inspection, either as an inspector or as an inspectee, is also an exercise in communication. Skills and experience in both asking questions and listening to responses are important.
- An inspection is a stressful situation, especially for the inspectee, and anything the inspector can do to alleviate that stress will help to improve the effectiveness of the whole process.
- There are three distinct phases to an inspection: conducting the inspection; participating in the inspection; and preparing the inspection report.
- While every company and every situation is different, there are some elements of the process that will be common to all inspections and lessons learned from one inspection can be applied to future ones.
- While many parts of the world have well-developed inspection routines, GMP certification in the developing world is still evolving.

6.8 Questions/problems

1. You are appointed to the role of QA manager in a small tablet manufacturing facility in Spain. List the different types of inspections and audits you might expect to be involved in.
2. How would your list differ if your factory was located in Chile?
3. What are the different types of inspections undertaken by a regulatory inspector?
4. You are a regulator at the FDA. You receive notification of a raised level of customer complaints relating to a product imported from a recently-licensed factory in Belgium. What would you do?
5. You are the head of the inspection department in the regulatory authority in a small country in Central Europe. You are finding it impossible to inspect all the factories on your list every year. What do you do?
6. You are a new inspector in the MHRA. You were previously employed in the production department of a multinational company. What knowledge, skills, and experience can you already demonstrate? What training needs do you have in your first year in the new role?

References

International Council on Harmonisation (ICH), n.d. About ICH\Mission. <https://www.ich.org/page/mission> (accessed 21.05.21).
International Council on Harmonisation (ICH), n.d. Home\organisation\members & observers. <https://www.ich.org/page/members-observers> (accessed 21.05.21).
Pharmaceutical Inspection Co-operation Scheme (PIC/S), n.d. Members. <https://picscheme.org/en/members> (accessed 21.05.21).
Pharmaceutical Inspection Co-operation Scheme (PIC/S), n.d. Publications. <https://picscheme.org/en/publications> (accessed 22.05.21).

Pharmaceutical Inspection Co-operation Scheme (PIC/S), n.d. Strategic development. <https://picscheme.org/en/activites-strategic-development> (accessed 20.05.21).

United States (US) Food and Drug Administration (FDA), n.d. Home\inspections, compliance, enforcement, and criminal investigations\inspection references\inspection guides. <https://www.fda.gov/inspections-compliance-enforcement-and-criminal-investigations/inspection-references/inspection-guides> (accessed 22.05.21).

World Health Organization (WHO), 2002. WHO technical report series, No. 902, 2002. Annex 7 Guidelines on pre-approval inspections. <https://www.who.int/medicines/areas/quality_safety/quality_assurance/PreapprovalInspectionsTRS902Annex7.pdf?ua = 1> (accessed 22.05.21).

CHAPTER 7

Quality improvement programs

7.1 Introduction

Throughout the pharmaceutical industry (and this book), there is a consistent focus on quality. This chapter provides an in-depth view of quality improvement programs in the pharmaceutical industry. The chapter begins with a general overview of the evolution of quality and then ties in the evolution of quality in pharmaceuticals. Next, a few of the key quality figures who laid the foundation for quality around the world are discussed. This section is followed by a lengthy discussion of quality management techniques and methodologies, including Total Quality Management, Cost of Quality, Lean Six Sigma, and Quality by Design. The chapter ends with a brief discussion of benchmarking. This chapter is essentially a theoretical overview of quality and quality improvement programs and is probably most relevant to someone who wants to understand the historical context of quality in the pharmaceutical industry. Chapter 8 deals more with the practical application of quality tools and techniques.

7.1.1 Evolution of quality

Before jumping into a discussion of quality programs and methodologies, it is prudent to provide a general overview of the evolution of quality including the evolution of quality in the pharmaceutical industry. Documentation has shown the existence of quality efforts dating back thousands of years. Egyptian wall paintings (c.1450 BCE) show evidence of both measurement and inspection. In his book *A History of Managing for Quality*, Dr. J.M. Juran provided examples of quality in ancient China (11 to 8 BCE), Greece, Israel, Rome, Scandinavia, Germany, and France. These examples demonstrated that the concept of quality has been important for thousands of years.

During the Middle Ages (typically the period between the 5th and 15th century) in Europe, quality was the responsibility of the skilled craftsperson. Craft guilds were developed to provide a distinction between the skills levels, that is from apprentice to journeymen to master. This type of skill designation is still actively used in many countries.

The next major period in the evolution of quality was 18th century Industrial Revolution. Honoré Le Blanc, a French gunsmith, was a pioneer of the use of interchangeable parts in the development of a process for manufacturing muskets using a standard pattern. Le Blanc shared his concept with Thomas Jefferson, and Jefferson brought the idea back to America. In 1798 the US government awarded Eli Whitney with a 2-year contract to use Le Blanc's concepts to develop 10,000 muskets for the armed forces. Unskilled workers made the parts according to a fixed design and compared the completed parts to a model. Previously, the muskets were developed individually with the stock, barrel, firing mechanism, and other parts fabricated for a specific musket. The significance of the concept of interchangeable parts led to this first Industrial Revolution and created the need for quality control and quality assurance.

The second Industrial Revolution which began early in the 20th century focused on mass production and manufacturing. In the early 1900s, the work of Frederick W. Taylor led to the separation of jobs into specific work tasks with a focus on increasing efficiency. With this approach to manufacturing, quality assurance became the responsibility of inspectors and inspection became the primary means of quality control. Eventually, manufactures created separate quality departments and made quality the responsibility of the quality department. Other notable quality occurrences during this century included:

- Henry Ford developed the concept of assembly-line production.
- Bell Systems created inspection departments at its Western Electric Company and ushered in the era of Statistical Quality Control (SQC).
- The United States began using statistical sampling procedures to control quality during World War II.
- After the war, Dr. Joseph Joran and Dr. W. Edwards Deming introduced statistical quality control techniques to the Japanese.
- During the 1980s and 1990s, the United States refocused its awareness of quality and began to embrace the concept of Total Quality Management (TQM).
- Other quality initiatives were developed, that is, Statistical Process Control (SPC), Continuous Improvement, quality standards, Lean, and Six Sigma.

In the 21st Century, the focus on quality is evolving into a collaborative focus on quality intertwined with technology. The term Quality 4.0 is used to reference quality and organizational excellence within the context of Industry 4.0. Industry 4.0, often referred to as the fourth Industrial Revolution, focuses heavily on computer and machine interconnectivity, automation, machine learning, and real-time data. The concept will marry physical manufacturing and production with smart digital technology, machine learning, and big data to create a holistic ecosystem for companies. Under the Quality 4.0 umbrella, the approach to quality for processes, people, and technology will differ from earlier centuries. People will need to become quality professionals who will use digital tools to manage quality. More and more processes will become automated, and the focus of the quality professional will transition from process operators to process designers. Technology will be used to optimize signal feedback and process adjustments, and to teach machines how to self-regulate and manage their own productivity and quality.

7.1.2 Quality definitions

Quality is a word with many meanings and definitions. There are almost as many definitions of quality as there are books written about the subject. The definition of quality will vary by industry, profession, and by context in which the word is used. This section provides a few definitions but is by no means an exhaustive list.

The American Society for Quality (ASQ) defines quality as: "A subjective term for which each person or sector has its own definition. In technical usage, quality can have two meanings: (1) the characteristics of a product or service that bear on its ability to satisfy stated or implied needs; (2) a product or service free of deficiencies." Later in this chapter, we will see that the different quality gurus had their own definitions of quality.

ISO 9000 defines quality as "the ability of a set of inherent characteristics of a product, system or process to fulfill requirements of customers and other interested parties."

Juran defines quality as "fitness for purpose," while Crosby talks about "conformance to requirements." Feigenbaum emphasizes that quality is not an absolute as in "the best" but relates to "best for the customer use and selling price." All these definitions are similar in that they relate to continually conforming to clearly understood and agreed customer requirements at the lowest overall cost.

There are, however, some quality terms with fairly consistent definitions. Relevant quality terms for the pharmaceutical industry include:

- Inspection: The activities designed to detect or find a nonconformance that exists in an already completed product and service (Summers, *Quality*, 6th Edition).
- Quality Control (QC): The use of specifications and inspection of completed parts, subassemblies, and products to design, produce, review, sustain, and improve the quality of a product or service (Summers, *Quality*, 6th Edition).
- Statistical Quality Control (SQC): Statistical data is collected, analyzed, and interpreted to solve problems and monitor production and parts inspection (Summers, *Quality*, 6th Edition).
- Statistical Process Control (SPC): The use of statistical methods to prevent defects and control the process (Summers, *Quality*, 6th Edition).
- Quality Assurance (QA): Is planned and systematic activities directed toward providing customers with goods and services of appropriate quality (Summers, *Quality*, 6th Edition).
- Total Quality Management (TQM): A management approach that emphasizes continuous process and system improvement as a means for achieving customer satisfaction and to ensure long-term company success (Summers, *Quality*, 6th Edition).

- Continuous Improvement (CI): A philosophy that focuses on improving processes to enable a company to give customers what they want the first time, every time (Summers, *Quality*, 6th Edition).

7.1.3 Elements of TQM

It is impractical to write about quality management techniques without discussing the concept of TQM. It is within the context of TQM that most of the quality techniques have been used in the past 40 years or so.

TQM is the management of all aspects of the quality of service provided to the customer—not just the product itself. It is recognized by many organizations as one of the most significant factors involved in gaining a competitive advantage in business.

Since most quality initiatives primarily focused on reducing defects and errors in the products and services, companies began to realize that a more comprehensive systems approach was needed to sustain lasting improvement. Therefore companies gravitated toward TQM as a strategic approach to producing the right quality of product consistently through a process of continuous improvement and innovation. Over the years, different types of TQM programs have been established; however, there are a number of elements that are common to all of them. The American Society for Quality lists the following primary elements of TQM:

1. *Customer-focused*: This involves recognizing the exact needs, requirements, and expectations of the customer in all aspects of the product or service and satisfying them effectively and profitably. The customer ultimately determines the acceptable level of quality.
2. *Total employee involvement*: All employees must participate in and be committed to working toward common goals. The employees must also be empowered to make decisions without constantly seeking management approval.
3. *Process-centered*: A fundamental element of TQM is process-focused thinking. A *process* is a series of steps that transforms inputs from suppliers into outputs.
4. *Integrated systems*: Horizontal processes must interconnect vertically structured departments. This integrated system approach will connect business improvement elements to continually improve and exceed the expectations of customers, employees, and other stakeholders.
5. *Strategic and systematic approach*: Strategic planning or strategic management is the strategic and systematic approach to achieving an organization's vision, mission, and goals. This approach includes the formulation of a strategic plan that integrates quality as a core component.
6. *Continual improvement*: Also called continuous improvement, is characterized by an emphasis on determining the best method of operation for a process or system.
7. *Fact-based decision-making*: TQM requires an organization to continually collect and analyze data (on performance measures) to improve decision-making, achieve

consensus, and allow prediction on current and future performance based on past history.

8. *Communications*: As part of day-to-day operations, effective communications play a large part in maintaining morale and in motivating employees at all levels.

The term TQM has become rather discredited in recent years, due to problems experienced in some companies with TQM programs that failed. The TQM philosophy provided a comprehensive approach to building excellence in an organization, but management often had difficulty implementing it. As a result, many companies shy away from using the term.

In some cases, alternative labels are applied such as World Class Manufacturing or Business Process Reengineering. In other cases, there is no high-profile program being run within the company. Many companies, however, continue to use some or all the elements of traditional TQM, but without labeling them as such. Quality improvement has become incorporated into the normal operations of the business—which is exactly where it should be.

7.1.4 Total quality management and the pharmaceutical industry

Pharmaceutical companies may not officially use the term TQM in their efforts to maintain quality, but the elements of TQM are evident in their everyday operations. Because of the primary customers served, the pharmaceutical industry has always placed high importance on quality. The employees must be committed to and involved in quality at every level of the product life cycle. This is evident in the application of Good Manufacturing Practice, the adherence to principles of Quality Assurance and Quality Control, and adherence to regulatory requirements. The entire pharmaceutical life cycle is process-centered with a quality focus throughout the life cycle. The processes and systems are integrated as demonstrated by the quality management system. Strategic planning or strategic management are demonstrated continuously. Fact-based decision-making in combination with continuous improvement are core components of the entire product life cycle. Decisions made during preclinical studies through clinical studies and final product approval are based on data. Additionally, a continuous improvement approach is maintained throughout the life cycle. Good communication must be maintained within the facilities, with the regulatory agencies, and with the customers to ensure the quality and efficacy of the products. Since the primary aspect of quality within the pharmaceutical industry is the quality of the product, there must be a continuous effort to ensure that the drug does what it is supposed to do (and no more) and that the drug is efficacious and safe.

Total Quality differs from the traditional definition of quality in at least two areas: firstly, it considers all aspects of the service to the customer, not just the product; secondly the emphasis is a commercial one, that is, quality as a means of gaining competitive advantage.

Total Quality does not in any way detract from or compromise the traditional quality focus of the pharmaceutical industry. Rather it seeks to build on the excellence of the product by achieving the same standard within all aspects of the service to the customer.

7.2 Key figures in the history of quality

In the Evolution of Quality section, there was some mention of key figures in the history of quality management, but there are many people who have contributed to the thinking and body of literature. This section provides more details of a few of these key figures.

7.2.1 Dr. Walter Shewhart

Dr. Shewhart's most important contributions to the quality body of knowledge were the Shewhart Plan-Do-Check-Act (PDCA) problem-solving process, the identification of two sources of variation in a process, and control charts. While working at Bell Laboratories in the 1920s and 1930s, Dr. Shewhart was the first to encourage the use of statistics to identify, monitor, and eventually remove the sources of variation. The two sources of variation identified by Dr. Shewhart were controlled variation and uncontrolled variation. Controlled variation, also termed common cause or chance cause, was defined as a variation that is present in a process due to the very nature of the process. Common causes are defined as problems that can be attributed to underlying causes that are present in any process. Uncontrolled variation, also known as the special or assignable cause, was defined as a variation that comes from a source external to the process. Special causes are recognized as the problems attributed to one-off causes such as operator error or machine breakdown. Dr. Shewhart also developed the formulas and table of constants used to create the Xbar and R control charts that were the foundation for SQC. He promoted control charts as a tool for distinguishing between assignable and common cause variation.

7.2.2 Dr. W. Edwards Deming

Dr. W. Edwards Deming was an American physicist who worked many years for the United States government in the area of statistical sampling techniques. In the late 1940s and early 1950s Dr. Deming spent a lot of time working with industry in Japan, via the Union of Japanese Scientists and Engineers (JUSE). It was Dr. Deming who is largely credited with the introduction and development of statistical quality control within Japan, at a time when the industry in that part of the world had yet to gain its reputation for world-class quality. Along with his mentor, Dr. Walter Shewhart, he promoted the use of the PDCA cycle and later changed it to the Plan-Do-Study-Act (PDSA) cycle. Dr. Deming encouraged management to get involved in creating an environment that supports continuous improvement and believed that process improvement activities were the catalyst needed to start an economic chain reaction.

7.2.2.1 Fourteen points of management

Dr. Deming's philosophy was primarily encapsulated in a list of 14 points for management. He believed that they were not set in stone (and in fact, he was continuously adjusting them) and they were not a set of rules. They were merely to be used as triggers for changing the way management thinks. His 14 points of management are summarized as follows:

1. Create constancy of purpose to ensure that products and services are continually improved.
2. Adopt the new philosophy that rejects "acceptable quality levels and poor service as a way of life." The responsibility of management to learn and to provide leadership must be appropriate for the economic circumstances of the times.
3. Cease dependence on inspection to achieve quality. Statistical measurement should be used to build quality into the product and thus reduce the need for high levels of inspection at the end of the process.
4. End the practice of awarding business based on price tag alone. Instead, the goal should be to minimize total cost and to develop good relationships with suppliers, where possible.
5. Constantly and forever improve the system for planning, production, and service. There should be an ongoing drive to improve quality, which leads to higher productivity and lower costs.
6. Institute training on the job for all. Skills need to be continually updated to keep in line with changes in the workplace. This training should extend to managers, to ensure that they use the workforce most effectively.
7. Institute leadership aimed at helping people do a better job. The responsibility of management must be to help the workforce carry out their duties more effectively. Leadership must focus on quality rather than quantity.
8. Drive out fear. There should be open, two-way communication across the organization to reduce any feelings of fear that may exist among the workforce.
9. Break down barriers between departments and staff areas. These barriers must be eliminated and cross-functional teamwork encouraged.
10. Eliminate exhortations for the workforce that may create adversarial relationships. Deming believed that poster campaigns, numerical targets (such as zero defects) and exhortations to the workforce to work harder are meaningless since most of the problems are outside the ability of the workforce.

11. Eliminate arbitrary numerical targets. Numerical goals tend to focus on quantity rather than quality and hence can be counterproductive. They should not be allowed to replace leadership with management.

12. Remove barriers that rob workers of pride in workmanship. By reducing the problems that cause people to produce poor quality work, there will be a tendency to increase the pride that they feel in the results they achieve.

13. Encourage education by instituting a vigorous program of education, retraining, and self-improvement for everyone.

14. Clearly define top management's commitment to improving quality and productivity. Any improvement activity will only last as long as the support that it receives from the senior management of the company.

7.2.2.2 Seven deadly diseases

Dr. Deming also identified "Seven Deadly Diseases of Management" which he observed to be prevalent in Western management and believed were the most serious barriers that management potentially faces within an organization. These needed to be overcome if the objective of continuous improvement is to be attained. The deadly diseases are as follows:

1. *Lack of constancy of purpose to plan product and service*: Companies tend to fail to plan for the future and maintain programs on an ongoing basis.

2. *Short-term profits*: The inability of companies to invest in quality for the future, due to things such as the behavior of funding organizations can lead to a short-term approach.

3. *Performance appraisal*: The use of performance appraisals, merit systems, and management by objectives can be detrimental if they create an atmosphere of fear and blame within the organization.

4. *Job-hopping*: The tendency of management to move between jobs after relatively short periods (every 3—4 years) causes instability in the organization and continuous improvement efforts will be broken and disjointed as new leaders come on board.

5. *Use of visible targets only for management*: The use of only obvious (primarily financial) measures do not give the whole picture. That is why it is important to use statistics to measure the things that are generally not known.

6. *Excessive medical costs*: Healthcare as a percentage of overall expenditures has steadily risen for decades. These costs will gradually push businesses into a state of crisis.

7. *Excessive costs of liability*: Deming blamed America's lawyers in part for the problems plaguing American business. The United States has more lawyers per capita than any other country in the world, and these lawyers spend much of their time trying to find someone to sue.

7.2.3 Dr. Joseph M. Juran

Dr. Joseph Juran was an American, born in Central Europe. He was an engineer by profession and first became famous with the publication of the *Quality Control Handbook* in 1951. He understood the link between money and quality, which formed his theory on the economics of quality. It was in this book that he first discussed the concept of Quality Cost. This concept was further expanded by Armand Feigenbaum who introduced the Four Quality Cost Categories (see Section 7.3).

Dr. Juran went to Japan in the early 1950s, following in the footsteps of Deming. He also worked with JUSE, but his lectures were also disseminated to more junior levels of management and triggered the development of internal training courses in some of the larger companies.

Dr. Juran focused on management much more than process. He believed that quality control is a key part of management control. His emphasis was on planning, organizational issues, management's responsibility for quality, and the importance of setting goals and targets for improvement.

7.2.3.1 Dr. Juran's philosophy

Juran's key message was that quality needs to be planned; it cannot just happen by accident. He defined a quality trilogy of quality planning, quality control, and quality improvement. With an emphasis on goal setting and a drive for error reduction, there is some conflict between his work and that of Deming. However, they did both agree that the vast majority of variations within a process are within the responsibility of management, rather than the individual operators. In Juran's case, he estimated the level to be over 80% (as opposed to 94% for Deming).

7.2.3.2 Quality trilogy

- Quality planning is defined as the activities used to create the processes that will enable one to meet the desired goal. It includes activities such as: establishing quality goals, identifying the customer and the customer needs, developing product features, developing a process that can produce the needed product features, and establishing process controls.
- Quality control is defined as the activities used to run, monitor, and adjust the process. It includes activities such as choosing control subjects and units of measure, setting goals, measuring actual performance, and interpreting the difference between the actual and standard performance.
- Quality improvement is defined as the activities used to reduce losses and move the process to a better and improved state of control. It includes activities such as identifying projects, organizing project teams, diagnosing the causes of losses or

poor control, providing remedies, dealing with resistance to change, and providing control mechanisms to hold gains.

Juran defined a "quality planning road map" to describe the steps that need to be taken to improve the quality of the operation.

- *Identify who are the customers*: This introduces the concept of both external and internal customers. Every person within an organization is a customer of the preceding person in the process flow and a supplier to the succeeding person. This holds true, not only within a manufacturing environment but also in other technical areas such as the QC laboratory and the administration areas such as finance or order processing.

- *Determine the needs of those customers*: In many cases, this is not just a case of the "supplier" not knowing what the "customer" wants. Often, the "customer" has not defined exactly what is required. With such a lack of clarity, it is not surprising that needs are not satisfied.

- *Translate those needs into our language*: In many cases, particularly in the case of an external customer, the requirements will be expressed in layman's terms that need to be converted into the more appropriate terminology for the specific process.

- *Develop a product that can respond to those needs*: Having defined the needs, it is important that the "product"—whether it is a physical product or an intangible service—satisfies the requirements of the customer. It must have "fitness for purpose." Optimize the product features to meet the company's needs as well as customers' needs.

To ensure that the product is both effective (i.e., does the right thing) and efficient (i.e., does things in the right way), it is important to ensure that all stakeholders' requirements are considered, not just the end customer.

- *Develop a process that can produce the product*: It is important that once the product has been designed, there is a consistent process in place to ensure that the product can be produced to order and on time.

- *Optimize the process*: Having designed the process that will produce the product effectively, it is then necessary to optimize that process so that it operates efficiently as well.

- *Prove that the process can produce the product under operating conditions*: Producing a product under special conditions, such as in a test laboratory, is the starting point. However, the process must also operate effectively under normal working conditions.

- *Transfer the process to operations*: Once all the optimization and proof of operation has been completed, then the process can be transferred to the operations department and full-scale production can begin.

While the above "road map" was described in terms of a manufacturing process, the same principles can easily be applied to an administrative operation or any service activity.

This quality planning road map very well describes the stages that the pharmaceutical industry goes through to research and develop a new drug and validate its manufacture before releasing it to the manufacturing department for normal production.

7.2.3.3 The quality crisis

Juran believed that while many companies from the 1980s onwards developed an increased awareness of the need for improved quality, there was less success when it came to the need to change behavior. This failure was attributed to a lack of planning and substance within improvement programs.

It appears that the programs did not progress from the original communications exercise to plan the specific tasks that needed to be completed. Nor were there any responsibilities allocated for completing those tasks. Also, there was no structured process for completing the tasks—the tools and techniques were missing. Finally, there was no reward system for management related to the required activities.

Juran was particularly insistent that the training for quality improvement should start at the very top of the organization. However, this view was not well received by many senior management teams who felt that "it was everyone else who had to learn and change."

7.2.4 Armand Feigenbaum

Armand Feigenbaum is an American quality control expert and businessman and was the originator of the Total Quality movement. He defined quality based on the customer's actual experience with a product or service, that is, only the customers can decide if and how well a product or service meets their needs, requirements, and expectations. As noted earlier Feigenbaum introduced the Four Quality Cost Categories in his 1956 *Harvard Business Review* essay Total Quality Control.

7.2.5 Phillip B. Crosby

Phillip Crosby is an American who spent his early career in quality control before moving into consultancy. Although he agrees that more than 80% of problems need management involvement to be solved, he differs from Deming and Juran, in that his approach majors on slogans, exhortations, and getting all the workforce involved in identifying causes of problems. Crosby authored several books including *Quality is Free, Quality Without Tears, Let's Talk Quality*, and *Leading: The Art of Becoming an Executive*.

7.2.5.1 Crosby's philosophy

Crosby's definition of quality is "conformance to the requirements which the company itself has established." He believed that most companies expect things to go wrong during any process and hence build in an allowance for these problems. Crosby developed the concepts of doing things "Right First Time" and "Zero Defects." He suggested that if the company does not start off expecting mistakes—and thereby implicitly accepting errors as okay—quality will be improved.

One of the problems with this approach relates back to the statistic, already stated, that more than 80% of problems within a process are fundamental ones that require management intervention. It was found that problems were highlighted by the workforce, but the management team could not react quickly enough and hence the program would grind to a halt in disillusionment.

7.2.5.2 Crosby's four absolutes of quality

The four absolutes of quality that Crosby defined are as follows:

1. Quality is defined as conformance to requirements, not as "goodness" nor "elegance."
2. Quality comes from prevention and not from quality inspection or appraisal.
3. The quality performance standard must be zero defects.
4. The measurement of quality is in monetary terms, that is, the price of nonconformance.

One of Crosby's famous quotes was "Quality is free. It's not a gift, but it is free. What costs money are the unquality things—all the actions that involve not doing jobs right the first time."

By comparison with previous sections in this chapter, it can be seen that there is a great similarity between these absolutes and the conclusions of Deming and Juran. The main difference appears in the methods that Crosby recommends for achieving quality improvement.

7.2.5.3 Crosby's 14 steps to quality improvement

Crosby identifies the following steps that need to be taken to improve the quality of the organizational performance:

1. *Management commitment*: It has already been stated that any sort of activity within an organization needs leadership and commitment from top management if it is to succeed.
2. *Quality improvement teams*: Organize Quality Improvement Teams with senior representatives from all departments. It is important that all parts of the organization are involved, to establish "ownership" of the program.
3. *Quality/process measurement*: If something is not measured, there is no way of knowing the current situation and hence it is not possible to develop targets for improvement or chart progress toward the targets. Crosby encouraged the measurement of defects and the posting of charts in the workplace so that improvements could be monitored visually over time.

4. *Cost of quality*: Calculate the cost of (poor) quality and use it as a management tool. This concept is fully reviewed later in this chapter. Crosby emphasizes that this measurement should be available so that everyone is aware of the price of nonconformance.

5. *Quality awareness*: For a quality improvement program to have any chance of success, it must involve all members of the organization. Hence any program should start with a good communications exercise to ensure that everyone understands the purpose and the objectives.

6. *Implement corrective action*: This requires the identification of problems and the positive action that needs to be taken to ensure that problems are corrected.

7. *Monitor progress of quality improvement*: Establish an ad hoc zero defects committee. This would be a cross-functional committee with responsibility for monitoring the zero defects program, facilitating its activities, and publicizing its successes.

8. *Train supervisors and employees*: Supervisors and employees need to be trained in the tools and techniques that are used for problem-solving and corrective action projects. Additionally, supervisors need to be trained in running and/or facilitating teams.

9. *Hold a zero defects day to establish the new attitude*: This would be a symbolic activity to aid the communications effort and emphasize the message that a culture change is expected to occur.

10. *Establish improvement goals*: This is usually done on a 30, 60, and 90-day basis. It would be tied to the quality measurements referred to earlier in this list of steps.

11. *Encourage employee communication with management about obstacles to improving quality*: Once problems and their fundamental causes have been identified, they should be eliminated. As already stated, this will place a heavy load on the management team, to correct fundamental underlying problems that are not attributable to individuals.

12. *Recognize participants' efforts*: Individuals or teams who achieve their goals or perform very well should receive appropriate recognition. Crosby recommends that this should be a nonfinancial award. (This differs from the traditional suggestion scheme where a financial award is presented, commensurate with the value to the company of the implemented suggestion.)

13. *Establish a quality council*: This is a steering committee for the entire quality improvement program. It can be composed of a mixture of functional quality specialists and project team leaders.

14. *Do it all over again*: This is recognition of the message, common to all the quality "gurus," that the journey toward quality improvement is a never-ending one. Every time the process is reexamined, it will be possible to find improvements. It is also a recognition of the fact that improvement tends to be brought about by many small incremental steps, rather than a few large strides.

7.2.6 Dr. Kaoru Ishikawa

Dr. Ishikawa was a Japanese engineer who is credited with the establishment of the Quality Circle movement in Japan. (Quality Circles are discussed more fully later in Chapter 8.) Dr. Ishikawa is also known for his development and the use of statistical techniques and for ensuring that the quality control culture spread throughout the organization within Japanese companies. He encouraged participation in quality improvement activities at all levels, from top management downwards.

In addition to Quality Circles, Dr. Ishikawa was most known for the development of the cause-and-effect diagram, also called the Ishikawa diagram (in honor of its creator) and the fishbone diagram (because of its shape), in the early 1950s.

Ishikawa emphasized the use of many statistical tools in the determination, evaluation, and analysis of causes of problems. He believed that "As much as 95% of quality-related problems in the factory can be solved with seven fundamental quantitative tools." The seven tools are as follows:

1. Check sheet
2. Pareto diagram
3. Flowchart
4. Histogram
5. Cause-and-effect diagram
6. Scatter diagram
7. Control chart

All of these tools are discussed in detail in Chapter 8.

7.3 Prerequisites for successful quality improvement programs

Reading the views of the various quality "gurus" as a prelude to establishing a quality improvement program could be confusing, as there is no one clear view on how to go forward. However, some consistent messages are coming out of their words.

These messages are presented here, reinforced by the experience gained by the author in quality improvement programs.

7.3.1 User-driven

A successful quality improvement program must be user-driven if the people within the organization are to take ownership of it and achieve good results. It is not uncommon for companies to use consultants to help introduce the program, particularly if it is a completely new approach for the company. However, these consultants should be used as facilitators and trainers only; they should advise on how the program should operate, based on their experience of the tools and techniques. The people working within the company are the experts on their own particular organization and are therefore best placed to decide how the tools and techniques can be applied in practice.

There are cases where consultants have been engaged by companies to "get ISO 9000 accreditation" for them. The consultant has written the quality manual and procedures and presented them to the company. However, without detailed knowledge of the particular company, it is very difficult to provide a set of documents that the workforce can commit to and take ownership of.

7.3.2 Management support

This point has already been made; however, it is so critical that it can certainly bear repeating. Support for quality improvement (or indeed for any other activity that the company wants to succeed) must start at the very top of the organization and cascade down to middle and junior managers. This requires good communication at the start of any program. There have been cases, for instance, where senior managers have involved the shop-floor workers in a quality circle program without ensuring full involvement at the supervisory level. This can cause a conflict of interest when pressure is applied to workers to attend meetings during their working hours and have to justify their absence to their supervisor.

7.3.3 Management commitment

There is a subtle difference between showing support for activity and being committed to its success. The best way that a senior management team can demonstrate its commitment to quality improvement is to take part in activities themselves. For example, company awareness training on the satisfaction of customer requirements should be presented to mixed groups, including board members. As shown in Chapter 3, the pharmaceutical industry has now embraced the quality management system approach. Senior management commitment is a key pillar of this approach.

7.3.4 Teamwork

The process of teamwork will be dealt with in much more detail later in Chapter 8. At this point, it is sufficient to say that the most successful improvement activities are those where people work in teams. These may be from within a single area, as in a Quality Circle, but are particularly effective when they are cross-functional. They provide an opportunity for people to get together that might normally never meet, let alone work on joint projects. They also allow people to pool knowledge and abilities to get sight of "the bigger picture."

7.3.5 Asking the right question

It has already been stressed that prevention is better than detection and correction. An increase in prevention costs can result in a drastic reduction in failure costs and also a lowering of appraisal costs on some occasions. This requires a shift in the way people think about their jobs and the questions they ask.

Instead of asking whether something has been done correctly (appraisal, after the event) it is better to question whether the capability is there to do the job properly. This brings into focus such things as process design, raw material specifications, and training of workers.

As an adjunct to this, once it has been determined that customer requirements can be satisfied, the next thing to question should be whether the job is consistently done correctly and whether there are ways of doing it better. This moves the action firmly toward quality improvement.

7.3.6 Breaking out of the silos

In the traditional company, walls tend to build up between different functions within the organization. If not checked, these "functional silos" can become isolated from one another and see their objectives only in terms of the immediate task of the department. In such cases, there can be suboptimization of performance, since what is best for the performance of one department might not be the best for the whole company.

A classic example of this is the old-fashioned approach to purchasing of raw materials. When the purchasing department was judged solely on the total budget for purchases and rewarded for buying cheaply, there was no incentive to liaise with the production department on the quality of the material being delivered and the impact that it had on the running of the process machines. However, by breaking out of the silos and considering purchasing as a horizontal process across the organization, with the involvement of several different functions, a much more effective operation can be achieved.

7.3.7 Acceptance of change

This aspect has two parts to it. First, it is important to accept that change is necessary. If people feel that everything is okay and there is no need for improvement, there will be a level of complacency built up which means that the company will lose its edge with regard to the competition.

There is a view that quality improvement programs should be established while things are going relatively well because once there are real problems, it is probably too late to do anything about it. However, this can be hindered by the "if it ain't broke, don't fix it" mentality, which needs to be overcome.

Secondly, changes can be very threatening for some people within an organization. They believe that changes will make their jobs bigger, harder, less stable, or less secure. The right messages must be given in the first place to ensure that people understand that the changes will make their jobs more effective, more value-adding, and more stable (assuming that the latter is true of course).

7.4 Cost of quality

As mentioned earlier Dr. Joseph Juran expressed the link between money and quality when he introduced the concept of Quality Cost in 1951. In 1956, Armand Feigenbaum expanded on the concept and introduced the Four Quality Cost Categories that are commonly referred to today. The "quality costs" concept has been assigned different meanings. It is sometimes equated with the costs of attaining quality. Others equate the term with extra costs incurred because of poor quality. This section will initially discuss the four quality cost categories. It then moves on to review how quality costs can be measured and will end with a discussion on the Cost of Poor Quality (COPQ). In the end, there are case studies of applications of the Cost of Quality within the pharmaceutical industry.

7.4.1 Definitions of cost of quality

The Cost of Quality is a concept that is embraced by many industries, usually within a TQM or performance improvement program. Total Quality Cost is the sum of costs associated with the Four Quality Cost Categories. Total Quality Cost can also be summarized as the total investment into the prevention of defects, the testing of the product to assure quality, and the failure of a product to meet the customer requirements. The Four Quality Cost Categories are prevention costs, appraisal costs, internal failure costs, and external failure costs.

7.4.1.1 Prevention costs

Prevention costs are the costs associated with making sure that things are done right the first time. These costs are investments made by the company to keep the nonconforming product from occurring and reaching the customer.

Examples of prevention costs are training, validation procedures, quality planning, procedure writing, market research, applicant screening, quality system audits, quality improvement projects, process monitoring and control (to determine status of the process), and design reviews. Some authorities contend that every dollar spent on prevention will save seven dollars in failure costs.

7.4.1.2 Appraisal costs

Appraisal costs are those associated with efforts to ensure conformance to the quality requirements, generally through measurement and the analysis of data. Examples of appraisal costs are raw material testing, in-process and finished product testing, laboratory testing, audits carried out by the company—whether internal self-inspections or supplier audits, equipment calibration, and personnel testing. Inspection costs, which includes the fee for a visit from the regulatory authorities also fall under this category of quality costs.

7.4.1.3 Internal failure costs

Internal failure costs are the costs incurred as a result of unsatisfactory quality found before the delivery of the product to the customer. Included in these are costs associated with avoidable process losses and inefficiencies that occur even when requirements and needs are met. Examples of these costs are rework, scrap or sorting, excess inventory, repair work, design changes, unplanned downtime, redundant operations, internal corrective action, root cause investigation costs, or employee turnover.

7.4.1.4 External failure costs

These are costs that occur after a poor quality product reaches the customer. Included with these costs are lost opportunities for sales revenue. Examples of external failure costs are product recalls, product returns, customer complaints, liability suits, lost sales, damage to image, customer defections, or problems with regulatory authorities.

A prime example of failure costs, covering several of these categories occurred in India some years ago. At least one multinational company had failed to validate its method for the destruction of waste packaging materials. A pirate company retrieved some waste material from the disposal area and used it to package and sell counterfeit material. When the regulatory authorities found out what was happening, the multinational company was shut down for 10 days, resulting in failure costs in all these categories

7.5 Calculating the cost of poor quality

Having defined the four types of quality costs, this section will explain how the analysis of these costs can be used to calculate Total Quality Costs oftentimes referred to as the COPQ. All the activities related to quality are measured and categorized as appraisal, prevention, internal failure, or external failure costs.

For each cost, regardless of the cost category, a dollar amount can be determined. After the dollar amounts are determined the total COPQ can be calculated.

Fig. 7.1 provides a generic table that can be used to calculate the COPQ for a pharmaceutical manufacturing process.

By highlighting the various costs in this way, it makes it easy to determine where to focus efforts to improve performance and reduce costs.

Studies of quality costs across many different countries have determined the costs result in an average of between 15% and 30% of total sales. Of this, it is estimated that up to 75% will be accounted for by failure costs.

Fig. 7.2 shows what happens when a company starts to evaluate and improve its quality costs.

The "Initial %" bars represent the typical situation in a company that is not controlling its quality costs. After evaluating and shifting its costs of quality, the

Cost Category	Activity	Number of People Involved per week (A)	Total People Hours Taken to Complete the Activity (B)	Average Cost/Pay per Hour (C)	Total People Cost (D) (D = A*B*C)	Number of Pieces of Equipment Used to Complete Activity Involved per week (E)	Average Equipment Utilization Cost per Hour (F)	Total Equipment Cost (G) (G = E*F)	Total Cost (H) (H = D+G)
Prevention Costs	Quality system development/revision								
	Process monitoring/control								
	Quality system audit								
	Supplier evaluations								
	Training								
Appraisal Costs	Vial inspection								
	Raw material testing								
	Lab testing								
	Internal audits								
	Maintaining test machines/equipment								
	Equipment calibration								
Internal Failure Costs	Retesting								
	Scrap								
	Rework								
	Failure analysis								
	Reinspection								
	Expediting								
	Time away from development or manufacturing								
External Failure Costs	Providing a customer interraction								
	Nonbillable consulting time								
	Cancelled orders								
	Making allowances for orders								
	Investigation								
	Reshipping								
	Lost sales								
	lost goodwill								
	Liability costs								
	Government investigations								
	Resorting returned goods								
	Disposal of returned goods								

TOTAL COST OF QUALITY =

Figure 7.1 COPQ example for a pharmaceutical manufacturing process.

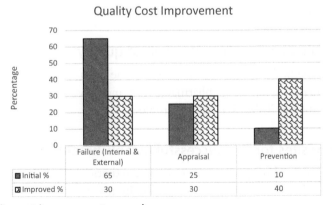

Figure 7.2 Quality cost improvement example.

Quality Cost Improvement

	Failure (Internal & External)	Appraisal	Prevention
Initial %	65	25	10
Improved %	30	30	40

Figure 7.2 Quality cost improvement example.

distribution of the costs is shown by the "Improved %" bars. In the pharmaceutical industry appraisal costs may increase initially, since it is necessary to ensure that any changes made were not detrimental to the processes. However, in the longer term, the appraisal costs will be reduced. For example, by instituting a supplier audit system (increasing the prevention costs), it should be possible in the medium to long term to reduce or eliminate raw material testing (reducing the appraisal costs). The more significant improvement is the reduction in failure costs. In the example above, an overall goal of a supplier audit system should be to reduce problems with deliveries, improve the quality of the raw materials, and reduce the level of waste produced when the material is processed (reducing failure costs). This example demonstrates Philip Crosby's statement that "Quality is Free."

There are a variety of ways in which a Cost of Quality measurement can be used within a company. First and foremost, it can be used as a communication tool to make people aware of costing issues and thereby influence company strategy. Cost of Quality measurements can be part of the decision-making process, as an adjunct to discounted cash flow or sensitivity analyses for project evaluation.

Cost of Quality measurements can be used to monitor performance across an organization, to identify priorities for improvement and to set cost-reduction targets. Once the Cost of Quality activities are conducted, the results can be used to monitor progress toward the target. The results can also be used as a basis for cost-benefit analysis against specific quality-related activities such as quality management programs or ISO certification. Finally, Cost of Quality measurements can be used in the development of budgets and product costing. In this context, it can be a complementary tool to Activity-Based Costing.

The Cost of Quality tool can be used as a one-time measurement to provide information about a specific activity, or it can be used continuously as part of the normal performance monitoring of the company. It is most effective in the latter case if the measurement is presented as one of the regular indices presented as part of the management accounts.

7.5.1 An applied approach to the cost of quality

The following methodology has been used by the author in unpublished studies of the Cost of Quality within the pharmaceutical industry. It consists of several steps which are described in Table 7.1 with examples.

7.5.2 Prerequisites for the successful establishment

Many programs related to quality improvement activities have been established within companies over the past decades and many of them have not been successful, due to an inappropriate culture or the failure to comply with prerequisites for success.

Table 7.1 Stages in a cost of quality project.

Stage	Example
Establishment of a project team, encompassing the departments in the company involved in the process under discussion.	QA officer–team leader TQM manager–facilitator Manufacturing supervisor Purchasing operative Warehouse manager Packaging operative
Identification of the scope of the project	Entire product pipeline for product X from raw material purchasing through manufacturing and packaging to release for sale.
Identification of stages in the product pipelines	Purchase of raw materials QC approval of raw materials Manufacture of bulk product QC approval of bulk product Packaging of finished product QC release of finished product

Identification of key steps in each stage	Manufacture of bulk product
	   Engineering set up
	   Routine maintenance
	   Training
	   Storage of raw materials
	   Manufacturing
	   Reject material
	   Sampling and testing
	   Approval for packing

Grouping of steps into Cost of Quality categories	Basic processes
	   Manufacturing
	Prevention costs
	   Training
	Appraisal costs
	   Sampling and testing
	Failure costs
	   Reject material

Assignment of units of measure for each step	Training: man-hours Sampling and testing: man-hours and cost of material Reject material: cost of material
Measurement and estimation of the activity associated with each step	Sampling and testing: x man-hours; a kg
Identification of costs	Sampling and testing: x man-hours at £y per hour; a kg at £b per kg
Analysis and interpretation of results	Total sales = S Total quality costs = T % Cost of Quality = T/S × 100
Derivation of useful information	Main source of reject material is machine M in process step 3. This would be a priority area for investigation.

However, this section deals with the issues that need to be anticipated and dealt with in the context of Cost of Quality.

One of the biggest barriers to a successful measurement could be the mismatch between the company's current financial monitoring system and the items that need to be measured to calculate the Cost of Quality. To prevent this barrier from arising, it is important to involve the finance department from the outset.

Any activity which focuses on problems with the way that people carry out their jobs can be seen as a process of criticism and blame if not presented correctly. It is important that the individuals concerned fully understand that the process is not personally based and can be beneficial to them in the long-term.

A Cost of Quality project will tend to be time-consuming in the initial stages. Inevitably, the members of the team will have other "real" jobs that they will have to continue to perform in parallel. Sufficient resources must be provided to ensure that team members are not overwhelmed with conflicting priorities.

One of the main ways of ensuring that these barriers will not arise is to provide an on-going, very visible project championship from a senior manager. The support from such a person will disseminate the message that the company is serious about this activity and is not going to let it slip quietly into oblivion after a respectable interval of time.

Apart from the project champion, there must also be a project manager who will run the activity. This person will need to meet with the senior management team to determine who are the most appropriate team members. These people will come from a variety of parts of the company and will be chosen for various reasons: obviously, these need to be people who understand the process and can explain the detailed steps. However, it is also important to have people who are creative in their thinking and are willing to consider doing things differently. These people can also be useful in presenting a "fresh pair of eyes" to the process. Sometimes, the process experts are too close to the detail to be able to see things clearly.

Once the team has been chosen, the project manager will need to establish the requirements in terms of time and agree on this with the members' managers so that they do not have problems in attending meetings or carrying out allocated tasks in between.

Finally, the team should meet to agree on its objectives and modus operandi. Depending on how large the company is and how well the members know each other, it could be beneficial to have some sort of ice-breaker or another team-building exercise at the start to ensure that the team operates effectively and efficiently during the course of the project.

The project manager should ensure that appropriate communication mechanisms are established, so that the project champion and other senior managers are aware of what is happening.

7.6 Lean techniques

Lean, the shortened version of Lean Manufacturing or Lean Production is a catchphrase that describes a philosophy, methodology, techniques, and tools. Until the late 1980s, when the term Lean was coined, the lean principles and practices were known only to specialized manufacturers, some academic researchers, and quality gurus. The Toyota Production System (TPS), cofounded and made famous by Taiichi Ohno, is the foundation for Lean. As a business philosophy, the Lean focus is to "do more with less" and covers the total enterprise. As a business practice, The Manufacturing Extension Partnership (MEP) Lean Network defines Lean as "A systematic approach to identifying and eliminating waste (non-value-added activities) through continuous improvement by flowing the product at the pull of the customer, in pursuit of perfection." Lean uses an integrated system of principles, practices, tools, and techniques focused on reducing waste, synchronizing workflows, and managing variability in production flows.

In the MEP Lean Network's definition are key components of the practice of Lean Production and Lean Thinking. Value-added refers to an activity that transforms inputs to meet customer requirements. These are activities that the customer is willing to pay for and are done right the first time. Examples of value-added activities are: a patient receives treatment, an employee puts parts together on the assembly floor, raw material is added to the manufacturing batch. Non-value-adding is the opposite of value-adding and refers to any activity that takes time, resources, or space but does not add to the value of the product or service. These activities should be eliminated, simplified, reduced, or integrated; however, sometimes the non-value-adding is necessary and/or regulated. The testing conducted during preclinical studies, the clinical trials application, and the new drug application could be categorized as non-value-adding activities, however, they are required by the regulatory agencies.

The ultimate goal of Lean is to eliminate waste. Waste, the equivalent of the Japanese term Muda, can be defined as any activity that consumes resources and produces no added value to the product or service a customer receives. Taiichi Ohno identified seven waste categories as part of TPS. In the 1990s when TPS was adopted in the Western world, an eighth category was added. The eight waste categories, which are often referred to by the acronym TIMWOODS, are as follows:

1. *Transport*: Unnecessary movement of resources, such as work-in-progress (WIP), people, tools, equipment, material, documents, and information.
2. *Inventory*: More materials or items on-hand than needed. Includes excess product that is not directly required for current customer orders, for example, excess raw material, WIP, and finished goods.
3. *Motion (or Movement)*: Extra steps, bending, turning, reaching, or lifting completed by employees and equipment to accommodate inefficient process layouts, defects, reprocessing overproduction, or too little or too much inventory.

4. *Waiting*: Idle time is created when people, information, equipment, materials, or services are not readily available. Also known as queuing and refers to the periods of inactivity in a downstream process that occurs because an upstream activity doesn't deliver on time

5. *Overproduction*: Redundant work or efforts. Making more product or an element of the product before it is required by the next process.

6. *Over-processing*: Doing more work, making more product than is immediately required, or having more steps in a product or service than what is required by the customer. Includes extra operations, such as unnecessary levels of decision-making, rework, reprocessing, handling and storage, that occur because of defects, over-servicing, overproduction, or too many or too few resources.

7. *Defects*: Products or aspects of a service that do not conform to specification or to the customer's expectations, thus causing customer dissatisfaction.

8. *Under-utilized people or unused talent (or skill)*: The mismatch of skills to the task required; not seeking, capturing, or using knowledge of employees to improve processes or underutilizing capabilities.

In the application of Lean Manufacturing or Production, many of the original TPS tools continue to be utilized. These tools include:

- Value stream mapping;
- Five S;
- Kanban (pull inventory management);
- Error proofing (Poka-yoke);
- Setup time reduction [single minute exchange of dies (SMED)];
- Reduced lot sizes (single piece flow);
- Line-balancing;
- Schedule leveling;
- Standardized work;
- Visual management.

As noted by many of the examples provided, lean tools and techniques can be used throughout the drug life cycle, to reduce waste and cost.

7.7 Six sigma methodology

Like Lean, Six Sigma has multiple definitions. It is a methodology that blends together many of the key elements of past quality initiatives, that is Juran's Quality Trilogy, Feigenbaum's TQM, Deming's Economic Chain Reaction and PDCA, Shewhart's PDSA and SQC, Crosby's zero defects, Ishikawa's seven tools for improving processes, Taguchi's Design of Experiments, and Continuous Improvement. It is a data-driven methodology that uses a specific problem-solving approach and specialized tools to improve processes and products and reduce the occurrence of unacceptable products or events. As a statistical concept, Six Sigma represents the amount of variation present in a process relative to customer requirements or specifications. Sigma is the Greek symbol used to represent variation. When a process is running at the six sigma level, the variation is so small that the resulting products and services are 99.9997% defect-free. This level is equivalent to the process delivering only 3.4 defects per million opportunities (DPMO).

The Six Sigma concept was originally formulated and coined in 1986 by Bill Smith, a reliability engineer for Motorola Corporation when he was investigating the number of repairs made in manufacturing related to the product failures in the field. The company discovered that products with a high first pass yield (i.e., products that made it through the production process defect-free the first time) rarely failed in actual use. Six Sigma emphasizes an increased focus on quality as defined by the customer, meeting and exceeding customer expectations, rigorous statistical methods, and the prioritization of improvement projects in alignment with an organization's resources to support the key strategic initiatives.

There are two basic Six Sigma models which are known by the acronyms DMAIC and DMADV. The five steps Define, Measure, Analyze, Improve, and Control form the DMAIC acronym and the steps Define, Measure, Analyze, Design, and Verify/Validate are represented by the DMADV acronym. The DMAIC model is used to improve current capabilities and existing processes and is the most commonly used model. The DMADV model, also known as Design for Six Sigma (DFSS) is used to help create a new process, product, or service to meet customer requirements or to completely redesign a process, product, or service that is consistently incapable of meeting customer requirements.

As noted earlier, Six Sigma uses a specific problem-solving approach and specialized tools to improve processes and products. This specific approach is structured through the work of a project team. As the DMAIC model is the most commonly used model, the next section will describe this model.

7.7.1 Define, measure, analyze, improve, and control model

7.7.1.1 Define
In the Define phase of the model, the project team is launched. The main goals of the Define phase include:
- to have the team and its sponsor reach an agreement on the scope, goals, and financial performance targets of the project;
- to define the project's purpose, scope, and charter;
- to define and validate the problem statement;
- to validate the financial benefits of the project;
- to identify, document, and validate the voice of the customer(s).

To achieve these goals, various Six Sigma tools are used and metrics are captured, for example, project charter, a high-level process map (called the SIPOC diagram), performance metrics, the voice of the customer (VOC), and cost/revenue implications.

7.7.1.2 Measure

The main goals of the Measure phase include:
- to thoroughly understand the current state of the process and collect reliable data on process speed, quality, and costs that will be used to expose the underlying causes of the problem;
- to gather data and information on the current performance of the process to determine the baseline performance;
- to determine the target performance of the process;
- to understand causal relationships between process performance and customer value.

To achieve these goals, check sheets are used to collect data to help the team understand how the current process operates and calculate the baseline process capability and process sigma.

7.7.1.3 Analyze

The main goals of the Analyze phase include:
- to analyze the data to pinpoint and verify the causes affecting the key input and output variables tied to the project goals;
- to establish the key process inputs that affect the process outputs;
- to identify and determine potential root cause(s) of the problem and confirm them with data.

To achieve these goals, the statistical analyses are performed on the process data and COPQ is calculated. The data are organized and summarized using applicable tools, for example, descriptive statistics, cause-and-effect diagrams, dot plots, frequency tables, bar charts, Pareto charts, frequency plots/histograms, box plots, scatter diagrams, and Design of Experiments (DOE). Many of these tools are described in detail in Chapter 8.

7.7.1.4 Improve

The main goals of the Improve phase include:
- to develop, try out, and implement solutions that address and eliminate the root cause(s) of the defects;
- to use data to evaluate, select, and optimize the best solutions;
- to develop and implement a pilot solution;
- to develop a full-scale implementation plan.
  Primarily, lean principles and DOE are used to achieve these goals.

7.7.1.5 Control

The main goals of the Control phase include:

- to complete the project work and hand off the improved process to the process owner, with procedures for maintaining the gains;
- improved mistake proofing;
- to develop Standard Operating Procedures, training plans, and process controls;
- to implement solutions and ongoing process measurements;
- to review before and after data on the process metrics;
- to implement a system for monitoring the consistent use of the new method(s), that is, a Control Plan;
- completed documentation and communication of the results, lessons learned, and recommendations;
- transition of process monitoring and control to the process owner;
- to calculate the financial gains from the project improvement.

To achieve these goals control systems are developed to monitor the improvements. The control systems could include visual inspection, control charts, and a control plan to record, monitor, and maintain the project gains.

When done correctly and the structure is followed, Six Sigma is a very powerful methodology that can be used to significantly improve any process. In the completion of the projects, all the tools available are not typically required, only the tools that help the team complete the goals of the phases. Very few processes actually reach the six sigma level of improvement, that is, 99.9997% defect free; however, after successfully completing the project, every process should demonstrate significant improvement. The improvement can then be translated into a financial gain.

7.8 Quality by design

QbD is a concept that was formulated by Dr. Joseph Juran in the 1970s in his book *Juran on Quality by Design* and was later adopted by industries—that is, automobile, aviation, and telecommunications companies—who focused on the development of high-quality products and services. In the 1990s the concept was adopted by the healthcare industries, especially medical device manufacturers. The concept wasn't adopted by the pharmaceutical industry until late 2004 when the US Food and Drug Administration (FDA) encouraged the adoption of QbD principles in drug product development, manufacturing, and regulation. In 2006, the USFDA published a guidance for industry entitled "Quality Systems Approach to Pharmaceutical Current Good Manufacturing Practice Regulations." In the guidance, the USFDA emphasized that "*Quality should be built into the product and testing alone cannot be relied on to ensure product quality.*" In the specific section on QbD, the guidance stated

Quality by design means designing and developing a product and associated manufacturing processes that will be used during product development to ensure that the product consistently attains a predefined quality at the end of the manufacturing process. Quality by design, in conjunction with a quality system, provides a sound framework for the transfer of product knowledge and process understanding from drug development to the commercial manufacturing processes and for post-development changes and optimization.

Since 2006, QbD has evolved with the issuance of guidelines from the International Conference on Harmonization (ICH). ICH Q8 Pharmaceutical Development, ICH Q9 Quality Risk Management, and ICH Q10 Pharmaceutical Quality System worked collectively to promote quality into the practice of pharmaceutical development and manufacturing.

In the application of QbD, the authors of the article *Understanding Pharmaceutical Quality by Design* (Yu et al., 2014) listed four goals for QbD in pharmaceutical:

1. to achieve meaningful product quality specifications that are based on clinical performance;
2. to increase process capability and reduce product variability and defects by enhancing product and process design, understanding, and control;
3. to increase product development and manufacturing efficiencies; and
4. to enhance root cause analysis and postapproval change management.

These goals align with the elements of QbD as stated in the following excerpts from ICH Q8:

1. *Define the Quality Target Product Profile (QTPP)*: The QTPP forms the foundation for the development of the product. Items that should be considered for inclusion in the QTPP are as follows:
   a. intended use in a clinical setting, route of administration, dosage form, delivery systems;
   b. dosage strength(s);
   c. container closure system;
   d. therapeutic moiety release or delivery and attributes affecting pharmacokinetic characteristics (e.g., dissolution, aerodynamic performance) appropriate to the drug product dosage form being developed;
   e. drug product quality criteria (e.g., sterility, purity, stability, and drug release) appropriate for the intended marketed product.
   An example of a typical QTPP for an immediate release solid oral dosage form would include: tablet characteristics, identification, assay and uniformity, purity/impurity, stability, and dissolution (Gandhi and Roy, 2016).
2. *Identify the Critical Quality Attributes (CQAs)*: A CQA is a physical, chemical, biological, or microbiological property or characteristic that should be within an appropriate limit, range, or distribution to ensure the desired product quality.

CQAs are generally associated with the drug substance, excipients, intermediates (in-process materials), and drug products.

CQAs of solid oral dosage forms are typically those aspects affecting product purity, strength, drug release, and stability. The CQAs may include appearance, hardness, physical form, dissolution, water content, and assay. For drug substances, raw materials, and intermediates (in-process materials), the CQAs may include appearance, particle size, water content, organic and inorganic impurities, bulk density, etc.

3. *Perform a Risk (Assessment) Analysis*: Risk assessment is a science-based process used in quality risk management (reference ICH Q9) that can aid in identifying which material attributes and process parameters potentially affect product CQAs. Risk assessment is typically performed early in the pharmaceutical development process and is repeated as more information becomes available and greater knowledge is obtained.

The USFDA defines quality risk management as "a systematic process for the assessment, control, communication and review of risks to the quality of the drug product across the product lifecycle." This definition aligns with the ICH Q9 definition and the risk management process outlined in the guidance.

4. *Determine the Design Space*: A design space refers to the ranges of material attributes and process parameters or by more complex mathematical relationships. The design space can also be described as a time-dependent function (e.g., temperature and pressure cycle of a lyophilization cycle) or as a combination of variables such as components of a multivariate model. Scaling factors can also be included if the design space is intended to span multiple operational scales. Additionally, historical data can be used to help establish a design space; however, regardless of how a design space is developed, it is expected that operation within the design space will result in a product meeting the defined quality.

An important part of determining the design space is the identification of the critical process parameters (CPPs). A CPP is any measurable input or output of a process step that must be controlled to achieve the desired product quality and process consistency. A parameter is critical if a real change in that parameter can cause the product to fail to meet the QTPP. When classifying a critical parameter, the range of interest, also called the potential operating space (POS), must be defined. Examples of critical parameters include mixing time, drying time, temperature, milling speed, feed rate, milling time, compression force, dwell time, inlet air flow, and spray pattern and rate.

5. *Design and Implement a Control Strategy*: ICH Q10 defines a control strategy as "a planned set of controls derived from current product and process understanding that assures process performance and product quality." A control strategy is designed to ensure that a product of required quality will be produced consistently. The elements of the control strategy should describe and justify how in-process controls and the controls of input materials (drug substance and excipients), intermediates, container closure system, and drug products contribute to the final

product quality. These controls should be based on product, formulation, and process understanding. "The controls can include parameters and attributes related to drug substance and drug product materials and components, facility and equipment operating conditions, in-process controls, finished product specifications and the associated methods and frequency of monitoring and control."

A control strategy can include:

- control of input material attributes (e.g., drug substance, excipients, primary packaging materials) based on an understanding of their impact on processability or product quality;
- product specification(s);
- controls for unit operations that have an impact on downstream processing or product quality, for example, the impact of drying on degradation, the particle size distribution of the granulate on dissolution;
- in-process or real-time release testing instead of end-product testing, for example, measurement and control of CQAs during processing; and
- a monitoring program, for example, full product testing at regular intervals for verifying multivariate prediction models.

A control strategy can include different elements. One element of the control strategy could rely on end-product testing, yet another element could depend on real-time release testing.

6. *Manage Product Life Cycle and Continuous Improvement*: Process performance should be monitored to ensure that the process is working as anticipated and delivering product quality attributes predicted by the design space. This monitoring could include trend analysis of the manufacturing process as additional experience is gained.

Like the other methodologies covered previously, QbD is a structured approach for planning, measuring, and ensuring pharmaceutical product quality. In addition to specific goals, the methodology includes specific elements to reduce product variability and defects and to enhance product development and manufacturing efficiencies.

7.9 Benchmarking

A company that decides to embark on a benchmarking journey must be humble enough to admit that another company or department is better at something and wise enough to learn to match or even surpass the competitor. Put simply, benchmarking is the practice of identifying, measuring, and learning from best practices. With the benchmarking process, a company will observe how another performs a given task and then apply any learnings to improve how the task is executed at its company. Benchmarking can be used to measure and compare organizations, business units or functions, or business processes, products, or services.

Benchmarking studies have been conducted between different factories within the same group as well as between different companies within the same industry. For example, if several pharmaceutical companies carried out a study of manufacturing performance parameters, some would be able to demonstrate best practices in productivity while others would be better in terms of inventory stock-turn or speed of fulfilling customers' orders. Finally, benchmarking can be conducted between companies from completely different industries. For example, in a cross-industry study, a mail-order catalog company might be able to demonstrate best practices in the logistics of rapid delivery; a pharmaceutical company might be able to demonstrate best practices in the validation of production processes and an internet company might be able to demonstrate best practice in the use of e-commerce.

There is vast literature written about benchmarking and several institutes and organizations that specialize in the facilitation of the process. The two case studies later in this section will illustrate the use of benchmarking in the pharmaceutical industry.

7.9.1 Steps in a benchmarking study

There are several models that have been published for carrying out a benchmarking study. In general, they all follow a similar pattern.

1. *Identify parameters and comparators*: Advance planning is critical to the success of benchmarking. Clearly defined parameters and specific metrics must be defined in this step to ensure consistency in data collection.
2. *Preliminary data collection*: Collect data on companies in a similar industry or with similar processes. Also, collect detailed data on your processes.
3. *Determination of best practice*: Identify companies with best-in-class processes or practices.
4. *Best-in-Class data collection*: Collect and analyze business or process data pertaining to the measures for the best-in-class companies.
5. *Data analysis*: Analyze the data to ensure that similar, that is, "apples to apples" metrics were collected.
6. *Benchmark report*: A report will be compiled to summarize conclusions drawn from the data analysis, including best practices between the companies. The report will also include key findings determined from a gap analysis performed by the benchmarking team members. The gap analysis will detail its company's strengths, weaknesses, improvements suggestions, and priority recommendations.
7. *Setting of goals for improvement*: A study can then be made of how the best practices are achieved. The company will determine how its performance can be improved, using lessons learned from the benchmarking study.
8. *Action planning*: action plans to attain superior performance are developed, together with progress monitoring systems.

9. *Doing it again*: As performance improves across the company, the level of best practice will hopefully improve (and in fact, the best practice company may change). It is, therefore, useful to repeat the exercise after a time to see whether there are more lessons to be learned in a process of continual improvements.

7.9.2 Case study 1—benchmarking in research and development

The senior team of an R&D directorate of a major MNC recognized that to be successful in reducing the time that it took to get a new product to the marketplace, they would have to improve their ability to run projects via a matrix management system. They, therefore, decided to take part in a UK-wide, cross-industry study, involving 14 companies from diverse industries. (There were no other pharmaceutical companies within the study). The companies varied widely in their histories of project management: in terms of experience, there was an engineering consultancy with a long pedigree in project management and a public service retail organization to which the concept was new.

The R&D team found that they were able to contribute to the study of best practices in understanding risk and moving high-risk projects into development. Unlike many industries, pharmaceuticals have no guarantee of a product at the end of the development phase.

The study was carried out in three phases. In Phase 1, the scene was set. Data were gathered and used to identify ranges of performance and to position each company with respect to each parameter. This gave rise to a measurement of each system. In other words, current positions were defined and compared.

In Phase 2, the participants homed in on examples of best practices and reviewed their strengths and weaknesses. Ten major performance areas were focused upon.

Phase 3 was the implementation of best practices and reciprocal site visits. The whole study was based on the belief that all projects have common features and that hence a generic project model could be developed which would allow an analysis of the best use of resources. Several key performance areas were identified by the study. These are presented in full below since they could also be applied to the working of teams within a quality improvement program:

7.9.2.1 Integrating project work into the organization

It is necessary to reorganize the company along project-based lines, paying attention to management, culture, committees, and rewards. In particular, rewards must be geared to project success rather than individual success while at the same time accepting that a failed project may be a success (particularly in the pharmaceuticals industry).

7.9.2.2 Managing human factors in projects

Scientists, like many other professionals, do not make particularly good managers—nor are they very easy to manage. With matrix management, where there are in effect two "bosses"—the functional manager and the project manager—the problem can be compounded. Project management is not recognized by many others as a legitimate profession. The project manager will often only be respected if they can do the functional job better than the professional can.

7.9.2.3 Defining project "anatomy"

Any project will have several elements within it: risk, time, cost, and culture. The skill comes in recognizing the relative importance of each in different projects. For example, in the development of a new drug, risk, time and cost will be the key factors. On the other hand, in a project to computerize a documentation system, the main element may be culture.

7.9.2.4 Defining and executing projects

Any successful project will have control systems and review systems so that activities can be monitored throughout. A postproject appraisal system is critical for learning the lessons—both good and bad—from one project for application on all subsequent ones.

7.9.2.5 Estimating cost, time, and resource requirements

Construction companies have traditionally been very good at estimating resources since they operate on such tight margins. Within the pharmaceutical company in the past, the cost was not considered to be particularly important, and many R&D people had no idea of their budgets. This began changing in the 1990s and costs became more important. Time always was and will remain important. In general, a shortage of resources leads to a need for change in thinking, skills, and management style.

7.9.3 Case study 2—benchmarking in manufacturing

The previous case study was an example of functional benchmarking - looking at the same function, carried out in companies across a range of industries. This case study demonstrates the approach of internal benchmarking within a multisite company. The project studied a single process technology, being carried out on a number of sites in different countries. The main aspects that were initially studied were direct and indirect labor (direct filling, direct packaging, production support, QA/QC, and technical/engineering support.) A second phase was initiated later, looking at material wastage, in the form of rejects and samples.

The study was carried out using retrospective data, based on simple definitions. For example, for filling, the calculation was a total number of units filled divided into a total number of direct operator minutes used to give units per operator minute.

From the data, the best in class was identified for each of the parameters being measured. In each case, this factory then analyzed itself to explain why it was the most successful. Each of the other factories then had the opportunity to comment on this analysis and amend it. The lessons learned were then applied to all the factories and improvements measured by a continuation of the original measurement.

The first lesson that came out was the need to make sure that the comparison is apples and apples, not apples and pears. Although all the factories were working from the same process formulation and with the same equipment, they had up to twenty years for diversity to creep in. This underlined the importance of clear simple definitions.

It was found to be important to avoid going into too much detail initially; again, this could be controlled by good definitions at the start.

There is also a need to apply sanity checks to the process—and this is where a good facilitator is essential. If any results look too good or too horrendous, it is worth checking that everything is okay before going public with the results. Otherwise, the whole process could be discredited.

One of the benefits of such a detailed analysis of a process is that the obvious stupidities can be put right straight away—and there is a chance to get a series of "quick wins" which is good both for the morale of the group and the credibility of the program.

One clear message that came out of the exercise is that, as suggested earlier in this section, no one is the best of class for all activities. This helped to maintain everyone's confidence in themselves and the process and ensured that everyone felt they were both contributing to and gaining from the process.

7.10 Summary

- The existence of quality dates back thousands of years and continues to evolve.
- Quality has various definitions as noted by ASQ, ISO, and different quality gurus.
- TQM is defined as a management approach that emphasizes continuous process and system improvement as a means for achieving customer satisfaction and to ensure long-term company success. It is composed of the following primary elements: customer-focused, total employee involvement, process-centered, integrated systems, strategic and systematic approach, continual improvement, fact-based decision-making, and communications.
- Pharmaceutical companies may not officially use the term TQM in their efforts to maintain quality, but the elements of TQM are evident in their everyday operations.
- Some of the key figures, "gurus," in the foundation of quality include Walter Shewhart, W. Edwards Deming, Joseph Juran, Armand Feigenbaum, Phillip B Crosby, and Kaoru Ishikawa.

- A successful quality improvement program must be user-driven, have management support and commitment, and include acceptance to change.
- Quality costs are equated with the costs of attaining quality or extra costs incurred because of poor quality.
- The four Quality Cost Categories are prevention costs, appraisal costs, internal failure costs, and external failure costs.
- Lean is defined as a systematic approach to identifying and eliminating waste (non-value-added activities) through continuous improvement by flowing the product at the pull of the customer, in pursuit of perfection.
- Value-added refers to an activity that transforms inputs to meet customer requirements.
- Nonvalue-adding refers to any activity that takes time, resources, or space but does not add to the value of the product or service
- The eight waste categories are transportation, inventory, motion, waiting, overproduction, overprocessing, defects, underutilized skills.
- TIMWOODS is the acronym used to capture the eight Lean wastes.
- Six Sigma is a data-driven methodology that uses a specific problem-solving approach and specialized tools to improve processes and products and reduce the occurrence of unacceptable products or events.
- Six Sigma is also defined as the amount of variation present in a process relative to customer requirements or specifications.
- When a process is running at the six sigma level, the variation is so small that the resulting products and services are 99.9997% defect-free.
- The two basic Six Sigma models are the DMAIC model and the DMADV model.
- The USFDA defines QbD as designing and developing a product and associated manufacturing processes that will be used during product development to ensure that the product consistently attains a predefined quality at the end of the manufacturing process.
- The elements of QbD are: Define the QTPP, Identify the CQAs, Perform a Risk (Assessment) Analysis, Determine the design space, Design and implement a control strategy, and Manage product life cycle and continuous improvement.
- Benchmarking is the practice of identifying, measuring, and learning from best practice.
- Benchmarking can be used to measure and compare organizations, business units or functions, or business process, products, or services.

7.11 Questions/problems

1. List three definitions of quality.
2. Give a brief timeline of the evolution of quality.

3. What are the primary elements of TQM?
4. What are the primary contributions of the following quality "gurus": Walter Shewhart, W. Edwards Deming, Joseph Juran, Armand Feigenbaum, Phillip B Crosby, and Kaoru Ishikawa?
5. Are quality costs and the cost of poor quality the same thing?
6. What are the four Quality Cost Categories?
7. Define Lean.
8. What is the difference between a value-adding and non-value-adding activity?
9. Can all non-value-adding activities be eliminated?
10. What does TIMWOODS mean?
11. What are the eight Lean waste categories?
12. What are three different definitions for Six Sigma?
13. What is the defect level for a process running at the six sigma level?
14. When do most companies achieve the six sigma level?
15. What are the two basic Six Sigma models?
16. Which Six Sigma model is used to improve an existing process?
17. Define QbD.
18. When was QbD first introduced?
19. What are the goals of QbD?
20. List and describe the elements of QbD.
21. Define benchmarking.
22. What are the different types of benchmarking?
23. What are the steps for completing a benchmark?

References

Gandhi, A., Roy, C., 2016. Quality by design (QbD) in pharmaceutical industry: tools, perspectives and challenges. PharmaTutor 4 (11), 12–20.
Yu, L.X., Amidon, G., Khan, M.A., Hoag, S.W., Polli, J., Raju, G.K., et al., 2014. Understanding pharmaceutical quality by design. AAPS J. 16 (4).

Further reading

ASQ.org. What is total quality management (TQM)? <https://asq.org/quality-resources/total-quality-management> (accessed 20.05.21).
ASQ.org. Quality 4.0. Retrieved 5/19/2021. Available from https://asq.org/quality-resources/quality-4-0#Evolution.
CQE Academy, Cost of quality. Retrieved 5/25/2021. Available from https://www.cqeacademy.com/cqe-body-of-knowledge/quality-system/cost-of-quality/.
Dague, D.C., 1981. Quality — Historical Perspective, Quality Control in Manufacturing. Society of Automotive Engineers, Warrendale, PA.
DeFeo, J.A., 2015. Juran's Quality Management and Analysis, sixth ed. McGraw Hill Education, New York.

Epicor. What is Industry 4.0—the industrial internet of things (IIoT)? Retrieved 5/19/2021. Available from https://www.epicor.com/en-us/resource-center/articles/what-is-industry-4-0/#:~:text = Industry%204.0%20refers%20to%20a%20new%20phase%20in,on%20interconnectivity%2C%20automation%2C%20machine%20learning%2C%20and%20real-time%20data.

Evans, J.R., Lindsay, W.M., 2015. An Introduction to Six Sigma and Process Improvement, second ed. Cengage Learning, Stamford, CT.

Focus, 2016. Quality Gurus and their key contributions. Retrieved 5/19/2021. Available from https://www.focusstandards.org/quality-gurus-key-contributions/.

Kranzberg, M., Hannan, M.T., History of the organization of work. Encyclopedia Britannica. Retrieved 5/19/2021. Available from https://www.britannica.com/topic/history-of-work-organization-648000.

Lubrizol Life Science, 2019. Quality by design. Available from https://lubrizolcdmo.com/wp-content/uploads/2020/01/TB-36-Quality-by-Design.pdf.

Malchi, G., McGurk, H., 2001. Increasing value through the measurement of the cost of quality (COPQ) — a practical approach. Pharmaceutical Engineering 21-3, pp. 92—96.

Osgood, A., 2012. Quality management 2.0: Deming's 7 deadly diseases of management. Quality Magazine. Retrieved 5/25/2021. Available from https://www.qualitymag.com/articles/88324-quality-management-2-0-deming-s-7-deadly-diseases-of-management.

QG, Quality Gurus, Retrieved 5/19/2021. Available from https://www.qualitygurus.com/category/gurus/.

Sarwar, B., Hasnain, M.S., Rahman, M., Swain, S., 2019. Introduction to quality by design (QbD): fundamentals, principles, and applications from pharmaceutical quality by design: principles and applications. Elsevier Sci. Technol.

Sayer, N.J., Williams, B., 2012. Lean for Dummies, second ed. John Wiley & Sons, Inc, Hoboken, NJ.

Skhmot, N., 2017. The 8 wastes of lean. The lean way blog. Retrieved 5/27/2021. Available from https://theleanway.net/The-8-Wastes-of-Lean.

Summers, D.C.S., 2018. Quality, sixth ed. Pearson Education, New York.

The MEP Network, 2006. Lean and environment training modules, version 1.0. Retrieved 5/27/2021. Available from https://www.epa.gov/sites/production/files/2015-06/documents/module_1_intro_lean.pdf#:~:text = Lean%20is%3A%20%E2%80%9CA%20systematic%20approach%20to%20identifying%20and,Toolkit%20%20%7C%20January%202006%20%7C%20Slide%206.

United States Food and Drug Administration, 2006. Guidance for industry quality systems approach to pharmaceutical CGMP regulations. Available from https://www.fda.gov/media/71023/download.

United States Food and Drug Administration, 2009. Guidance for industry Q8(R2) pharmaceutical development. Available from https://www.fda.gov/media/71535/download.

CHAPTER 8

Corrective and preventive action

8.1 Introduction

This chapter provides a broad review of the application of corrective and preventive action (CAPA) in the pharmaceutical industry. The chapter begins with an overview and background of CAPA. It follows with a discussion about the different approaches for implementing a CAPA program, using as few as five steps or as many as nine steps. Then, the final and most comprehensive part of this chapter discusses and demonstrates various quality tools and techniques that can be used to implement a CAPA program. The tools and techniques discussed include brainstorming, check sheets, root cause analysis (RCA), Pareto diagram, flowchart, histogram, cause-and-effect (C&E) diagram, scatter diagram, run chart, control chart, Kepner–Tregoe (KT) problem analysis, nominal group technique (NGT), 5 WHYs, failure mode and effects analysis (FMEA), decision matrix, process capability, and descriptive statistics.

8.2 Overview of corrective and preventive action

CAPA can be viewed as part of a company's quality management system (QMS) as well as a system or program for correcting and preventing nonconformances. The United States Food and Drug Administration's (FDA's) Guidance for Industry, Quality Systems Approach to Pharmaceutical Current Good Manufacturing Practice (CGMP) Regulations define CAPA as "a well-known CGMP regulatory concept that focuses on investigating, understanding, and correcting discrepancies while attempting to prevent their recurrence." This quality system approach discusses CAPA as three separate concepts—that is, remedial corrections, RCA, and preventive action. The foundation for the guidance is the Code of Federal Regulations (CFR). For medical devices, the FDA has a dedicated CAPA section in the CFR, for example, 21 CFR Subpart J, Section 820.100. However, for the pharmaceutical industry, the CFR is not direct. It is vaguely referenced with records and corrective action in Subpart J, Section 211. Similarly, corrective action is mentioned in ISO 9001:2015. On the other hand, the Q10 Pharmaceutical Quality Systems guidance published by the International Council for Harmonization (ICH) of Technical Requirements for Pharmaceuticals for Human

Quality
DOI: https://doi.org/10.1016/B978-0-323-90815-3.00012-8

Use listed a CAPA system as one of the elements of a quality system. Moreover, the guidance states that:

The pharmaceutical company should have a system for implementing corrective actions and preventive actions resulting from the investigation of complaints, product rejections, nonconformances, recalls, deviations, audits, regulatory inspections and findings, and trends from process performance and product quality monitoring. A structured approach to the investigation process should be used to determine the root cause.

This guidance is much more direct than the CFR, and it also includes a table on how a CAPA system can be implemented throughout the product life cycle.

In general, these regulatory bodies will not dictate how companies must implement a CAPA system or program; however, they do expect companies to address how they will conduct investigations, determine probable root causes, and implement corrective actions. Corrective *action* is defined in several regulations and guidances:

- "action to eliminate the cause of a detected nonconformity or other undesirable situation" (ICH Q10).
- "a reactive tool for system improvement to ensure that significant problems do not recur" (Guidance for Industry, Quality Systems Approach to CGMP Regulations).
- "action to eliminate the cause of a nonconformity and to prevent recurrence." (ISO 9000:2015).

The corrective *actions* that may be taken can be defined as the process for reacting to the product problems, customer complaints, or nonconformances to eradicate the causes and prevent them from recurring.

The regulations and guidances also clearly define preventive *action*:

- "action to eliminate the cause of a potential nonconformity or other undesirable potential situation:" (ICH Q10).
- "action taken to eliminate the cause of a potential discrepancy or other undesirable situation to prevent such an occurrence" (Guidance for Industry, Quality Systems Approach to CGMP Regulations).

Preventive *actions* follow a proactive approach to detecting nonconformances and undesirable situations with the goal of preventing them before they occur.

8.3 Implementing corrective action and preventive action

As noted in Section 8.1, regulatory bodies will not dictate how companies implement a CAPA system or program. Research shows that the number of steps used to implement a CAPA program vary from five to nine. The following are some of the approaches:

- *Five-step approach*: 1. Identification, 2. Evaluation, 3. Investigation, 4. Implementation, and 5. Verification (Markins, 2014).

- *Five-step approach*: 1. Initiate CAPA, 2. Investigate, 3. Form solution, 4. Implement, and 5. Monitor effectiveness (https://www.pharmamanufacturing.com/articles/2019/perfecting-capa/).
- *Six-step approach*: 1. Analyze, 2. Investigate, 3. Identify corrective action (CA) and preventive actions (PA), 4. Verify and/or validate CA and PA, 5. Implement CA and PA, 6. Evaluate effectiveness (Rodriquez-Perez, J., 2010).
- *Seven-step approach*: 1. Identification, 2. Evaluation, 3. Investigation, 4. Analysis, 5. Action plan, 6. Implementation, and 7. Follow-up steps (https://pres.net.in/2012/10/31/7-steps-of-corrective-action-preventive-action-ca-pa/).
- *Seven-step approach*: 1. Identify, 2. Evaluate, 3. Investigate, 4. Analyze, 5. Create, 6. Implement, and 7. Evaluate (https://www.ptc.com/en/blogs/plm/what-is-capa-in-pharma).
- *Nine-step approach*: 1. Identification, 2. Risk/Impact assessment, 3. Evaluation, 4. Data gathering and analysis, 5. Investigation, 6. Root cause analysis, 7. Develop CA and PA, 8. Implement action plans, 9. Verify effectiveness (Rodriquez-Perez, 2010).

A detailed evaluation of these different approaches will reveal that they are all similar. The primary difference between them is the amount of detail or number of actions taken during the respective steps. Each company must decide which approach is the best fit for their organization.

8.4 Quality tools and techniques

This section will describe various tools and techniques that can be used to complete a CAPA program. A seven-step approach will be used to describe the tools. Any documentation associated with the CAPA must follow the guidelines established by the company's QMS.

8.4.1 Problem identification

As noted in Section 8.3, the first step of the CAPA process for most of the approaches listed is to identify the problem. In this first step, a detailed explanation of the problem must be developed. To enhance the potential for eliminating the problem, the explanation must include additional details that are not typically included with a customer complaint, product defect or recall, or a regulatory infraction.

A detailed description of the problem must be developed from a careful review of the difference between the ideal state and the current state. Questions that should be asked include:

- What is the actual problem?
- What product, process, system, piece of equipment, production line, service, etc. is not performing at the required level or is not meeting the expected goal?

- Where or in what department is the problem occurring?
- What product, process, piece of equipment, production line, or service is affected by the problem?
- When did the problem occur?
- How long has this problem been occurring?
- Who is the internal customer(s) most affected by this problem?
- Who is the external customer(s) most affected by this problem?
- What is the primary metric used to measure and/or track the problem?
- How and where are the metrics recorded or reported?

After these questions are answered, a concise but detailed problem statement should be developed. The problem statement:

- should be specific. For example, the statement "Defects are occurring in the production department" is not very specific.
- should state facts about the problem that are based on observation or data and not opinions or assumptions. For example, the statement "Line 2 failed validation because the operator didn't properly secure the door to the bioreactor" includes an assumption about the cause of the problem.
- should not be too narrowly defined (i.e., occurs only at Station B on Line 1) or too broadly defined (i.e., occurs each day throughout the facility).
- should not prejudge a root cause. For example, the statement "The problem focus is the fill defect caused by the nozzle on Line B." includes a root cause.
- should not include an implied solution. For example, the statement "The loose bracket of the vial spinner caused a decrease in throughput in finishing." includes a potential root cause and potential solution.

An important part of the investigation is to assign responsibility for conducting each aspect of the investigation. Any additional resources that may be required should also be identified and documented. For example, specific testing equipment or external analysis may be required. It is for this reason that the company should assemble a team to carry out the CAPA process. The development of the problem statement can be completed by management or by a team assembled by management. The next section discusses different types of teams.

8.4.2 Teams

A team can be defined as a small number of people with complementary skills who are committed to a common purpose, performance goals, and approach for which they hold each other mutually accountable. Depending on the focus of the project, several different types of teams can be assembled and the type of team may be called by different names within different organizations.

8.4.2.1 Quality task force

A quality task force is a cross-functional group, generally set up by a senior manager to examine a specific issue that the manager believes is important enough to be investigated by a dedicated team. Ownership, therefore, sits with the senior manager. The members will generally be made up of people who know the task at hand and the group leader will often be a person who has a vested interest in seeing a positive result. The membership will be appointed, rather than by volunteering.

8.4.2.2 Quality department group

This group is similar to a quality task force, except that they will be concerned with a single department and will mainly be made up of members of that department. A few "outsiders" may be drafted if additional expertise is needed. Once again, the task will tend to be set by a senior manager and the team members will be appointed.

8.4.2.3 Quality circle

These are groups of volunteers who meet regularly to identify, analyze, and solve problems related to their jobs. Quality circles are most widely found in Japan and are associated with the work of Dr. Ishikawa. Since the group is a collection of volunteers, the members have complete ownership of the process. The group is often, but not always, chaired by the supervisor of the area. The other main difference between quality circles and other types of quality teams is that they do not just form to look at one problem and then split up. They are ongoing as part of the continuous improvement program.

Another major difference between quality circles and the previous types of teams is that responsibility for implementing the improvements generally rests with the team itself. In the earlier groups, it is often necessary for other parts of the organization—and certainly for senior managers—to be involved in the implementation of recommendations.

8.4.2.4 Quality improvement or project team

These are similar to quality circles apart from the fact that they are cross-departmental and/or cross-functional. Once again, membership is voluntary. However, they are a temporary group of associates from appropriate functional areas with the necessary skills to work on a specific task. After the specific issue is addressed or eliminated, the group is disbanded.

8.4.2.5 Management team

The team is composed of department heads to develop strategic plans. This team may initiate the CAPA.

8.4.3 Quality tools for problem identification

A useful quality tool that can be used to help identify the problem and develop the problem statement is brainstorming.

Brainstorming is a creative method for helping people generate large numbers of ideas in a short space of time. It can be done in a structured way, in which each member of the team offers a suggestion in turn, or as an unstructured session, where everyone shouts out their ideas as they think of them. The process could include a facilitator who acts as a scribe and records all the ideas on a flip chart or board. On the other hand, the participants could write their ideas on a piece of paper or a self-stick note and place them in a predetermined location where they will be sorted according to similar ideas.

The basis of brainstorming is to encourage a group of people to provide a wide range of ideas around a specific topic. Data have shown that a group brainstorming session can generate far more ideas than the same number of individuals working independently.

There are a few rules that must be applied if brainstorming is to be successful:
- the question to be brainstormed is agreed upon in advance and written on the top of the flip-chart or a board;
- there should be no criticism or evaluation of ideas during the session;
- freewheeling—that is, wild ideas—are encouraged;
- the objective should be quantity not quality;
- every idea should be recorded, even repetitions;
- no discussion is allowed until all ideas are gathered;
- all ideas should be evaluated at the end of the session.

After the participants are out of ideas, the papers or self-stick notes are gathered, sorted, and categorized with similar ideas.

8.4.4 Problem evaluation

In this step the magnitude and impact of the problem are determined. To access the magnitude of the problem, various questions should be asked. These questions include:
- What is the estimated size or magnitude of the problem? (e.g., reject rate or percentage, rework percentage, recall percentage, minutes of downtime, percentage of product impacted, number of customers impacted, the scope of the regulatory infraction, scope of deviations, etc.)
- What risks are associated with the problem? (e.g., risks to end-users, regulatory impact, supply chain impact, etc.)
- What is the safety impact of the problem? (e.g., negligible impact, minor impact, moderate impact, critical impact as defined by the company)

- What remediation was implemented to minimize the impact of the problem?
- Which internal customer is impacted? The customer is the person, process, or organization that receives the output. An internal customer is a department or individual within the company who receives a product, service, or information from another department in the company.
- How was the internal customer impacted? (e.g., were they required to shut down a line or process, cancel orders, place the product on hold, recall the product, dispose of the product, etc.)
- Which external customer is impacted? An external customer is a department or individual external to the company who receives a product, service, or information from a supplier.
- How was the external customer impacted? (e.g., were they required to shut down a process or line, cancel orders, place the product on hold, recall the product, dispose of the product, etc.)
- What is the financial impact of the problem for the company?
- Has the problem increased or decreased over time? Are any trends apparent?

Answers to these questions will help determine the magnitude and impact of the problem and prepare the company to transition to the next step, Problem Investigation.

8.4.5 Problem investigation

After the problem has been clearly defined, a detailed problem statement has been developed, and the problem has been thoroughly evaluated, data should be collected to further investigate the problem. All actions taken to resolve or eliminate the problem should be data-driven.

During this step, an exhaustive list of reports, data records, and data sources should be identified. These data sources may include:

- Product and quality data
- Process control records and data
- Process testing records and data
- Device testing records and data
- Equipment records and data
- Inspection reports and data
- Yield reports and data
- Rework records and data
- Returned product reports and data
- Internal and external audit reports
- Customer complaints
- Warranty claims
- Legal claims

- Field service reports
- Deviation reports
  Any specific data storehouses should be included with the listed sources.

8.4.6 Quality tools for problem investigation

A check sheet is an ideal tool for collecting data to support the problem investigation. The check sheet is a data collection form used to systematically collect and compile data so that patterns and trends can be detected and shown. Check sheets use a simple columnar or tabular format to record data. The data collected may be interpreted directly on the form without additional processing.

The check sheet can be used throughout the CAPA process. Initially, it can be used to tabulate high-level data to provide a summary for the problem investigation. Later in the process, the sheet can be used to capture detailed data about processes. An example of a check sheet is shown in Table 8.1. A quick review of the data shows that "Underweight" was the main defect for the week and most of the defects occurred on Monday.

Table 8.1 Check sheet for a vial finishing line.

Defect description	Monday	Tuesday	Wednesday	Thursday	Friday	Saturday	Sunday	Total
Under weight	23	12	27	14	9	21	13	119
Over weight	7	10	5	9	15	8	8	62
No stopper	5	0	0	8	3	2	2	20
Dirty	0	3	1	3	3	1	2	13
Total	35	25	33	34	30	32	25	214

8.4.7 Problem analysis

The primary goal of this step is to identify the root cause of the problem identified in the previous steps. The root cause is the condition or interrelated set of conditions that caused or allowed a defect to occur. It is the thing or condition that sets into motion the C&E chain that causes the problem. If the root cause is corrected or eliminated, recurrence of the defect can be permanently prevented. A general definition of analysis is the examination of processes, facts, and data to gain an understanding of why a problem occurs and where opportunities for improvement exist. When the analysis is combined with the pursuit of a root cause, RCA results. The Institute for Safe Medication Practices Canada defines RCA as "a structured process for reviewing an event, with the goals of determining what happened, why it happened and what can be done to reduce the likelihood of recurrence."

Andersen and Fagerhaug (2006) depict the root cause chain as a hierarchy showing the root cause as "the evil at the bottom." That root cause sets into motion the cause-and-effect chain that causes the problem. The root cause sits at the lowest level with three other levels above it, for example, the higher-level cause, the first-level cause, and the symptoms, respectively. The symptom reflects the visible results of a cause, and the downward chain will lead to the actual root cause.

This RCA approach combined with several tools can be used to complete the CAPA process. The next section will list some of the tools that can be used.

8.4.8 Quality tools for problem analysis

In Chapter 7, it was noted that Ishikawa emphasized the use of many statistical tools in the determination, evaluation, and analysis of causes of problems. He believed that "As much as 95% of quality-related problems in the factory can be solved with seven fundamental quantitative tools." Those seven tools (check sheet, Pareto diagram, flowchart, histogram, C&E diagram, scatter diagram, and control chart) as well as a few others (except for the check sheet which was discussed in Section 8.4.6) will be discussed in this section.

8.4.8.1 Flowchart

Before using any of the quality tools in this section, the CAPA team should develop a flowchart of the process where the problem occurs. A flowchart, also called a process map or process flowchart, displays a graphic pictorial representation of all the steps involved in an entire process or a segment of a process. It is useful for examining the sequence of tasks or steps in a process and how the various steps relate to one another.

Flowcharts are drawn using symbols that represent different types of activity within the process. At the simplest level, a rectangle is used to denote a process step, whereas a diamond is used to denote a decision point. It is important that the boundaries of the process are clearly defined from the start and that arrows are used to show the direction of flow. The following steps can be used to develop a flowchart:
1. Define the process boundaries
2. Define the process steps
3. Sequence the steps
4. Place the steps in appropriate flowchart symbols
5. Evaluate the steps for completeness

Fig. 8.1 shows a simple flowchart describing the process of moving from customer inquiry, via purchase order to manufactured and approved product for dispatch.

8.4.8.2 Kepner—Tregoe problem analysis

In the late 1990s the Kepner—Tregoe (KT) Institute introduced a problem analysis approach that utilized a matrix to capture the details of a problem in four dimensions.

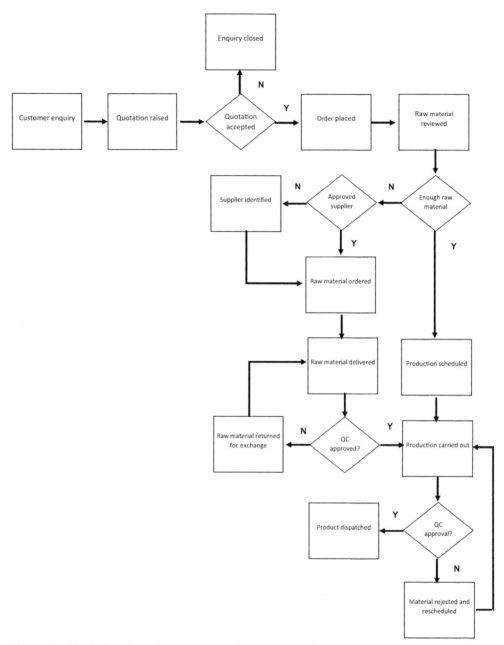

Figure 8.1 Simple flowchart of customer enquiry to product dispatch process.

Table 8.2 Example of Kepner–Tregoe problem analysis table.

Is	Could be but is not
What: Where: When: Extent:	

The approach analyses a problem using an "Is" and "Is Not" column and the following four dimensions:

- Identity—"What is it we're trying to explain?"
- Location—"Where do we observe it?"
- Timing—"When does it occur?"
- Magnitude—"How serious? What is the Extent?

After Table 8.2 is populated, potential causes of the problem can be identified and ranked as to whether the cause is likely the root cause.

8.4.8.3 Cause-and-effect diagram

The C&E diagram, also called the Ishikawa diagram (giving homage to its developer) and fishbone diagram (because it resembles the bones of fish), is an effective tool for displaying the possible causes of a problem (the effect). The diagram is also used to sort the possible cause into useful categories. Free templates for this diagram are readily available online or the team can easily develop the diagram using standard software. The following steps can be used to create the C&E diagram:

1. Identify the problem.
2. Write a short description of the problem on the right-hand side of the page or flip chart. This is considered the head of the fish.
3. Draw a horizontal line (the spine of the fish), extending from the head, from right to left.
4. Write cause categories as lines extending from the spine of the fish and label each category. The categories may vary according to the process diagramed; however, the categories should be generic to maximize the likelihood that all causes will be listed.
   a. The recommended categories for a manufacturing process are:
      i. Machine (equipment),
      ii. Method (how things are done),
      iii. Material (components or raw material),
      iv. Measurement (equipment or manual measurements),
      v. People or Manpower (any person involved with the process),
      vi. Environment (buildings, logistics, space, atmospheric environment) or Information if the problem relates to a digital process.

   b. The recommended categories for a service process are:

     i. Policies,

     ii. Procedures or Methods,

     iii. People or Manpower,

     iv. Measurement,

     v. Information.

5. Use brainstorming to identify possible causes and place them under the applicable category. If necessary, subcategories may be listed under the primary category.

6. After an exhaustive list of possible causes have been identified and the diagram is completed, the team should rank each cause for its perceived impact on the problem. The likelihood that a cause is the root cause can be used to rank the perceived impact on the problem. The following categories can be used:

   a. High (most likely the root cause),

   b. Medium (somewhat likely the root cause),

   c. Low (least likely the root cause).

7. After ranking of the causes, the team can proceed with investigating the "High" potential causes.

Fig. 8.2 shows a C&E for hair in vial problem at the manufacturer of a sterile product. The six recommended categories for manufacturing were used to capture potential causes of the hair problem.

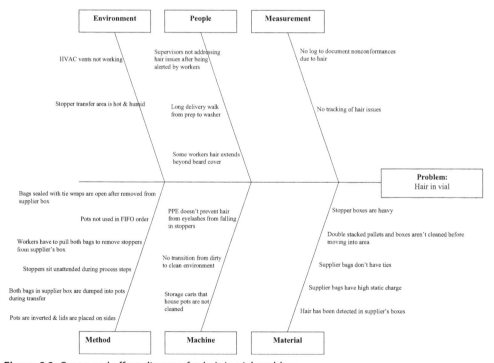

Figure 8.2 Cause-and-effect diagram for hair in vial problem.

8.4.8.4 5 WHYs

This tool, also called the WHY–WHY diagram, is another one that can be used to identify the root cause of a problem. The tool organizes the thinking of a group and illustrates them as a chain of symptoms (similar to the C&E chain discussed in Section 8.4.8.3) leading to the true cause of the problem. When using this tool, the causes identified are written on the diagram in single, clear statements. Each cause should be supported by facts as much as possible. The investigation and chain of causes are continued through as many levels as needed until the root cause is found. It suggested that at least five causes are identified for each chain. The end of the chain will indicate areas that need to be addressed to resolve the original problem or the root cause of the problem. The following steps should be followed to use this tool:

1. On the left side or the top of a flip chart, board, or piece of paper, state the problem to be resolved or the cause to be evaluated.
2. Ask the group "Why does this issue or problem exist?"
3. To the right of the problem statement (or on the next level below), record the response as a short statement of a cause.
4. From the answers given, ask "Why does that issue or problem exist?"
5. Repeat Steps 3 and 4 at least five times or until the group agrees that the root cause of the problem is found or the group agrees that it's useless to go any further.

8.4.8.5 Failure mode and effects analysis

FMEA is a tool used to identify the ways that a product, process, or service can fail and the effects of the failure. A systematic approach is used to generate a list of potential failures, rank the critical characteristics, and generate a list of actions that can be taken to eliminate the causes of failures or reduce their rate of occurrence.

Different types of FMEAs can be used to address different issues. The different types and how they can be used are as follows:

- Systems FMEA:
  - Used to optimize a system design and determine the ways that the system can fail.
  - Used to study the functions of a system and reveal whether or not design deficiencies exist.
  - Used for service and manufacturing systems.
- Product or design FMEA:
  - Used during product development to identify potential product failure modes and their likelihood of occurring.
- Process FMEA:
  - Used to assist in the design or redesign of manufacturing, assembly, or service processes.
  - Used to identify the different ways that a process can fail and results of the failure.

Examples of how this tool has been utilized at a sterile products pharmaceutical manufacturing facility are:

- to evaluate potential failures of a glass washer,
- to evaluate potential failures of a sterilization conveyor,
- to evaluate potential failures of a liquid filler,
- to evaluate potential failures of a capper.

To complete an FMEA, a template must be used. There are many options for free downloads online or a template can easily be developed using Excel or similar software. An example of a template from https://goleansixsigma.com/failure-modes-effects-analysis-fmea/ is shown in Fig. 8.3 and a populated template for a vial washer is shown in Fig. 8.4.

The following steps should be followed to populate the template:

1. Study the process, system, service, or part:
   a. Review the flowchart, C&E diagram, 5 WHYs results, KT problem analysis results, the NGT results, and any other brainstorming ideas for the process or service.
2. Identify and record the process or system that the FMEA will focus on.
3. List process steps or inputs that are of concern for this process or system.
4. In the "Failure Mode" column, list one or more potential failures (one failure per row) for each key process step or input.
5. List the effect of each failure.
6. List potential causes of the failures.
7. On a scale of 1−10 (no effect to hazardous), rate how severely the customer, process, equipment, or operation will be impacted by the failure. The rating is recorded in the "Severity" cell for the applicable failure.

Figure 8.3 Copy of the free template provided at https://goleansixsigma.com/failure-modes-effects-analysis-fmea/.

FMEA														

Process/Product Name: Vial Washer _____   Prepared By: _____

Responsible: _____   FMEA Date (Orig.): _____   (Rev.): _____

Process Step/Input	Potential Failure Mode	Potential Failure Effects	SEVERITY (1 - 10)	Potential Causes	OCCURRENCE (1 - 10)	Current Controls	DETECTION (1 - 10)	RPN	Action Recommended	Resp.	Actions Taken	SEVERITY (1 - 10)	OCCURRENCE (1 - 10)	DETECTION (1 - 10)	RPN
What is the process step, change or feature under investigation?	In what ways could the step, change or feature go wrong?	What is the impact on the customer if this failure is not prevented or corrected?		What causes the step, change or feature to go wrong? (how could it occur?)		What controls exist that either prevent or detect the failure?			What are the recommended actions for reducing the occurrence of the cause or improving detection?	Who is responsible for making sure the actions are completed?	What actions were completed (and when) with respect to the RPN?				
Line 104 Washer	Belt Ripped (Setup 5mL to 2mL)	Downtime	10	Misaligned fingers	10	None	10	1000	Create STW for setup instructions	Improvement Team					0
Line 104 Washer	Elevator setup wrong	Vials fall before reaching grabber	8	Loose and wrong set	10	None	10	800	Verify belts are not Create STW for setup instructions	Improvement Team					0
Line 104 Washer	Scroll (Worm)	Stops production	1	Vial breakage	8	Adjust loading	10	80	Add Redundant Sensor to monitor impact	Maint / MS&T					0
Line 104 Washer	Scroll (Worm)	Stops production	1	Gaps in glass loading	4	Adjust loading	10	40	No action <100						0
								0							0
								0							0

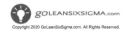

Figure 8.4 A completed FMEA for a vial washer issue.

8. On a scale of 1−10 (highly unlikely to almost inevitable), rate the likelihood that the failure will occur. The rating is recorded in the "Occurrence" cell for the applicable failure.

9. On a scale of 1−10 (absolute certainty the failure will be detected to absolute uncertainty that the current controls will detect the failure), rate the likelihood that the existing controls or control system currently in place will detect and/or prevent the failure. The rating is recorded in the "Detection" cell for the applicable failure.

10. Multiply the severity, occurrence, and detection ratings together to calculate a risk priority number (RPN) for each failure.
    a. The highest possible RPN would be 1000 and the lowest RPN would be 1.
    b. Low ratings indicate lower risk.
    c. If any process variable has a high rating of 9 or 10, the first focus should be on these variables.

11. Prioritize the RPN from highest to lowest and determine the recommended actions to take to minimize the risk to the customer.

Prior to using this tool, the company must develop the scale ratings for the severity, occurrence, and detection and use those ratings for any FMEA that is competed.

8.4.8.6 Nominal group technique

NGT is used to determine priorities among a list of problems that a team has identified. It is a structured method of brainstorming that encourages contributions from everyone and facilitates quick agreement on the relative importance of issues, problems, or solutions. This technique could be used at any time in the Problem Analysis step where a decision needs to be made about the importance of a problem, cause, or course of action. The steps for using this technique are as follows:

1. State the problem, issue, or cause that is the subject of the brainstorming session and ensure that everyone understands.
2. Each team member is asked to silently think of solutions or ideas that come to mind when considering the problem or issue and write down as many as possible. Five to ten minutes are typically given to complete this step.
3. Each member is asked to state aloud one idea. The facilitator records the idea on the flipchart or board.
   a. No discussion or questions for clarification are allowed during this step.
   b. Ideas stated can be taken from team members' written lists or ideas generated from others' ideas.
   c. During this process, a member may "pass" his or her turn and may then add an idea on a subsequent turn.
   d. Continue around the group until all members pass or until an agreed-upon length of time has passed.
4. The facilitator selects an item from the list and the team discusses the item.
   a. The wording of the idea may be changed only when the idea's originator agrees.
   b. An idea may be stricken from the list only when it is a duplicate or when there is unanimous agreement to remove it.
   c. The discussion may clarify meaning, explain the logic, raise and answer questions, or lead to agreement or disagreement.
   d. The group may also combine ideas into categories.
   e. This step is repeated until all the items are discussed.
5. The group prioritizes the recorded ideas about the original question using a point system.
   a. For small lists (up to 10 items), scoring is used for all items. For example, the most important item in a list of 5 items is scored as "5," the next is scored as "4" and so on.
   b. For a longer list, the "one half plus one" rule may be applied. For example, in a list of 20 items, the most important item is scored as "11," the next is scored as "10" and so on.
6. The individual scores are added up and the item with the highest score is the one of most importance to the group or is selected as the final decision.

Problem/team members	1	2	3	4	5	Total
A Equipment breakage	2	1	3	3	5	14
B Missing documents	5	4	2	5	4	20
C Due dates missed	3	5	1	4	3	16
D Sampling training	4	3	4	2	2	15
E Laboratory temperature	1	2	5	1	1	10

Figure 8.5 Nominal group technique example.

a. Other variations of this technique include estimating the amount of work required to implement each solution by assigning it a point value, where the higher the point value, the more work involved.

Fig. 8.5 shows an example of an NGT analysis carried out on a list of problems identified by a quality control laboratory quality team of five people. It can be seen that "missing documents" is the most important item, followed by "due dates missed."

8.4.9 Data analysis

As the team continues to analyze a problem, data will be collected and analysis of the data will be required. The best way to summarize, organize, or display the data will depend on the type of data collected. Data are an objective fact that describes people, objects, and events in an organization until it is organized in a form that humans can interpret.

There are two types of data:

- Attribute or qualitative (sometimes called categorical) data refer to those quality characteristics that are observed to be either present or absent, conforming or nonconforming or values that can only be placed into categories, that is, pass/fail, yes/no, stopper color, line number, and equipment type.
- Variable or quantitative (sometimes called numerical) data refer to those quality characteristics that can be measured. There are two categories of variable data:
  - Discrete data arise from a counting process, that is, defects per hour and vials per minute.
  - Continuous data arise from a measuring process, that is, temperature, pressure, and weight.
  - These data answer questions like "how much," "what volume," "how much time," and "how far."

The analysis of data is dictated by the data type. The next two sections discuss methods for analyzing the different data types.

8.4.9.1 Analysis of attribute (qualitative) data
8.4.9.1.1 Frequency table

One of the basic ways to analyze attribute data is with a summary or frequency table. Similar to the check sheet discussed in Section 8.4.6, a summary table tallies the

Table 8.3 Frequency table example.

Defect description	Number of occurrences	% of Defects
Hair in vial	7	14
Underfilled	11	22
Overfilled	1	2
Particles in liquid	3	6
No stopper	23	47
Incorrect label	4	8
Total	49	

frequencies or percentages of items in a set of categories so that differences between categories can be seen. This is an ideal tool for tallying defects.

After the table has been populated, frequencies or percentages for the different categories can be calculated. The frequency is calculated by dividing the number of occurrences for each category by the total number of occurrences. For example, in Table 8.3, the total number of defects recorded for a line was 49. The frequency (percentage) for each type of defect is found by dividing the number of occurrences by the total number of defects, for example, frequency of "Underfilled" defects = $11/49 = 0.22 \times 100 = 22\%$. After calculating the frequencies, it is clear that the "No stopper" defect occurred most frequently and "Overfilled" was the least occurring defect.

8.4.9.1.2 Bar chart

The data in Table 8.3 can also be displayed graphically using a bar chart. With a bar chart, each bar shows a category and the length of the bar represents the amount, frequency, or percentage of values falling into a category. Excel or most statistical software can be used to create a bar chart. Fig. 8.6A shows a bar chart for the number of occurrences, and Fig. 8.6B shows a chart for the frequencies for the data in Table 8.3. As shown, the bars in the chart can be displayed horizontally or vertically.

8.4.9.1.3 Pie chart

Another graphic that can be used to display attribute data is the pie chart. A pie chart displays a circle broken up into slices that represent categories. The size of each slice of the pie varies according to the count or percentage in each category. Excel or most statistical software can also be used to create this chart. Fig. 8.7 shows a pie chart for the number of occurrences and the frequencies for the data in Table 8.3.

8.4.9.1.4 Pareto chart

A Pareto chart, named after its creator Vilfredo Pareto, is a graphical tool that ranks the causes of problems from the most significant to the least significant. The chart

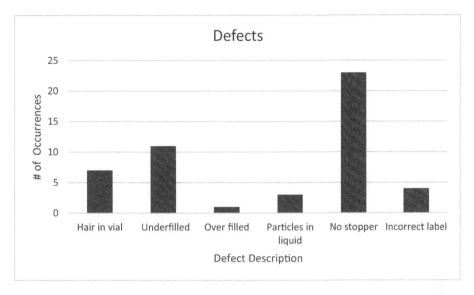

(A)

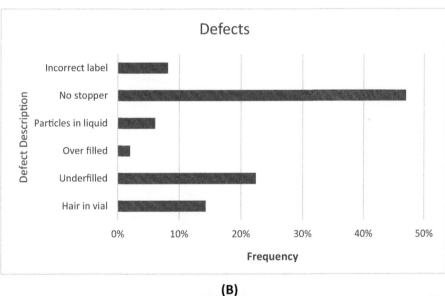

(B)

Figure 8.6 Bar chart showing (A) the occurrence of defects as vertical bars and (B) the frequency of defects as horizontal bars.

displays the categories of data with a vertical bar in the descending order of occurrence along with a cumulative frequency curve. The ultimate goal of the chart is to help identify the "vital few" from the "trivial many" causes of a problem. Fig. 8.8 shows a Pareto chart for the data shown in Table 8.3. The chart shows the count of

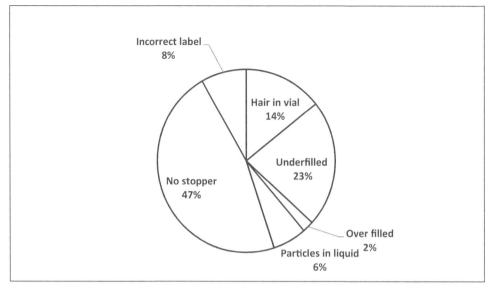

Figure 8.7 Pie chart showing the occurrence of defects.

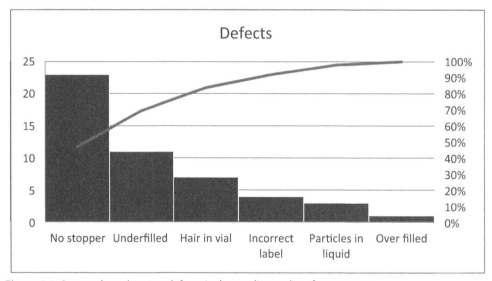

Figure 8.8 Pareto chart showing defects is descending order of occurrence.

defects on the left axis, the percentage of defects on the right axis, and the cumulative percentage is shown by the curve. Ideally, if the causes that fall under the 80% location of the curve can be eliminated, the majority of the problem will be eliminated. Excel or most statistical software can also be used to create this chart.

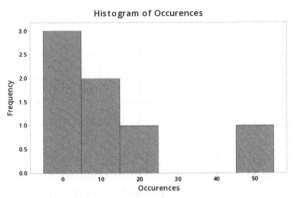

Figure 8.9 Histogram of defect data showing relative frequencies.

8.4.9.1.5 Histogram

The histogram is another graphic that can be used to display attribute data. The histogram is a vertical bar chart of the data in a frequency distribution. With a histogram, there are no gaps between adjacent bars, the class boundaries (or class midpoints) are shown on the horizontal axis, and the height of the bars represents the frequency, relative frequency, or percentage. The histogram can be used to display both qualitative and quantitative data. Excel or most statistical software can also be used to create this chart. Fig. 8.9 shows a histogram created with the data in Table 8.3.

8.4.9.2 Analysis of variable (quantitative) data

As noted earlier, quantitative or numerical data represent quantities that result from a counting or a measuring process. In addition to charts and graphs, the CAPA team should analyze any numerical data collected during their investigation.

8.4.9.2.1 Descriptive statistics

As a minimal, the team should calculate descriptive statistics (also called summary statistics) that characterize the central tendency and the variation of a collection of data. The central tendency describes the extent to which all the data values group around a typical or central value. The three measures of central tendency that will be discussed are the mean, median, and mode. Variation describes the amount of dispersion or scattering of the values. The three measures of variation that will be discussed are the range, variance, and standard deviation. Each of these statistics tells a story about the data.

- Mean, also called the average, is the most common measure of central tendency. It is the sum total of all data values divided by the number of data points. For example, if actual fill volumes were collected to better understand the extent of the under or over fill defects listed in Table 8.3, the average fill volume could be calculated.

- When the mean is calculated, the team should be cautious of extreme values that might distort the true mean; however, an extreme value should not be deleted from the data set unless an assignable cause is identified and eliminated.
- The average number of occurrences of defects for the Table 8.3 data is 49 divided by $6 = 8.17$.

- Median is the midpoint (50% above, 50% below) of the data after it is arranged in ascending or descending order. For an even number of values, the median is the average of the two middle values. The median is not affected by extreme values.
  - The median number of occurrences of defects for Table 8.3 data is 5.5.
- Mode is the most frequently occurring number in a data set. The mode is not affected by extreme values. The analysis may show that there are several modes or no mode.
  - There is no mode for the number of occurrences of defects for the Table 8.3 data because no value occurs more than once.
- Range is the simplest measure of variation and is found by calculating the difference between the largest and smallest value in a collection of data. The range can be displayed as one number or the spread between the largest and smallest number.
  - The range for the number of occurrences of defects for Table 8.3 data can be stated as 22 or from 1 to 23. This shows that the number of occurrences varied significantly.
- Variance is a measure of the amount by which a value differs from the mean. It is equal to the sum of the squared deviations from the mean, divided by the sample size or appropriate degrees of freedom. It is not a commonly used statistic. Variance is equal to the standard deviation squared.
  - The variance for the number of occurrences of defects for the Table 8.3 data is 64.97.
- Standard deviation is the average difference between any value in a series of values and the mean of all the values in that series. It is the square root of the variance and shows the variation about the mean. It also shows the dispersion of the data within the distribution. It is the most commonly used measure of dispersion.
  - The standard deviation for the number of occurrences of defects for Table 8.3 data is 8.06.

All these statistics can be calculated with a basic calculator, Excel, or most statistical software. If central tendency measures are calculated and reviewed, the team should also review the measures of variation (dispersion) because those values will provide important additional information about the collection of data.

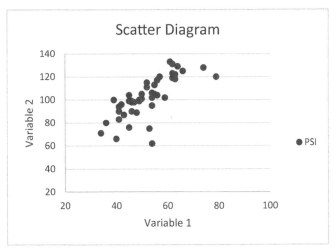

Figure 8.10 Scatter diagram example.

8.4.9.2.2 Scatter diagram

The scatter diagram (or plot) is developed from numerical data, consisting of paired observations of two numerical variables. The plot is used to examine possible relationships between two different numerical variables. The dependent variable (the variable being predicted) is shown on the vertical axis (the y-axis), and the independent variable (the variable that is manipulated) is shown on the horizontal axis (the x-axis). The primary purpose of this diagram is to display whether there is a visual relationship between the dependent and independent variable. Fig. 8.10 shows a positive relationship between Variable 2 and Variable 1. As Variable 1 increases, the pounds per square inch (PSI) for Variable 2 increases. This plot can be created with Excel or most statistical software.

8.4.9.2.3 Correlation

Correlation is a measure of a linear relationship between two variables. The scatter plot shows the visual of the relationship; however, the correlation coefficient should be calculated to quantify the strength of the relationship. The correlation coefficient "r" (also called the coefficient of correlation) can be calculated to determine the degree of association between two variables. The correlation coefficient (r) calculation produces a value between -1 and 1. This number indicates the degree to which the two variables are linearly related. The value can be interpreted as:

- $r = 1$, implies a strong positive relationship;
- $r = -1$, implies a strong negative relationship;
- $r = 0$, implies no correlation, the two variables are independent.

If the calculated correlation coefficient suggests there is a relationship between two variables, care must be taken regarding how changing the x-axis variable will affect the y-axis variable. For the data shown in Fig. 8.10, the calculated correlation coefficient is 0.75. This value agrees with the visual interpretation that there is a positive relationship between the two variables. The coefficient can be calculated with Excel or most statistical software.

8.4.9.2.4 Run chart

A run chart is a simple graph used to study patterns of a numeric variable over time. The chart is a good tool for charting progress, to show changes in a metric, or to show if a process is changing over time. A numeric variable is displayed on the vertical (y-axis), and a measure of time is displayed on the horizontal (x-axis).

Fig. 8.11 shows a chart of reject levels in batches of tablets compressed over a period of months, during which several improvements were made to the machine and its operation.

8.4.9.2.5 Control chart

Control charts were developed by Walter Shewhart in the mid-1920s. Control charts are used to display a series of measurements relating to an individual parameter (e.g., tablet weight on a compression machine), to determine whether the process is statistically under control. The control chart is a run chart with a statistically calculated upper control limit (UCL), lower control limit (LCL), and process average. Control charts are the most powerful tool for analyzing variation in most processes. There are two types of control charts: control charts for attribute or discrete data and control charts for variable or continuous data.

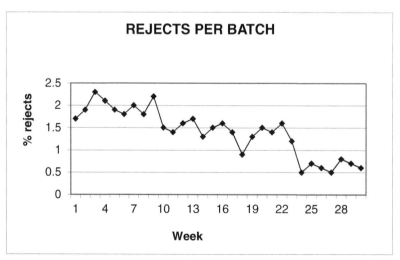

Figure 8.11 Run chart example of tablet rejects.

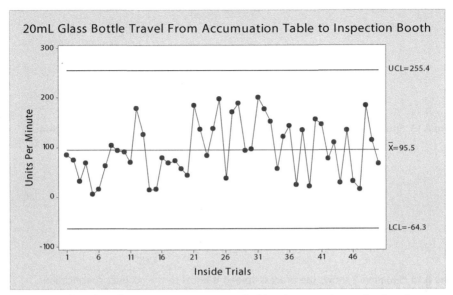

Figure 8.12 An Xbar chart for units per minute travel of bottles to an inspection booth.

Fig. 8.12 shows an Xbar control chart from an experiment on the units per minute travel of bottles to an inspection booth. The goal was 300 units per minute. The chart does not show any points outside the control limits; however, the majority of the data points for trials 21 to 34 are above the centerline. The points should oscillate above and below the line. Also, all the eight previous points are below the centerline. A review of Western Electric Company (WECO) rules will help determine if these points are indications of out-of-control conditions or process instability.

8.4.9.2.6 Process capability

Process capability is a measure of the ability of a process to produce a product or provide services capable of meeting customer specifications. In the assessment of the process capability, specification limits are compared with the six standard deviation (sigma) spread of the process to determine how capable the process is of meeting the specifications. It should be noted that specification limits are the agreed–upon limits with the customer. They are not the same as control limits which are calculated for control charts using process data.

Three different situations can exist when the specifications and the six sigma spread of the actual process data are compared:

- *Situation 1*: The process spread is within the specifications. This is the desired scenario and shows that the process is quite capable of meeting the customer's specifications (Fig. 8.13). LSL refers to the lower specification limit and USL refers to the upper specification limit.

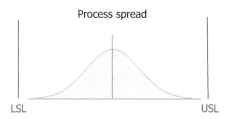

Figure 8.13 Situation 1 shows the process spread is less than the product specifications.

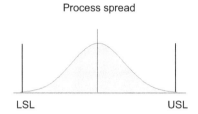

Figure 8.14 Situation 2 shows the process spread is equal to the product specifications.

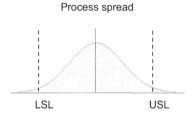

Figure 8.15 Situation 3 shows the process spread exceeds the product specifications.

- *Situation 2*: The process spread is equal to the specifications. Parts produced by this process will be produced within specification as long as the process remains in control and centered. Fig. 8.14 shows this situation.
- *Situation 3*: The process spread is greater than the specifications. This process is incapable of meeting the customer specifications. Fig. 8.15 shows this situation.

Process capability is quantified using calculated capability metrics. Process capability metrics are mathematical ratios that quantify the ability of the process to produce products within the customer specifications. The metrics are based on the performance of individual products or services against the specifications. Two types of metrics can be calculated:

1. C_p is an indicator of the process spread and is the ratio of tolerance. The formula for calculating this metric is:

$$C_p = \frac{\text{USL} - \text{LSL}}{6\sigma}$$

The following guidelines should be used to interpret this metric:
- $C_p > 1$ implies that the process is capable (as shown in Fig. 8.13).
- $C_p = 1$ implies process spread = specification spread and the process is barely capable (as shown in Fig. 8.14).
- $C_p < 1$ implies that the process is not capable and the product produced will not meet specifications (as shown in Fig. 8.15).

2. C_{pk} is another process capability metric. It is an indicator of process centering. The formulas for calculating this metric are:

$$C_{pk} = \min\left(C_{pl}, C_{pu}\right)$$

where $\quad C_{pl} = \frac{\overline{X} - \text{LSL}}{3\sigma} \quad$ and $\quad C_{pu} = \frac{\text{USL} - \overline{X}}{3\sigma}$

$\overline{X}$ = process average

The following guidelines should be used to interpret this metric:
- The goal is to have a C_{pk} 1.
- When $C_p = C_{pk}$, the process is centered.
- A C_{pk} value of zero indicates that the process average is equal to one of the specification limits.
- A negative C_{pk} indicates that the average is outside of the specification limits.

After the CAPA team has reviewed, plotted, and analyzed the data, action should be taken to address the problem(s) identified. The next section discusses how to develop action plans to move forward.

8.4.10 Action plan

Once the plots and data are analyzed, the best method for permanently eliminating the problem or for preventing future occurrences should be identified and an action plan should be developed. A decision matrix can be used to rank potential solutions.

8.4.10.1 Decision matrix

A decision matrix is a useful tool for mathematically ranking potential solutions. The following steps should be used for this tool:

1. Conduct a brainstorming session to identify three to five possible solutions that will provide corrective action for your problem.
2. Identify four general criteria for which the long-term solution should be judged. Examples are:
   - The solution's potential to prevent a recurrence of the problem.
   - If the solution addresses the root cause of the problem.
   - If the solution is cost-effective.
   - If the solution can be implemented in a reasonable amount of time.

3. For the four general criteria identified, assign a weight of its relative importance. The cumulative weight of the four criteria must equal 100%. For example, if the potential to prevent recurrence is the most important criterion, it could be assigned a weight of 35%. The other three criteria could be weighted as 25% for the addresses root cause, 25% for cost-effective, and 15% for implementation time.

4. In a table or spreadsheet, list the potential solutions in a column (one solution per row).

5. On the table or spreadsheet, list the four criteria identified in Step 2 as column headers to the right of the solutions column.

6. For the first potential solution, use a score of 1 (very low potential) to 10 (highly likely potential) to rank how well the solution will prevent the recurrence of the problem.
   - Repeat this ranking process for the potential to address the root cause and the implementation time criteria.
   - For the cost-effective criteria, a ranking of 1 implies that the solution will be the costliest and a ranking of 10 implies that the solution will be the least costly.

7. Repeat Step 6 for each potential solution.

8. Determine the mathematical rating for each solution by multiplying the ranking for each criterion by the decimal equivalent of the weight assigned to the criteria in Step 3. For example, if prevent recurrence was assigned 35% and the rank for a solution was 4, multiply 0.35 times 4 for that solution.

9. Repeat Step 8 for each solution and each criterion.

10. For each solution, calculate the cumulative sum for each criterion.

11. The best solution will be the one with the highest cumulative sum and the worst solution will be the one with the lowest overall sum.

Fig. 8.16 shows an example of a decision matrix for potential solutions to address the "hair in a vial" problem. In addition to a variety of potential solutions, the matrix

Decision Matrix Worksheet

	Criteria				Final Rankings				
	Prevent	Addresses	Cost	Timely					
	Prevent Recurrence (%)	Addresses Root Cause (%)	Cost Effective (%)	Timely Implementation (%)	Prevent Recur	Address Root Cause	Cost Effective	Timely Implement	Totals
	50	15	20	15					
Potential Solution									
Enforce employee hair netting	6	6	10	8	3	0.9	2	1.2	7.1
Incoming inspection of supplier's bags	3	3	2	3	1.5	0.45	0.4	0.45	2.8
Replace HVAC units	9	6	1	1	4.5	0.9	0.2	0.15	5.75
Clean storage carts	7	6	8	8	3.5	0.9	1.6	1.2	7.2
Put stoppers at point of use	8	7	8	8	4	1.05	1.6	1.2	7.85

Figure 8.16 Decision Matrix for "Hair in a Vial" Solutions.

shows the weights for the four general criteria and the rankings for each potential solution. The final rankings show that the best decision was "Put stoppers at point of use" followed by "Clean storage carts."

After a solution(s) has been chosen to address the problem, an action plan should be developed. The action plan should include:

- activities and tasks that must be completed;
- resources required (human, equipment, and information);
- new or revised documents;
- new or revised specifications;
- new or revised processes; and
- employee training.

All these thing actions could be summarized in a table or worksheet.

8.4.11 Implementation of action plan

In this step, the action plan is implemented. The team should use a project approach to implementing the plan. The implementation plan should list:

- the activities that must be completed;
- who will do each activity;
- how long each activity is expected to take; and
- when each activity should be completed to meet the organization's goals.

As the activities are completed, they should be summarized and documented in the final CAPA report. The summary should include:

- process, equipment, documents, or process control changes;
- training completed;
- preventive measures taken; and
- lessons learned.

8.4.12 Follow-up

The final step in the CAPA process is the follow-up step. In this step, an evaluation of the actions taken should be completed, similar to an audit. The evaluation should include:

- assessment of the effectiveness of the actions;
- verification that the tasks on the Action Plan have been completed;
- verification that the actions have no other adverse effects;
- validation of the results of the actions;
- verification that the problem has been eliminated or significantly reduced; and
- verification that adequate monitoring has been established.

Any new information found during this step should be added to the final CAPA report.

8.5 Chapter summary

- Corrective action is action to eliminate the cause of a nonconformity and to prevent recurrence.
- Preventive action is action to eliminate the cause of a potential nonconformity or other undesirable potential situation.
- CAPA is the acronym for corrective and preventive action
- A CAPA can be completed in five to nine steps.
- Brainstorming is a creative method for helping people generate large numbers of ideas in a short space of time.
- A check sheet is a data collection form used to systematically collect and compile data so that patterns and trends can be detected and shown.
- RCA is a structured process for reviewing an event, with the goals of determining what happened, why it happened, and what can be done to reduce the likelihood of recurrence.
- Pareto chart is a graphical tool that ranks the causes of problems from the most significant to the least significant.
- Flowchart also called a process map or process flowchart displays a graphic pictorial representation of all the steps involved in an entire process or a segment of a process.
- Histogram is a vertical bar chart of the data in a frequency distribution.
- C&E diagram also called the Ishikawa diagram or a fishbone diagram is an effective tool for displaying the possible causes of a problem (the effect).
- Scatter diagram is a plot used to examine possible relationships between two different numerical variables.
- Run chart is a simple graph used to study patterns of a numeric variable over time.
- Control charts are used to display a series of measurements relating to an individual parameter to determine whether the process is statistically under control.
- NGT is used to determine priorities among a list of problems that a team has identified.
- 5 WHYs is another tool that can be used to identify the root cause of a problem. The tool organizes the thinking of a group and illustrates them as a chain of symptoms leading to the true cause of the problem.
- FMEA is a tool used to identify the ways that a product, process, or service can fail and the effects of the failure.
- Decision matrix is a useful tool for mathematically ranking potential solutions.
- Process capability is a measure of the ability of a process to produce a product or provide services capable of meeting customer specifications.
- Descriptive statistics (also called summary statistics) are used to characterize the central tendency and the variation of a collection of data.

8.6 Questions/problems

1. What is CAPA the acronym for?
2. What regulations reference CAPA?
3. What is the difference between corrective action and preventive action?
4. How many steps are used to complete a CAPA?
5. What quality tool(s) should be used for each CAPA step?
6. What is RCA the acronym for?
7. How should RCA be used to complete a CAPA?
8. What is meant by descriptive statistics?
9. How should descriptive statistics be used to complete a CAPA?
10. How should process capability be used to complete a CAPA?
11. What tools can be used to make decisions for a CAPA?

References

Andersen, B., Fagerhaug, J., 2006. Root Cause Analysis: Simplified Tools and Techniques, second ed. ASQ Quality Press, Milwaukee, WI.

Markins, U., 2014. CAPA management in a GMP environment. SGS life science technical bulletin. <https://www.sgs.com/-/media/global/documents/technical-documents/technical-bulletins/sgs-lss-capa-management-in-a-gmp-environment-en-14.pdf> (accessed 08.07.21).

Rodriquez-Perez, J., 2010. CAPA for the FDA-Regulated Industry. ASQ Quality Press, Milwaukee, WI.

Further reading

ASQ, What is nominal group technique? <https://asq.org/quality-resources/nominal-group-technique> (accessed 14.07.21).

Evans & Linsey, 2015. An Introduction to Six Sigma Improvement & Process Improvement, second ed. Cengage Learning, Stamford, CT.

FDA, 2006. Guidance for industry, quality systems approach to cgmp regulations goleansixsigma.com. failure modes & effects analysis (FMEA). <https://goleansixsigma.com/failure-modes-effects-analysis-fmea/> (accessed 15.07.21).

ICH, 2009. Guidance for industry, Q10 pharmaceutical quality systems institute for safe medication practices Canada. <https://www.ismp-canada.org/index.htm>.

Kepner, C.H., Tregoe, B.B., 1981. The New Rational Manager. Kepner-Tregoe, Inc, Princeton, NJ.

Koziol, D., 2020. What is CAPA in pharma? <https://www.ptc.com/en/blogs/plm/what-is-capa-in-pharma> (accessed 08.07.21).

Levine, D.M., Stephan, D.F., Szabat, K.A., 2017. Statistics for Managers Using Microsoft Excel, eighth ed. Pearson Education, Inc, Boston, MA.

McCormick, K., 2002. Quality. Butterworth-Heinemann, Woburn, MA.

Oddo, F. (Ed.), 1994. The Memory Jogger II. Goal/QPC, Methuen, MA.

PRES, 7 Steps of corrective preventive action. <https://pres.net.in/2012/10/31/7-steps-of-corrective-action-preventive-action-ca-pa/> (accessed 08.07.21).

Rodriguez, J., 2016. CAPA in the Pharmaceutical and Biotech Industries, How to Implement an Effective Nine Step Program. Elsevier Ltd, Boston, MA.

Shafer, P., 2019. Perfecting CAPA. Pharma manufacturing <https://www.pharmamanufacturing.com/articles/2019/perfecting-capa/> (accessed 08.07.21).

Smith, K.A., 2004. Teamwork and Project Management, second ed. McGraw Hill, New York.

CHAPTER 9

Calibration

9.1 Introduction

Within the pharmaceutical industry, measurement is a major activity. Measurements are taken of time, linear dimensions, mass or weight, temperature, volume or capacity, velocity or speed, pressure, heat, electrical values such as current or resistance, and many other things.

Consequently, there is a high level of instrumentation used in the pharmaceutical industry. An instrument is defined as the device used to measure a parameter. It will typically display the value or condition of the parameter and/or feed a signal representing the value or condition to an alarm, controlling device or system.

This instrumentation has a number of uses:

- Monitoring and recording process parameters, for example, a pressure gauge on an autoclave.
- Monitoring and recording environmental conditions, for example, a particle counter.
- Controlling process equipment, for example, a temperature control on a manufacturing reactor.

In all cases, the accuracy of the instruments is a critical factor in ensuring manufacturing continues to take place in a controlled manner and hence the validated status of all processes is maintained.

The process of ensuring instrumentation maintains its accuracy is known as calibration. In this chapter, there is a review of the type of calibration program a typical manufacturing plant would have in place. This is followed by discussions of documentation, classification of instruments, and the calibration laboratory. The chapter closes with a section on training of calibration technicians.

9.2 Objectives of calibration

The definition of calibration is: "The set of operations which establish, under specified conditions, the relationship between values indicated by a measuring instrument or measuring system, or values represented by a material measure, and the corresponding known values of a reference standard" (EU Guide to GMP Glossary).

The objectives of calibration are twofold:

- To review the degree of error between a reading taken from an operational instrument and the same reading taken from a standard instrument.

Quality
DOI: https://doi.org/10.1016/B978-0-323-90815-3.00011-6

- To alter the operational instrument in order to reduce the degree of error to zero or an acceptable level.

Calibration should be considered as one part of the ongoing validation of a facility. It will cover both the production departments and the laboratories.

9.3 Calibration program

All companies should have a formal program for the calibration of their instruments. In summary, the program has a number of stages, all of which need to be addressed:
- All the pieces of equipment that can be defined as instruments are identified.
- A full list of these instruments is produced.
- For each one, the appropriate category is identified (critical, major or reference).
- For each one, tolerance and acceptance limits are determined.
- Written procedures are developed and authorized. These will vary depending on the category of instrumentation.
- The program is defined in terms of schedule and frequency.
- Responsibilities are assigned for the various calibrations.
- Contracts are set up for any calibrations that need to be outsourced.
- Resources, including manpower and equipment, are provided.
- Calibration is carried out and records kept.
- Calibration equipment is maintained in an appropriate manner.

There will be a number of elements to this program, each of which is considered in the following sections.

9.4 Calibration documentation

All companies prepare their documentation is a manner specific to their own policies and procedures. However, there will be a number of generic documents required for the calibration program. These will include:
- a master list or inventory of all instrumentation within the company;
- specifications relating to the performance of each instrument;
- standard operating procedures for the calibration of each type of instrument;
- a planning program listing the individual calibrations to be carried out (preferably as part of the formal planned preventive maintenance program of the company);
- the records of calibrations that have been carried out internally within the company;
- calibration certificates issued internally or by external bodies carrying out calibration on behalf of the company; and
- training plans and records for the calibration technicians.

All calibration records and certificates constitute good manufacturing practice (GMP) records and hence should be completed, stored, and archived in accordance with documentation procedures.

9.4.1 Instrument calibration index

The purpose of this document is to catalog all instruments on a calibration schedule and to trigger the execution of the calibrations at the predetermined times. It should contain a record for each instrument requiring periodic calibration. Each record should include:

- the last due date;
- the last calibration date;
- the expiry date;
- the (next) due date; and
- the calibration period.

Wherever possible, due dates should be planned to coincide with manufacturing plant's planned shutdown dates or preventive maintenance dates.

9.4.2 Specifications

The specification for calibration of an individual instrument is very important and requires appropriate authorization and control. In particular, there are a number of key factors:

- The category of the instrument (see below for full definitions of each category): a critical instrument will be treated significantly differently from a major or a reference instrument.
- Accuracy and range: these should be set to meet the minimum needs of the parameter being measured.
- Calibration period: this should be arrived at to give a reasonable balance between overfrequent calibration and "as found" failures. It may include consideration of, for example: the durability and stability of the instrument, the required accuracy, the nature of the environment and usage, and the degree of criticality of the measured parameter.

9.4.3 Calibration instruction sheet

The calibration instruction sheet is the standard operating procedure, which states how to calibrate an instrument. It should contain all the instructions necessary to ensure a competent craftsperson, following the instructions, will correctly calibrate the instrument. Each calibration instruction sheet should have a unique identity and the appropriate one for each instrument should be included on the instrument calibration index.

The calibration instruction sheet should be signed by the appropriate functions within the company to indicate acceptance of the calibration instructions, the category rating, the accuracy and range. These would include the instrument specialist, a product or process specialist and a representative of quality assurance.

Any changes to the format of the calibration instruction sheet should be authorized by the same signatories. The revisions should be recorded on a revision-tracking sheet, which should list all the material changes from the previous version and a rationale for each.

9.4.4 Worksheet log

The worksheet log is a record of every worksheet produced and should indicate the date it was created, the due date, and the date of completion.

9.4.5 Proforma worksheet

The proforma worksheet is a blank checklist containing instructions common to a particular type of instrument calibration and is used to produce individual, numbered worksheets.

It will contain sections for the technician performing the calibration to enter the following as necessary:
- responses to questions;
- test instrument numbers;
- deviation numbers;
- any other document references;
- results of tests; and
- spaces for indicating completion of tasks with initials and date.
  Proformas are needed for all types of calibrations, such as:
- "*in-situ*" calibration;
- bench calibration; and
- dispatch to external calibrating house.

9.4.6 Worksheets

The worksheet performs two separate functions. First, it is the instruction to carry out a calibration on a specified instrument in a specified time. As such, it is analogous to a works order. Second, after execution of the calibration, it is the record of the work carried out, including:
- the tasks performed;
- the person doing the work; and
- any unusual actions taken.
  Once completed, it will become part of the service history of the instrument.

Worksheets should be generated when the instrument calibration index is reviewed. They are generated from the proforma worksheet appropriate to the type of calibration. Each worksheet needs to have a unique number taken from the worksheet log; in effect a works order number. The number should be clearly marked on each page of the worksheet. The worksheet should also reference:

- the tag number of the instrument;
- the calibration due date; and
- the appropriate calibration instruction sheet.

9.4.7 Generating worksheets

The instrument calibration index should be reviewed at intervals no greater than monthly to determine all instruments with a due date before the end of the following month.

For each calibration identified, a worksheet should be produced, which is given a unique number and recorded in the worksheet log. At the same time, the instrument calibration index should be updated to flag the existence of the worksheet.

9.4.8 Calibration certificates

Calibration certificates should only be issued, or adopted if externally generated, for calibrations that meet the accuracy requirements laid down in the appropriate specification.

Calibration certificates should have a unique certificate number and give a clear indication of the tag number and plant number or manufacturer's serial number of the instrument.

Certificates should be traceable to a national standard, by detailing the identity of the test equipment used or derived from acceptable values of natural physical constants. These can be found in British Standard BS EN ISO 10012: 2003, *Measurement management systems—requirements for measurement processes and measuring equipment*. Alternatively, they can be identified via the National Institute of Standards and Technology, within the US Department of Commerce. The certificates should contain the date calibration was carried out, together with the next due date and date of expiry of the calibration.

There should also be an indication of the person who carried out the calibration and that person's signature to indicate responsibility for the accuracy of the information on the certificate.

Externally produced calibration certificates may not have all the above information. To be adopted they must have the missing information added by hand to complete the minimum requirements. This should be added by a member of the company's internal instrument group and signed and dated.

9.5 Instrument tagging

An instrument tag is the unique identifier applying to each instrument located within the manufacturing plant. Each instrument should be labeled with such a tag carrying a summary of the calibration history of that instrument. The tag should include:

- the ID number of the instrument;
- the date of the previous calibration;
- the due date for the next calibration; and
- the signature of the calibration technician.

9.6 Carrying out calibration

The calibration should be carried out following the instructions in the appropriate calibration instruction sheet, and all appropriate information recorded on the worksheet as each step is completed.

First of all, the "As Found" condition is determined. This is defined as the accuracy of the instrument over the required range before any calibrating adjustment or repairs are made. If the accuracy is outside the limits specified on the calibration certificate, it may indicate faulty product has been produced since the instrument was last known to have been correct. To address this possibility a deviation should be raised in accordance with procedure. It may also be necessary to place on "hold" any product batches which consequentially have suspect quality, depending on the nature of the instrument in question.

The instrument is then calibrated and a final "As Left" condition determined. This is defined as the accuracy of the instrument over the required range after calibration. If the "As Left" condition meets the accuracy requirements, the calibration certificate is completed, and a calibration sticker indicating the calibration date is affixed in a prominent position.

If the "As Left" condition does not meet the accuracy requirements, the technician raises a deviation. The deviation shall address the controls to be used to ensure the instrument is not used for drug products and the actions to repair or replace it. The technician shall therefore in conjunction with departmental personnel, establish if it is necessary to put the associated manufacturing plant on "hold" to prevent inadvertent use on drug products.

When the calibration is carried out and the worksheet is completed, the worksheet log is updated to show the completion date and the instrument calibration index is updated to the new calibration date.

All instruments covered by the calibration program should be calibrated prior to the expiry date. If a critical instrument were used on drug products when its calibration has expired, a deviation would need to be raised which would address the risk to product quality of the batches made during the time since the calibration of the instrument expired. If such an instrument cannot be immediately calibrated or replaced by one that is calibrated, the part of the manufacturing plant to which it relates should be shut down to prevent inadvertent usage on drug products unless an approved deviation allows continued use.

Recalibration may be carried out as part of preventive maintenance procedures in which case a calibration instruction sheet and worksheet would not be needed. However, a calibration certificate should still be generated.

External parties, whether individuals or organizations, may be used for calibrating or repairing instruments. Where they are used, they should be monitored by internal personnel in order to ensure the company's procedure for the control of external parties is met.

9.7 Review of data

When a calibration is carried out, the data obtained should be reviewed. There should be communication at this point between the calibration department and the relevant operational department, whether in production or the laboratories. If the calibration is carried out successfully, it may only be necessary to confirm that the calibration program is up to date. However, if there is a problem with any of the instruments, more detailed information should be provided.

9.8 Different types of standards

There is a hierarchy of standards used within calibration. The following sections provide details on the different standards and their uses.

9.8.1 Absolute standards and international standards

These are the ultimate standards against which all reference equipment is calibrated. For example, all temperature measuring equipment such as thermometers and thermocouples must be traceable to the International Temperature Scale of 1990 (ITS-90). Developed as a practical solution to the difficulties of working with the thermodynamic temperature scale, ITS-90, together with reference thermometers and calculations, provides an accurate basis against which reference and working instruments can be calibrated.

9.8.2 Primary standards

A primary standard is the main equipment used to calibrate the rest of the instrumentation. It is usually maintained at the appropriate National Testing Laboratory or other accredited laboratory and is used as the reference standard against which the company's reference standards are calibrated. It is generally four times more accurate than the secondary standard.

9.8.3 Secondary or reference standards

The secondary standard is the reference standard maintained within the company, which is used to carry out routine calibrations. It is generally four times more accurate than the working instrument.

9.8.4 Measuring standards

The measuring standard is the working instrument used for routine measurement and control within the company. It would be the temperature gauge on an autoclave, for example, which records the temperature during a production cycle.

9.9 Different types of calibration equipment

The types of equipment found in a calibration laboratory will vary with the type of operations the company is carrying out and the types of instrumentation installed around the premises. However, the sort of equipment required will include those shown in Table 9.1.

9.10 Maintenance of calibration equipment

It is important that the calibration equipment is stored and handled in an appropriate manner. As a minimum, the temperature and the humidity of the calibration laboratory should be controlled. The influence of other environmental conditions such as vibrations should also be considered.

9.11 Categorization of instrumentation

The frequency of calibration of individual instruments will vary depending on circumstances such as the pattern of usage, the sensitivity of the process being controlled and/or monitored, the recommendations within the manufacturer's operation and

Table 9.1 Different types of calibration equipment with the relevant instrumentation.

Calibration equipment	Relevant instrumentation
Universal calibrator	Digital equipment
Stable thermobath	Temperature gauge
Dead weight tester	Pressure gauge
Vacuum gauge	Pressure and vacuum gauges
Multipoint temperature scanner and printer	Autoclaves, ovens and sterilizing tunnels
Conductivity calibration jig	Conductivity meter
Standard solution kit	pH meter

maintenance manual, and the history of previous calibration performance. For example, an instrument that has been shown to maintain its previous calibration state over a period of more than 6 months would not necessarily need to be calibrated on a quarterly basis.

However, the key point to be considered in determining frequency of calibration is the process being controlled and/or monitored and in particular, the importance of the level of accuracy obtained. There are three categories of instrumentation: critical, major, and reference instruments.

9.11.1 Critical instruments

Critical instruments are those whose performance will affect both the process and the product. An example of such an instrument would be a temperature control on an autoclave. These instruments would generally be calibrated at least every 6 months.

9.11.2 Major instruments

Major instruments are those whose performance will affect either the process or the product. An example of such an instrument would be a balance in the dispensary. These instruments (and in the context of calibration, a balance may be considered as an instrument) would generally be calibrated at least annually.

9.11.3 Reference instruments

Reference instruments are those installed as reference points only and whose performance do not affect either the process or the product. An example of such an instrument would be a thermometer in an ambient condition warehouse where temperature is monitored, but not controlled. These instruments would generally be calibrated on installation but not afterwards.

9.12 Purchase of new instruments

When a new instrument is purchased, there are a number of steps to be taken as follows:
- First, the instrument should be identified, and the instrument group be informed so they can issue a tag number.
- Second, it must be categorized as critical, major, or reference.
- Finally, this categorization and the rationale behind it is recorded and authorized, ensuring the decision is consistent with company policy.

All critical instruments should be purchased with current calibration certificates that cover appropriate accuracy and range and state a specific expiry date. These certificates must be traceable to national standards. If certificates cannot be supplied with the instrument, there will be a need to carry out initial calibration.

9.13 Review of calibration program

On an annual basis, it is a good idea to review the calibration program to ensure it is still appropriate and effective. There are two key elements that should be reviewed:

- First, the frequency of calibration of individual instruments. As mentioned above, the history of previous calibrations should be taken into account when determining the most appropriate frequency of calibration. There may be some instruments for which a recategorization is appropriate.
- Second, this would be the time to review standard operating procedures to determine whether they need to be amended. For example, the procedure is generally written such that the instrument is tested across the whole of its operational range. However, if an instrument is normally used to measure around one focal point in the range, it may be more appropriate to concentrate the taking of readings around this point.

9.14 Training of calibration technicians

It is necessary to have in place a training program which covers not only the people carrying out the calibration, but also the people reviewing the data to ensure there is full understanding. Like any other part of the training program, there should be a written training plan and full records of all the training already completed. In this way, the company is able to monitor the available skills pool and the ongoing plans to maintain that pool.

Training should be carried out when a person commences a role and also on a regular basis thereafter. Refresher training on at least an annual basis is recommended to ensure standard operating procedures are carried out in the correct manner and no bad habits have been learned over time.

When a new piece of instrumentation is purchased and installed, it is important to ensure all relevant personnel are trained in the new methodology relating to calibration.

9.15 Calibration in good manufacturing practice guidelines

The references to calibration in the international GMP standards are relatively minor. In the EU guidelines, there is a statement that all "Measuring, weighing, recording, and control equipment should be calibrated and checked at defined intervals by appropriate methods. Adequate records of such tests should be maintained" (EU GMP guidelines Chapter 3 paragraph 3.41).

Similarly, there is a statement in the US Code of Federal Regulations:

"automatic, mechanical, or electronic equipment or other types of equipment, including computers, or related systems that will perform a function satisfactorily, may be used in the

manufacture, processing, packing, and holding of a drug product. If such equipment is so used, it shall be routinely calibrated, inspected, or checked according to a written program designed to assure proper performance. Written records of those calibration checks and inspections shall be maintained"

(Title 21 > Chapter I > Subchapter C > Part 211 > Subpart D > Section 211.68). Additionally, the FDA guide to inspection of computer systems in drug processing states sensors on I/O devices: "should be systematically calibrated and checked for signal outputs" (Computerized Systems in Drug Establishments 2/83, Section III B 3).

The Code of Practice for Qualified Persons (see Chapter 5 for more details) specifies that calibration records is one of the items a QP must ensure are in existence before certifying a batch of product for release onto the marketplace.

9.16 Chapter summary

- Measurement is a major activity in the pharmaceutical industry; instrumentation is therefore a critical element.
- An instrument is any device used to measure a parameter. Instruments are used for monitoring, recording and controlling.
- Calibration is the process by which the ongoing accuracy of an instrument is maintained and assured.
- The purpose of calibration is to measure the degree of error in an instrument's reading, relative to a standard instrument, and to adjust that degree of error to an acceptable level.
- All companies must have a formal documented calibration program. There are a number of steps involved in setting up and implementing that program.
- Documentation is prepared in compliance with the company's policies and procedure, but there are a number of different types of documents that should be present.
- The calibration index catalogs all instruments and triggers individual calibrations according to a predetermined schedule.
- The calibration specification identifies the category of the instrument, the accuracy and range, and the calibration period.
- The calibration instruction sheet is the standard operating procedure for a given instrument.
- The worksheet log is a record of every worksheet produced, with dates of creation and completion.
- The worksheet is the checklist used to record the completion of an individual calibration. It is produced from an appropriate template and generated in response to a due date on the calibration index.

- A certificate must be generated for each successful calibration. They must contain sufficient information to identify the specific instrument to which they relate. This will include the instrument tag, its unique identifier.

- Calibration is carried out in a number of steps. The "As Found" condition must be recorded to ensure all batches produced to date are of the correct quality. Following calibration, the "As Left" condition is recorded. Data recorded at both stages should be communicated with the relevant operational department.

- There is a hierarchy of standards used within calibration, with varying degrees of accuracy. All must be traceable back to the relevant national or international standard. All must be stored in appropriately controlled conditions.

- Instruments are categorized as critical, major, or reference depending on their use and impact on the product and/or the process.

- When new instruments are purchased, they should be formally assessed and inserted into the calibration program based on their categorization.

- It is good practice to review the calibration program on an annual basis to ensure it is still appropriate and effective.

- There must be a training program in place for all people involved in calibration, either as technicians or as reviewers of the data.

- There are no guidelines specifically dealing with calibration, but the requirement for calibration is a stated requirement within GMP guidelines.

9.17 Questions/problems

1. What is calibration and why is it a critical part of the control of pharmaceutical manufacturing?

2. You have just been appointed to the role of an Engineering Manager at a small factory producing tablets and capsules. The company has been criticized by the regulators for having an inadequate calibration program. What steps would you take to correct the situation?

3. You are the calibration technician with responsibility for a manufacturing suite producing terminally sterilized injections. List ten instruments you would expect to find on your calibration index.

4. Taking your list of instruments from question 3, categorize them as critical, major, or reference; and identify appropriate frequencies at which each would be calibrated.

5. You are calibrating a balance in the manufacturing suite. The "As Found" condition is outside the permitted range. What actions would you need to take?

6. You are recruiting a new technician for your team. Define the training program you need to have in place.

Further reading

British Standards Institute (2003). BS EN ISO 10012:2003, Measurement management systems—requirements for measurement processes and measuring equipment.

Electronic Code of Federal Regulations Title 21, Chapter 1, Sub-chapter C, Part 211, Subpart D, Section 211.68 *Automatic, electronic and mechanical equipment.* <https://www.ecfr.gov/cgi-bin/text-idx?SID=1d28ece5b89fc653d9ae1d92790f2f95&mc=true&node=se21.4.211_168&rgn=div8>. Accessed 08.09.08.

European Commission Health and Consumers Directorate-General. (2015). EudraLex *The rules governing medicinal products in the European union volume 4 EU guidelines for good manufacturing practice for medicinal products for human and veterinary use Part 1 Chapter 3: premises and equipment.* <https://ec.europa.eu/health/sites/default/files/files/eudralex/vol-4/chapter_3.pdf>. Accessed 09.06.21.

European Commission Health and Consumers Directorate-General. (2015). EudraLex *The rules governing medicinal products in the european union. Volume 4. EU guidelines for good manufacturing practice for medicinal products for human and veterinary use. Glossary.* <https://ec.europa.eu/health/sites/default/files/files/eudralex/vol-4/pdfs-en/glos4en200408_en.pdf>. Accessed 08.06.21.

Royal Pharmaceutical Society, Royal Society of Biology & Royal Society of Chemistry. (2015). *Qualified persons in the pharmaceutical industry code of practice.* <https://www.rsb.org.uk/images/QP_Code_of_Practice_2015v1.pdf>. Accessed 17.05.21.

US Food and Drug Administration. (1983). *Computerized systems in drug establishments.* <https://www.fda.gov/inspections-compliance-enforcement-and-criminal-investigations/inspection-guides/computerized-systems-drug-establishments-283>. Accessed 09.06.21.

CHAPTER 10

Validation

10.1 Introduction

This chapter reviews validation for pharmaceutical manufacturing with a primary focus on process validation. After a brief overview of validation in Section 10.2, the chapter presents definitions of validation and definitions of qualification from various national and world guidances in Sections 10.3 and 10.4. Section 10.5 briefly compares and contrasts validation and qualification to demonstrate how they are different concepts. Section 10.6 discusses the four different types of process validation, namely prospective, concurrent, retrospective, and revalidation. In Section 10.7, the three phases of process validation, namely Stage 1: Process Design/Development, Stage 2: Process Qualification, and Stage 3: Process Verification are discussed. Finally, Section 10.8 ends with a discussion of validation documentation.

10.2 Overview of validation

The topic of validation is a very important one that deserves a lot of careful thought. This section presents an overview. From the simplest definition, validation refers to "the act of confirming something as true or correct" (reference Dictionary.com). In the pharmaceutical industry, this confirming act can include a broad scope, that is, manufacturing operations or processes, instrumentation, product design, equipment, facilities, cleaning, raw materials, packaging materials, test methods/procedures, computerized systems, etc. The primary focus of this chapter is process validation.

The concept of validation was first suggested by two United States Food and Drug Administration (USFDA) officials, Ted Byers and Bud Loftus, in the mid-1970s to address the issues of safety relating to sterility of the large volume parenteral (LVP) market. The first testing activities focused on the processes involved in the manufacture of the LVPs but quickly spread to other related products. Beginning in the late-1970s, the concept of process validation began appearing in good manufacturing practice (GMP) documents and current GMP (CGMP) documents. Validation of manufacturing processes is a requirement of the CGMP regulations for finished pharmaceuticals.

Quality
DOI: https://doi.org/10.1016/B978-0-323-90815-3.00008-6

10.3 Definitions of validation

Today, validation is clearly referenced and defined in national and international GMP guidances including those published by the USFDA, the European Commission, the International Council for Harmonization (ICH), the World Health Organization (WHO), and Pharmaceutical Inspection Co-operation Scheme (PIC/S). The following are a few of the definitions:

- *USFDA*: "Process validation: The collection and evaluation of data, from the process design stage through commercial production, which establishes scientific evidence that a process is capable of consistently delivering quality products." (Reference USFDA Guidance for Industry—Process Validation: General Principles and Practices.)
- *European Commission*: "Process Validation: The documented evidence that the process, operated within established parameters, can perform effectively and reproducibly to produce a medicinal product meeting its predetermined specifications and quality attributes." (Reference EU Guidelines for Good Manufacturing Practice for Medicinal Products for Human and Veterinary Use.)
- *ICH*: "Process Validation (PV) is the documented evidence that the process, operated within established parameters, can perform effectively and reproducibly to produce an intermediate or API meeting its predetermined specifications and quality attributes." (Reference Good Manufacturing Practice Guide for Active Pharmaceutical Ingredients Q7.)
- *WHO*: "Validation: Action of proving, in accordance with the principles of GMP, that any procedure, process, equipment, material, activity or system actually leads to the expected results." (Reference Good Manufacturing Practices for Pharmaceutical Products: Main Principles.)

10.4 Definitions of qualification

Validation and qualification are often mentioned together; however, they are not the same. Validation is defined by the preceding definitions and is sometimes extended to include qualification, whereas qualification typically refers to the ability of a process and its components to produce the specified product. A few definitions of qualification are as follows:

- *USFDA*: "Process qualification: Confirming that the manufacturing process as designed is capable of reproducible commercial manufacturing."
- *European Commission*: "Performance Qualification: The documented verification that systems and equipment can perform effectively and reproducibly based on the approved process method and product specification."

- *ICH*: "Qualification: Action of proving and documenting that equipment or ancillary systems are properly installed, work correctly, and actually lead to the expected results. Qualification is part of validation, but the individual qualification steps alone do not constitute process validation."
- *WHO*: "Qualification: Action of proving that any premises, systems and items of equipment work correctly and actually lead to the expected results."

As the preceding definitions show, validation and qualification are separate concepts, but they are often discussed simultaneously. In practice, qualification of processes is typically required prior to validation and other times it is included as a part of process validation.

10.5 Validation versus qualification

Since validation and qualification are often discussed simultaneously, it is prudent to clearly differentiate how the two are approached. Table 10.1 captures key differences between the two concepts. The lists of differences demonstrate how qualification is primarily equipment focused and validation is primarily process focused.

10.6 Process validation

Process validation requires the identification of critical elements and includes equipment qualification. There are four different types of process validation that can be performed.

1. Prospective validation (premarketing) is completed prior to the distribution and sale of a new drug product or a product made under a modified manufacturing process that is significant enough to potentially affect the characteristics of the product. Included are preplanned tests with acceptance criteria that are measurable and prove that the production is reproducible. It is generally considered acceptable that three consecutive batches or runs within the finally accepted parameters, yielding product of the desired quality, would constitute a proper validation of the process. The preferred validation batches should be of the same size as the intended production scale batches. When this is not practical, a reduced batch size corresponding to at least 10% of the intended batch size for full scale production can be considered.
2. Concurrent validation is completed during normal production where current batches of production are used to monitor process parameters. It includes a preplanned test with acceptance criteria that are measurable. It also involves very close monitoring of at least the first three production-scale batches. This method provides limited assurance of the consistency of quality from batch to batch following the current batch being studied. The FDA prefers this type of validation

Table 10.1 Key differences between validation and qualification.

Category	Qualification	Validation
Primary focus	Refers to objective evidence that equipment or ancillary systems are properly installed, work correctly, and actually lead to the expected results.	Refers to the collection and evaluation of data, from the process design stage through commercial production, which establishes scientific evidence that a process is capable of consistently delivering quality products.
Scope	Qualification is required prior to validation or is included in the validation process.	Validation includes the qualification of equipment and systems, cleaning, analytical methods, computerized systems, raw materials, packaging materials.
Approach	Design qualification (DQ), performance qualification (PQ) or process performance qualification (PPQ), operational qualification (OQ), installation qualification (IQ), equipment, facilities, utilities.	Completed in stages: Process design, process qualification, and process verification, or prospective, retrospective, and concurrent.
Target	Equipment, instruments, and systems.	Processes.
Performance target	Equipment.	Entire manufacturing process.
Outcomes	Main concern is proper functioning of the system and subsystems. Reproducible outcome isn't demanded.	Goal is consistent reproducible outcomes and products.
Manufacturing support	Ensures equipment or systems are installed correctly, operate as required, and perform as intended.	Ensures the process is capable of producing consistent results according to the customer specifications.
Requalification/ revalidation requirements	Requalification needed if: • modifications made to critical systems, • relocation of systems, or software • control system modification.	Revalidation needed if changes to: • process or its environment; • starting material; • packing material; • process steps or procedure; • equipment.

approach to be rarely used. In special situations the product will be released prior to demonstrating full reproducibility. Situations when concurrent validation may be the practical approach include:

- when a previous approved process is moved to the contract manufacturer of a third party to another location;
- when the drug with the same active or inactive ingredient ratio is a different intensity when compared to the previously tested product;
- when the number of lots produced is limited;
- when the process has low volume of output per lot;
- when the manufacturing process is urgently needed due to a shortage of the drug or lack of supply;
- when there is a preapproved protocol for concurrent reasonable validation;
- when a deviation is justified and accepted by the owner, head of quality of the facility, and head of the process;
- when concurrent validation batches are collected in the report and all core disciplines are accepted.

3. Retrospective validation uses extensive data collected over several lots and over time to assess the consistency of a process. This type of validation may be used for older products that were not validated by the manufacturer when they were first marketed and are now being validated to confirm regulatory requirements. This validation is only suitable for well-established comprehensive processes and is unacceptable if recent changes have been made to the composition of the product, the operating procedures, equipment, or facilities.

4. Revalidation is necessary only when a product is made in one facility and transferred to another or if there is a change in the CPPs, composition, primary packaging, raw materials supplier, major equipment, or modification of premises.

Revalidation is divided into two categories: revalidation after a specific change and periodic revalidation. In the former category, typical changes that require revalidation include changes in a raw material or packaging material, changes in the process parameters, changes to equipment, including major repairs and changes to the premises. Additionally, revalidation is required for any changes resulting from a failure investigation. Corrective actions deemed necessary after such an investigation must be brought under the change control procedure, which will determine what aspects of revalidation are required.

A periodic revalidation is the opportunity to check that the systems are still operating as originally validated and that no "drift" (unobserved or unintentional process changes) has taken place over time.

Currently, the FDA expects that all validations are to be prospective with preplanned acceptance criteria that must be met before the validation is considered complete and successful.

10.7 Stages of process validation

Process validation involves a series of activities taking place over the lifecycle of the product and process. The activities of the process validation are divided into three stages: Stage 1: Process design/development, Stage 2: Process qualification, and Stage 3: Continued process verification.

10.7.1 Stage 1: Process design/development

In this stage of process validation, the commercial manufacturing process is defined based on knowledge gained from development and scale-up activities. This is the process that will be reflected in planned master production and control records. The main deliverables from this phase include planned commercial production and control records, which contain the operational limits and overall strategy for process control. Creation of the commercial process includes activities related to: product research and development, formulation pilot batch studies, scale-up studies, transfers of technology to commercial batches, establishing stability conditions and storage, handling of in-process and finished dosage forms, and certification of equipment. In addition to information about the drug product, the validation approach is developed in this stage. Included in the approach are: the validation master plan (VMP), vendor selection, equipment specification, critical process parameter (CPP) selection, critical quality attributes, and development of other quality systems or programs. All of these things should be carried forward to the next stage for confirmation.

10.7.2 Stage 2: Process qualification

During this stage, the deliverables from the process design phase are evaluated to determine whether the process is capable of reproducible commercial manufacturing. The manufacturer is required to run the process developed in the process design phase several times to prove that the process can be maintained in control over time and verify that all established limits for the CPPs are valid and will produce product that meets specifications. This phase is typically the most documented stage since it captures the qualifying of existing products. This phase has two elements: (1) design of the facility and qualification of the equipment and utilities and (2) process performance qualification (PPQ).

In the qualification of the equipment and utilities subphase, the manufacturer should undertake activities that demonstrate equipment and utilities are suitable for their intended use. The activities generally include selection of equipment for the construction of materials and performance characteristics, verification of equipment for installation in compliance with design specifications, and verification that the equipment operates in accordance with anticipated operational ranges and in accordance with the process requirements.

The approach to PPQ subphase should be based on thorough science and the manufacturer's overall level of process and product understanding. The execution of qualification may be as individual plans or as part of an overall project plan and may include:

- Design qualification (DQ) is the process of completing and documenting design reviews to illustrate that all quality aspects have been fully considered at the design stage. The purpose is to ensure that all the requirements for the final systems have been clearly defined at the beginning. In other words, has it been designed and selected correctly?
- Installation qualification (IQ) is the process of checking the installation to ensure that the components meet the approved specification and are installed correctly and how that information is recorded. The purpose is to ensure that all static aspects of the facility or equipment are installed correctly and comply with the original design. In other words, has it been built or installed correctly?
- Operational qualification (OQ) is the process of testing to ensure that the individual and combined systems function to meet agreed performance criteria and recording the results of that testing. The purpose is to ensure that all the dynamic attributes comply with the original design. In other words, does it work correctly?
- Performance qualification (PQ), also called process qualification, is the process of testing to ensure that the individual and combined systems function to meet agreed performance criteria on a consistent basis and how the result of testing is recorded. The purpose is to ensure that the criteria specified can be achieved on a reliable basis over a period of time. In other words, does it produce product correctly?

10.7.3 Stage 3: Continued process verification

In this final validation stage, the goal is continual assurance that the process remains in a state of control (the validated state) during commercial manufacture. This should include adherence to the CGMP requirements, specifically, the collection and evaluation of information and data about the performance of the process which will allow detection of undesired process variability. The assurance of process control should also include strict compliance with the master batch record and a written plan. An ongoing program to collect and analyze product and process data that relate to the product quality must be established. The performance data should be statistically trended and reviewed by trained personnel to verify that the quality attributes are appropriately controlled throughout the process. Evaluation of the performance of the process will identify problems and determine if action must be taken to correct, anticipate, and prevent problems to keep the process in control. In addition to statistical analysis, other process monitoring tools that may be used are control charts and process capability analysis.

10.8 Validation documentation

Documentation at each stage of process validation is essential for effective communication and to establish, monitor, and record all aspects of quality. Documentation serves as an effective method for capturing knowledge gained about a product and process. It should be accessible, comprehensible, and provide transparency about the methods used so the organization units responsible and accountable for the process can make informed science-based decisions that support the release of a quality product.

There are three types of documents related to validation: master plans, protocols, and reports.

10.8.1 Validation master plans

Each company should have a VMP, which describes its overall philosophy, intention and approach to establishing performance adequacy.

It also identifies which items are subject to validation and the nature and extent of such testing. It defines the applicable validation and qualification protocols and procedures.

The VMP is the overall planning document that details what should be covered during the program. It covers who, what, where, when, why, and how. It includes a breakdown of the process, plant or equipment into separate parts. It also determines which are critical to the quality of the product and therefore require validation, and at which stages. For example, in a project to commission a sterile manufacturing suite, the operation of the sterilizers are critical and will require IQ, OQ, and PQ; the operation of the ventilation system is critical and will require IQ, OQ, and PQ; the layout of the suite is important, but could only require IQ.

The VMP should be a concise and easy to read document which will serve as a guide to the validation committee and personnel who are responsible for implementing validation protocols. The VMP should also be viewed as a source document for use by regulatory auditors.

The VMP will always be a brief overview, as well as being a dynamic document, as many details are not finalized at the start of a project. However, if the plan is changed, it must be done under an effective change control procedure.

10.8.2 Validation protocols

A validation protocol is a detailed document relating to a specific part of the validation process, for example, the OQ for a manufacturing vessel. It outlines the tests that are to be carried out, the acceptance criteria and the information that must be recorded. It will also define the approval process for the validation.

The protocol should clearly describe the procedure to be followed for performing validation. The protocol should include at least the objectives of validation and qualification study, site of the study, the responsible personnel, description of instrumentation to be used (including calibration before and after validation), SOPs to be followed, standards and criteria for the relevant products and processes, the type of validation and time/frequency should be stipulated. The processes and/or parameters to be validated (e.g., mixing times, drying temperatures, particle size, drying times, physical characteristics, and content uniformity) should be clearly identified.

10.8.3 Validation reports

The validation report is the final collection of test results and other documents such as instrument calibration certificates. This report will be used to determine whether a particular process is judged to be valid. A written report should be available after completion of validation. The results should be evaluated, analyzed, and compared with acceptance criteria. All results should meet the criteria of acceptance and satisfy the stated objective. If necessary, further studies should be performed. If found acceptable, the report should be approved and authorized (signed and dated).

The report should include the title and objective of the study, refer to the protocol, details of material, equipment, programmes and cycles used, together with the details of procedures and test methods. The results should be compared with the acceptance criteria.

Included in the final report should be recommendations on the limits and criteria to be applied to all future production batches. The report could form part of the basis of a batch-processing document.

It is a common practice in many companies for the protocol and the report to be combined into a single set of documents. The protocol is approved as a proforma into which the test results are recorded as they become available. This reduces the amount of paperwork that needs to be stored and makes an overall assessment of the validation results easier to carry out.

10.9 Chapter summary

- Validation refers to "the act of confirming something as true or correct."
- Process validation is defined as the collection and evaluation of data, from the process design stage through commercial production, which establishes scientific evidence that a process is capable of consistently delivering quality products.
- Process qualification is defined as confirming that the manufacturing process as designed is capable of reproducible commercial manufacturing.
- Validation and qualification are different concepts.
- Qualification of a process is typically required prior to validation and other times it is included as a part of validation.

- There are four different types of process validation, namely prospective, concurrent, retrospective, and revalidation.
- There are three phases of process validation, namely Stage 1: Process design/development, Stage 2: Process qualification, and Stage 3: Process verification.
- There are different types of qualification, such as DQ, IQ, OQ, and PQ.
- Validation documents that should be developed include: VMP, validation protocols, and validation reports.

10.10 Questions/problems

1. What is the difference between validation and qualification?
2. What are the four types of process validation? How are they different?
3. What are the process validation phases? How do they differ?
4. What are the different types of qualification that may be completed as a part of validation?

Further reading

Dictionary.com. https://www.dictionary.com/.

European Commission, 2015. EU guidelines for good manufacturing practice for medicinal products for human and veterinary use.

Ghagare, P.M., Patil, A.R., Deshmane, B.J., Kondawar, M.S., 2020. Review on pharmaceutical validation. Res. J. Pharma. Dos. Forms Tech. 12 (1), 17–26.

International Council for Harmonisation, 2000. Good manufacturing practice guide for active pharmaceutical ingredients Q7.

McCormick, K., 2002. Quality. Butterworth-Heinemann, Woburn, MA.

Ostrove, S.A., 2016. How to Validate a Pharmaceutical Process. Academic Press, New York.

Raul, S.K., Padhy, G.K., Mahapatra, A.K., Charan, S.A., 2014. An overview of concept of pharmaceutical validation. Res. J. Pharm. Tech. 7 (9), 1081–1090.

Riley, C.M., Rosanske, T.W., Riley, S.R.R., 2014. Specification of Drug Substances and Products. Elsevier, Ltd, Waltham, MA.

Rodríguez-Pérez, J., 2014. The FDA and Worldwide Current Good Manufacturing Practices and Quality System Requirements Guidebook for Finished Pharmaceuticals. American Society for Quality, Quality Press, Milwaukee, WI.

USFDA, 2011. Guidance for industry—Process validation: General principles and practices.

World Health Organization, 2003. Good manufacturing practices for pharmaceutical products: Main principles. https://gmpua.com/World/WHO/Annex4/trs908-4.pdf (accessed 06.04.21).

CHAPTER 11

Technology transfer

11.1 Introduction

Technology transfer is the process of commissioning and installing a new product or process in a manufacturing facility. It involves the transfer of documented knowledge and experience, built up during development and/or previous full-scale production, and requires a demonstration by the receiving facility of their ability to achieve all the critical parameters of the process. It is a major project activity and needs to be managed carefully to be successful.

This chapter starts by reviewing some of the reasons why technology transfer is required. It then looks at the ways companies choose where to relocate a production process or facility. This is followed by consideration of both the hardware (i.e., equipment) aspects of technology transfer and the software aspects (processes and people). Issues such as validation and registration are discussed. A technology transfer guide, developed from within the industry, is then introduced. Finally, there is a section on the need to maintain the quality during a technology transfer program triggered by a factory closure.

11.2 Reasons for technology transfer

Technology transfer of manufacturing processes and analytical methodology occurs within the pharmaceutical industry for many different reasons, often very positive ones. When a multinational company develops a new product and the demand exceeds the capacity at the original manufacturing site, it often transfers the product to other factories within the organization. When a product is nearing the end of its product life cycle, it may be moved from one of the strategic sites to other regional or local factories. When a company decides outsourcing is a preferable alternative to refurbishment or expansion, it needs to transfer the technology to the contract manufacturer. Finally, if a factory is being closed, there will be a need to transfer the production processes to other manufacturing sites before that closure takes place.

This section reviews each of these reasons in a little more detail.

11.2.1 Scale-up and product launch

The early stages of product development are carried out at the laboratory scale in the Research and Development (R&D) department. This tends to be true, both for

Quality
DOI: https://doi.org/10.1016/B978-0-323-90815-3.00005-0

products being developed under patent, using a new chemical entity, and for generic products taken from the national pharmacopeia.

In some companies, there is an intermediate stage, where pilot-scale production is carried out. Typically, this would be at a one-tenth full production scale. To be truly effective, the equipment should be as close as possible to the type used in production.

The final stage of product development will always be carried out on the production equipment since it is only at this point that the process parameters can be refined and confirmed.

At this point in the life cycle of the product, the development personnel will be the ones who have the most knowledge of the product characteristics, while the production personnel will generally be the experts in the use of the production equipment.

Technology transfer would typically take place during any experimental batches and the first few full batches produced in the plant. During this technology transfer, an effective handover of knowledge is important, if ongoing production is going to be problem-free.

11.2.2 Extension of manufacturing base

This is based on where the products will be marketed. With economic organizations such as the European Union, or free trade agreements such as the United States—Mexico—Canada Agreement or the Southern Common Market in South America, significant tax and pricing advantages may be gained by manufacturing in one country for the whole of the region. On the other hand, there might be trade barriers that can affect decisions. Some countries impose high import duties on finished pharmaceuticals to protect their own manufacturing industry. Such a situation tends to shape manufacturing strategy with respect to that country. Also, some countries' agreements on pricing may be affected significantly by whether products are manufactured in the home market or not.

Another issue to be considered is in relation to pack requirements. Where markets are relatively small and have specific pack requirements, such as language, it may be sensible to decouple bulk manufacturing and packaging. For example, a single strategic site could be used to produce the global supply of a particular tablet, which could be shipped in bulk to individual markets for local packaging.

When relocating product manufacture from one country to another, it is important to consider the registration restrictions relating to third countries that currently provide a market for the product. In Case study 1, discussed in Section 11.8, a major market for one of the products was not prepared to purchase from the new manufacturing country. Any potential loss of market has to be factored into the decision to move the product to a new location.

11.2.3 Contracting out or licensing of product

These two options have been used by companies over the years, often as a first step into a new marketplace. They can be alternatives to building a new facility in countries where having local manufacture is a prerequisite for doing business.

Many companies also contract out—termed more frequently as outsourcing—to supplement their own manufacturing capacity. This might be in the case of a company that wishes to move older products, in order to free up capacity for the new drugs. Alternatively, a company might have a product requiring specialized technology which is not part of their expertise.

In these situations, there needs to be close communication between the technical team in the receiving factory and the staff from the company itself. The latter would either be from the development function or from the manufacturing departments, depending on the age of the product and the resources available.

11.2.4 Sale of the product

When a product reaches the end of its product lifecycle, in most industries it would be discontinued. However, in the pharmaceutical industry, this may not be possible, or indeed desirable. Markets mature at different rates and some countries have fewer resources to spend on new drugs than others. Hence, there will be cases where there is a small, ongoing need for a product. In this case, an option is to sell off the product to a local company. The process for technology transfer should be the same in this case as in contracting or licensing out.

11.2.5 Closure of a factory

It is an inevitable fact of pharmaceutical manufacturing at some point in the industry's history that multiplant companies will decide to close one or more of their plants. This has been the case with every merger over the years. At the same time, some companies are deciding manufacturing is no longer a core part of their business and are moving from in-house production to contract manufacturing.

Whatever the reason for the closure, it is preceded by a transfer of some or all of the products to alternative manufacturing sites. If this process is to be achieved in a satisfactory manner without severe consequences for quality in one or both of the plants, a number of key issues need to be addressed.

A factory closure with ongoing manufacture at an alternative location is a project divisible into three main phases:
- the preannouncement planning phase;
- continuation of production in the closing facility from the time of announcement to the date of closure;
- transfer of production from the closing facility to an alternative manufacturing site.

Each of these phases has their own issues and management implications that must be dealt with if the project is to be successful.

11.3 Choosing the receiving site

The decisions to be taken as to where a company will transfer products are often considered during the development of a manufacturing strategy.

In the author's experience, there are a variety of issues considered during strategy development, some technical and some financial. On the technical side, issues such as proximity to development resources, an ability to meet the required quality standards, and the opportunity for standardization and pack rationalization rank highly. On the financial side, aspects such as the ability to cut fixed costs, the minimization of capital expenditure, an ability to service key markets, and the existence of tax advantages were important.

Some organizations define individual factories as strategic, regional server, or local server. These definitions specify the level of autonomy in standard setting and relationships with R&D. They also set the tone for the type of product and packs to be made.

11.3.1 Available capacity

In broad terms, there needs to be sufficient capacity of the right type in the receiving site to cover the current workload and potential growth throughout the life of the plant. This is not to say that capital expenditure will not occur in the future, but any expenditure directly resulting from the transfer project must be factored into the cost-benefit analysis. Consensus will have to be obtained on capacity measurement particularly on the number of shifts to be used. Experience has shown this will generally be dictated by a central group. The number of shifts to be used will typically be two or three per day and either 5 or 7 days per week, according to local custom. A manufacturing plant that is only utilized on a single shift basis is less likely to be cost-effective.

11.3.2 Quality standards

In the 1970s and 1980s there was a proliferation of construction projects and/or development of contract manufacturing relationships by the multinationals, resulting in an overcapacity situation and a swing in the opposite direction with rationalization beginning in the 1990s and still continuing. Inevitably, facilities in different countries will have different quality standards, even within the same companies, although this is not to suggest a double standard exists in terms of the final product.

A technology transfer project is therefore an opportunity to ensure optimal quality standards are maintained. Note the use of the word "optimal," rather than "maximum." Certain markets place additional requirements for quality onto the factories supplying to them. However, to suggest imposing the requirements of the United States Food and Drug Administration (US FDA) or the European Union in all factories around the world, serving all markets, would be as inappropriate as aiming for lowest cost across the board at the expense of quality.

11.3.3 Product costing

When comparing candidates for receiving product transfer, there is a temptation to compare product costing as an absolute measure of performance. This is only valid if the entire company has a single, rigidly-applied costing system. This is rare, particularly in the pharmaceutical industry.

Thus the use of existing product costing data should be treated with caution. It may be worthwhile to recost the affected products against common criteria. A simpler alternative could be to guarantee to the markets served by the closing site that products will be made available at a cost no greater than the existing source of supply or even that they would be cheaper by x%.

11.3.4 Geopolitical considerations

This point has already been discussed in Section 11.2.2. It will be briefly presented again, as it is relevant here too. This is based on where the products are going to be marketed. Economic organizations such as the European Union, or treaties such as the United States—Mexico—Canada Agreement can provide significant tax and pricing advantages for manufacturing within the region without being in the same country.

Other geopolitical issues include countries with high import duties of finished pharmaceuticals or pricing agreements between governments and companies which manufacture in a local facility.

Where markets are relatively small and have specific pack requirements, a single strategic site could be used to produce the global supply of a particular tablet, which could be shipped in bulk to individual markets for local packaging.

And finally, registration restrictions relating to third-party countries that currently provide a market for the product need to be taken into account. Any potential loss of market must be factored into the decision to move the product to the new location.

11.3.5 Market perceptions

Company rationalization programs are often carried out on a regional basis. When considering using a particular country to supply other countries within a region, it is important to consider the perception of that country throughout the rest of the region. For example, in the early 1990s, any Latin American strategy that centered on using Mexico to supply other parts of the region was faced with the issue that poor quality packaging materials had traditionally led to Mexico having a reputation for poor quality products across the region. Even today in parts of the developing world, products produced locally will be considered as inferior to imports, even in cases where the perception is incorrect.

11.4 Evaluating the hardware and software issues

In some technology transfer projects, it is a case of moving the products only from their existing manufacturing site to an alternative one. In this case, it is better where the equipment in the receiving site is the same, or very similar to that in the originating site. If this is not the case, a degree of reformulation is likely to be necessary.

However, there are some projects where the existing production line is to be relocated to the new site or where a new line is to be installed. This adds a whole new dimension to the situation.

11.4.1 Identifying costs

In the case where a production line is being transferred into a new manufacturing plant, there is likely to be a certain amount of refitting. It is essential this is recognized at the cost-benefit analysis stage and included in the calculations.

In the case of a project involving a factory closure, it is likely that initial discussions will take place over a period of time prior to the announcement and these discussions will involve very few people. As a result, the planning phase can suffer from a lack of accurate data and costs in particular. In this case, the perceived need for secrecy can result in a loss of quality information.

11.4.2 Attention to detail

Consideration of product transfer requires close attention to detail. In comparing product listings between factories, it may appear at first sight the same products are being made. However, in the author's experience, examination of each product in detail is necessary as early as possible:

- Even if the formulation is theoretically the same, has there been any drift since launch?
- Is the tablet design identical?
- Are the packaging details the same?

Once differences are detected—and there will be differences—the implications for registration and refitting can be determined.

11.4.3 Asking for help

It has to be recognized by the new site of manufacture, that in the case of an old, established product, there is a high level of knowledge within the previous production team, and it is not a sign of weakness to ask for and utilize this knowledge. In two different cases observed by the author, this was handled differently with interesting results. In one project, full discussions took place with the product experts from the handover site and the plant design benefited from this. The handover was smooth and everyone felt their experience and expertise had been recognized. In the second project, there was virtually no discussion and the plant was redesigned without taking into account the lessons learned over a 20-year period. Whether through ignorance or arrogance, the original staff was completely alienated by the process and handover was much more protracted and problematical as a result.

11.4.4 Soft systems

Refitting might involve not only the physical plant but the soft systems as well.
- Can the logistical software handle the products?
- Are changes needed to the software?
- Do the new markets require specific packing, shipping details or documents?
- Are there limitations on payment from the new market that can affect the operating systems of the new location?
- Finally, what impact will there be on training requirements and staffing levels?

For example, a smooth transfer of production will be hampered at the last minute if the contractor's software cannot handle the new product range. This could result in stock-outs in the marketplace, despite product being approved and available for dispatch from the warehouse.

11.5 Validation and registration

11.5.1 Validation

In terms of validating the product transfer, the level of work required will depend on a number of things:
- Does the transfer involve a range of new products or simply an increase in volume of an identical range?
- Is it an additional set of products for an existing range?
- Is it alternatively a completely new type of production?
- Finally, what level of validation has already been carried out in the original site of manufacture?

There is also a temptation to use the opportunity of product transfer to improve the processes in some way. However, this should be balanced against the validation implications of making too many changes at one time. If the speed of transfer is critical, then the number of changes should be kept to an absolute minimum. In some closure projects, entire manufacturing suites may be transferred from the closing site to the factory taking on the products. By restricting any process changes, the validation requirements are limited and hence do not take up too much time.

Frequently there may be regulatory reasons why the existing product has to be manufactured in the same way as previously. The new location needs to understand these reasons and continue to adhere to them even if there is a corresponding increase in costs or complexity.

11.5.2 Registration

There are two main areas of consideration in terms of registration, particularly if the transfer of production is across international boundaries:
* the needs of the new manufacturer; and
* the needs of the final marketplace.

In terms of the new manufacturer, registration requirements should have been considered at the time of the assessment. For example, the use of a factory in the United States to supply other parts of the world will have implications for cost and timescales as all products have to be registered for sale in the United States as well as in all final markets, even if the product is only to be exported. On the other hand, products manufactured in the European Union only have to be registered for the countries in which they are to be sold.

In terms of the marketplace, there may be a need for understanding local requirements, even if these seem unreasonable to the receiving site. It can become very frustrating for the people in each of these markets when the facilities that are going to take over manufacturing fail to accept the need for things they do not supply to other countries. For example, the Medicines Control Council in South Africa is very strict about notification of process changes, even down to requiring information of one-off process deviations. This is not common in other countries and hence some sites would find it difficult to comply with such a request.

Extra requirements must be accepted by the new site of manufacture as a necessary result of the transfer decision. Identification of such requirements early in the process is essential as registration can be protracted and is frequently on the critical path of the project plan.

11.6 The technology transfer guide

When the first edition of this book was published in 2002, there was a huge amount of technology transfer being carried out within the pharmaceutical industry and very little guidance on how to do it effectively. Therefore the International Society for Pharmaceutical

Engineering (ISPE) created a user-friendly document presenting a clear and concise general process for transferring technology between two parties. The document was produced in collaboration with the US FDA and the American Association of Pharmaceutical Scientists (AAPS). Input was received from the European regulatory authorities and submission made to the Japanese Ministry of Health and Welfare (MHW). Hence, while having no regulatory power, it represented industry best practice, with a standardized process and a recommended minimum base of documentation in support of the transfer request. (Good Practice Guide: Technology Transfer.)

In December 2018 the third edition of the guide was published. As with the previous two editions, it looks at three main topics:

- Technology transfer of analytical methods
- Technology transfer of drug substances or active pharmaceutical ingredients
- Technology transfer of drug product or dosage forms manufacturing processes

The guide is written: "to achieve a balance between risk management and cost-effectiveness while aligning with applicable regulatory expectations." In doing so, it aligns with the key topics discussed throughout this book such as Quality by Design, Quality Risk Management, Critical Quality Attributes, and Process Validation.

11.7 Planning for a successful technology transfer

The process of technology transfer between two sites may be defined as a project and like any other project, the key to success lies in the planning stage. There needs to be an overall project plan, covering all aspects of the transfer. In particular, there should be a detailed training plan to ensure the receiving site will, by the end of the project, be able to demonstrate competence in manufacturing the product in question.

Of particular importance is the product information dossier that will contain the accumulation of data regarding the product from development onward. This dossier will include information on at least the following items:

- product characteristics;
- packaging specifications;
- formulation rationale;
- stability data;
- raw materials, both actives and excipients;
- process details and critical process parameters;
- product performance report (if the product has already been manufactured elsewhere);
- facility and equipment requirements;
- qualification and validation reports;
- analytical test methodology; and
- environmental and safety assessments.

11.8 Maintaining quality during a factory closure

This section draws on observations made and lessons learned by the author during a number of factory closures. In particular, it deals with the closure of three factories in different parts of the world:

1. *Case study 1*: It relates to a closure of an entire factory in mainland Europe, with transfer of production to factories around Europe, including the United Kingdom. The sales and marketing operation, plus quality assurance functions were retained at the original site.

2. *Case study 2*: It relates to the closure of a plant in the United Kingdom, with transfer of production to other European sites, mainly in the United Kingdom, but also in mainland Europe, at a time when the United Kingdom was a member state of the European Union. All functions on the original site were shut down and the site was disposed of.

3. *Case study 3*: It relates to closure of a factory in South Africa, with production being split between a local contract manufacturer and other plants belonging to the parent company all around the world.

There are obvious cultural differences between the cases, and these should be taken into consideration in drawing conclusions. However, there were a number of generic messages coming out of each project applicable to future rationalization activities.

11.8.1 Retaining the support of the existing workforce

11.8.1.1 Openness versus secrecy

A potential factory closure is obviously a highly sensitive subject. At the point where an assessment of the situation is still being made, the desire to keep the discussions as secret as possible is understandable. However, this secrecy will have implications that must be recognized.

In Case study 1, the discussions took place between senior managers from the head office and the local team, together with internal consultants. At some point, external consultants were also involved, but not all the team was aware of this. Hence, the secrecy extended even to the assessment team in part. This had to be properly managed to meet the requirements of the national social legislation.

In Case study 3, only a small number of senior managers were involved in the preannouncement discussions. This was a high-risk strategy for the company, as, by South African law, any decision on retrenchment should be preceded by a chance for the workforce to offer an alternative solution. To get around this problem, the management came to an agreement with the workforce with implications for subsequent stages of the process, as will be discussed later.

The decision on when to "go public" is one of balance, timing, local legislation, and Trade Union relations. Who are the right people to involve and when? However, there are examples of when everyone was aware of what was being discussed, and it was not necessarily a major problem. In fact, in the postmerger situations experienced within major multinationals such as GlaxoWellcome and SmithKline Beecham, everyone knew their positions within the new company were being assessed, so in theory, there should be no major surprises. This is not to trivialize the potential personal trauma experienced by an individual who finds their services are no longer required by an organization. It merely questions the validity of keeping the discussions secret for a long period prior to announcements being made.

11.8.1.2 Expectations versus reality

Notwithstanding the wish to keep discussions secret, rumors spread very quickly, particularly if there is an unusually high incidence of visits from head office personnel or external consultants. Not knowing is often worse than knowing, even when the knowledge is bad. When the announcement was made in Case study 3, the general reaction was "at least I now know what's going to happen and can start planning the rest of my life accordingly."

Once the announcement has been made, there is no going back. In Case study 3, the decision to close the plant was a side effect of an ongoing program of collaborations between two companies. In the event, the negotiations on collaboration within Southern Africa broke down some weeks after the closure announcement had been made. Hence, the original cause of the closure had gone away. However, by that time it was too late to reverse the closure—it had already started to become a reality.

It is not only the people in the factory itself who are affected by a closure decision. In both Case studies 1 and 3, there were examples of senior managers on secondment overseas at the time of the announcement. Immediately, their obvious return routes home were eliminated. In a case like this, it is the responsibility of the human resources (HR) function at the head office to ensure such individuals are looked after, particularly if the local HR function is a casualty of the closure. The trauma of losing one's position is greatly intensified if one is working in a foreign country at the time, without obvious support mechanisms.

In general, it is better for very short, demanding timescales to be set for implementation. The reason for this is to fully engage the existing staff in the project but for the shortest time possible, to allow them to plan for their own futures.

11.8.1.3 Incentives

In order to keep the plant running to the end, some, if not all, of the workforce will need to be employed until the closure date. In a situation where everyone is inevitably putting their own interests before those of the company, this may be difficult to achieve. In Case study 1, an agreement was reached, in the form of a generous severance package, but only if the staff stayed until the end. As a result, there were virtually no staff losses prior to the closure date.

In Case study 3, as a result of the secrecy issue discussed earlier, an agreement was made that all contracts would be terminated, and severance packages made available from 6 months prior to closure. Staff members were than reemployed on 6-month temporary contracts. Consequently there was no incentive for people to stay with the company once they had found alternative employment. The loss of staff, particularly in the middle management levels was considerable, just at the time when extra resources were needed to keep things going smoothly.

The receiving plant personnel also need to have some incentives. This may sound surprising, but they need to understand their future is also not guaranteed as a right. They have to be able to deliver what the new customer wants.

11.8.1.4 Technical support

It was necessary with both Case studies 1 and 3 to provide technical support from other parts of the main companies. In Case study 1, a senior technical manager left 6 months prior to closure. An experienced production manager from the head office internal consultancy group was seconded to the post for 6 months. This had the advantages of putting in position someone who was committed to making the project successful, with no fear for his own future adversely affecting his performance and also created a bridge with the main site in the United Kingdom where much of the production was being transferred to. The individual also had an awareness of the issues involved in the closing factory and was able to understand what was needed to support them.

In Case study 3, the senior managers remained in post, but many of the junior and supervisory staff left at the early stages. This resulted in a requirement for considerable input of technical support to keep the factory going on a day to day basis. A permanent presence in the laboratory was provided by the company's central quality assurance (QA) function and at various times, supervisory support was provided from the United Kingdom, Pakistan, and Australia. For many of these individuals, it was an ideal career development opportunity. For the company itself, it was a timely reminder that not all the talent and experience resides in the country where the head office is located.

One further opportunity is provided by the need for support in the closing unit: it can be used to help the production transfer process. In Case study 3, one of the people who spent time working in the closing plant came from the manufacturing area in Australia which was due to take on many of the products. While providing support, he was also learning about the products for the future. Again, the importance of a bridge with the receiving plant is critical.

11.8.1.5 Improvement versus maintenance

The following points are to a certain extent culture-dependent. However, it is likely they will apply to a degree in any factory being closed down. Once the announcement had been made in Case study 3, all improvement activities stopped immediately. In fact, it was difficult to obtain maintenance of basic systems such as procedure writing. The role of QA became particularly vital at this point. They increased the frequency of joint production/QA self-inspections, which ensured the processes continued to operate effectively. In the final months, these self-inspections were moved from a monthly to a weekly cycle.

11.8.1.6 Management versus policing

It is also possible the style of management may need to change to a more policing style. In factory closure projects, there sometimes occur a number of security incidents that can be directly related either to people taking less responsibility for their actions or deliberately causing problems as a way of expressing their frustration. It may be necessary to increase the level of supervision to prevent this sort of incident continuing.

On the other hand, in other closure projects, the workforce maintain their pride in the job and hence their responsibility for their actions until the end. This was particularly evident with some teams in Case study 2. In many respects this is due to the way in which the total project is managed.

11.8.1.7 Continuity

In each of the closures being discussed, anyone who has a guaranteed role in the future organization is key to the success of the transfer phase of the project.

The situation with technical staff in Case study 3 has already been referred to. In Case study 1, the QA manager was to stay on as the only technical representative after the factory closed. In Case study 2, one of the senior technical managers was transferred to one of the receiving sites to run the areas that had taken on the work. All these people played a significant role in seeing the projects through.

11.8.1.8 Cannibalization

If a factory is closing down, inevitable decisions are taken about disposal of equipment, whether to the new site of manufacture or elsewhere in the company. An element of sensitivity should be exercised in dealing with this. People walking around the production areas with tape measures, as happened in Case study 1, can cause a high degree of resentment if not handled properly.

11.8.2 Stock building versus rapid closure

Given the difficulties experienced in keeping a factory running once the closure announcement has been made, there is a case for implementing the closure as quickly as possible. In Case study 1, the General Manager wanted to implement the closure over a period of 3 months. This was found to be impossible; however everything was completed in 9 months. In Case study 2, the whole project took 2 years; and towards the end of that period, there were only a few people left, keeping the last few processes running. For these people, the atmosphere was poor, and the working environment left much to be desired.

The decision to close a factory is obviously a tough one. However, once it has been taken, it is advisable to implement it as humanely as possible, not only for the obvious humanitarian reasons but also because a closure takes a finite period of time (from experience, at least 6–9 months) and production needs to be maintained during that time.

It is possible to make allowances for a delay in start-up by increasing the level of stock-build prior to closing. In fact, if the transfer of production is to be accompanied by a transfer of critical plant or machinery, a stock-build is essential. In Case study 1, despite a stock-build exercise, some stock-outs did occur. All delivery promises from new manufacturing sites must be kept, otherwise, logistics will fall apart. The new site must understand the consequences for them of failure to maintain agreed schedules. Changes in requirements must be negotiated with the marketing organization and the receiving location.

It should also be remembered that building stock over and above normal production levels is difficult at the best of times, assuming the plant is operating at anywhere near full capacity. It requires hard work and goodwill among the workforce and frequently results in significant amounts of overtime being worked. To achieve this in the context of a closure situation could be even more difficult.

Finally, it should be made clear to the sales and marketing departments why the stock-build is taking place. The manufacturing staff of a factory in Latin America once made the mistake of not explaining the situation. They had worked very hard to build up stock in advance of a major project to refurbish parts of the factory, a much more positive reason to build stock than as a precursor to closure. However, the sales representatives observed the stock levels rising in the warehouse and went out to their customers with special sales drives. As a result, sales rose considerably, and the refurbishment was delayed while production did it all again!

11.8.3 Management of the implementation

11.8.3.1 Management commitment

The decision to close a factory is taken at the highest level in the company, although hopefully with the full knowledge and agreement of the senior management within the unit. However, once that decision has been taken, it must be implemented by the local management. In Case study 1, the general manager was far from happy with the decision, but once it had been taken, he was fully committed to carrying it through successfully, without damaging the business in the country. His involvement in, and sponsorship of, the latter stages of the project were invaluable. In fact, it can be concluded that if the senior management team is not committed to making the closure happen effectively, they should be replaced by a team that is. Anything less will frustrate the ability of the company to meet its objectives for the closure.

11.8.3.2 Priorities
To the closing unit, activities associated with the transfer of production constitute the number one priority, albeit in parallel with keeping the market satisfied in the interim. However, for the new site of manufacture, this is not likely to be the case. It is often a much larger site, with many products, both new and old. The activities such as registration and pack design may come way down the priority list. Reconciling these differences of approach is very much a people issue—and one to be addressed at an early stage, so sufficient resources can be allocated. A neutral, knowledgeable individual who can work in both units is most helpful, some would say essential, in ensuring the receiving unit understands the priorities of the closing unit and responds appropriately.

11.8.3.3 Deadlines
Following on from the previous point about priorities, the transfer project will encompass a series of deadlines. There is a tendency for these to be set by the closing unit, based on their view of the appropriate closing date. However, this can then require amendment as other aspects are taken into account. For example, in Case study 3, the closure date was calculated on the basis of registration lead-times and then agreed with the workforce as part of the severance negotiations. Once delays were apparent with certain aspects of registration, the date for the start-up of production was seen to be slipping back. A decision was needed on whether the closure date should also be amended. It is however vital that delay is not just accepted as something about which nothing can be done. Otherwise, the project will never be completed. Good relationships with Government can assist in the process.

11.8.3.4 Divided attention
Transferring production from one pharmaceutical factory to another is a major project and can be a full-time job, at least for part of the time period. Running a factory is also a full-time job. Trying to combine these two roles could be a recipe for disaster.

In Case study 1, an internal consultant from head office was drafted in to provide the resource necessary. In Case study 2, the transfer project was split into a number of subprojects, each led by a different person. In Case study 3, a slightly different approach was taken. A consultant was employed from the start to handle the legal and other commercial aspects of the project. The technical director maintained control of much of the rest of the transfer. However, recognizing this could lead to him taking his eye off the ball in the old factory, he appointed one of his senior managers to stand in for him on a day-to-day basis.

11.8.3.5 New products versus old

During all phases of a closure project, business must carry on as usual. Not only will the old products need to be supplied to the marketplace but launch of new products may also be occurring. The resource implications of this should be recognized and allowed for.

11.8.3.6 Low-demand products

In any manufacturing site, the product listing will include a number of "old favorites" which for various reasons are still produced, even though the commercial case is weak. A closure project is an opportunity to revisit this issue and the discussion should be held early in the process with finance and marketing, to avoid unnecessary waste of time and resources later on.

In Case study 2, a particular product was identified for which special equipment was required. The sales were quite low, but marketing insisted the product should remain in the range. A new site was identified, but due to the weight of the equipment, some structural alterations to the building were required. Transport was costed and planned, as was the construction. At the last minute, marketing changed their minds, and the product was dropped from the range. If the original decision had been challenged more vigorously at the start, much time and money could have been saved.

11.8.3.7 Project management

Throughout this section, closures have been referred to as projects, and like any other project, its management is critical. In the closing site, a project manager is required, as has been discussed previously, and the use of project management software may be found to be advantageous. In addition, the receiving site will require someone responsible for making things happen. With each of the closures described here, there was a significant amount of work for a number of departments in the receiving sites, such as registration and pack development. In Case studies 1 and 3, in particular, it was necessary for a project manager to act as a link between the closing unit and the receiving site.

11.8.3.8 Project sponsorship

Finally, each project requires a sponsor who in the final analysis can bring pressure to bear if things are not happening. This will often be a member of the executive who authorized the closure in the first place. In Case study 1, the local general manager and the main board director for the region jointly took this role. Since the latter was also responsible for all the receiving sites, he was able to resolve issues of conflict very quickly.

In Case study 3, the local general manager and the regional manager at the head office jointly took the role. However, as neither of these had responsibility for any of the receiving sites, there was less strength in their position and issues still took time and influencing skills to resolve on occasion.

The overall message of this section is that closing a factory down is neither easy, quick nor cheap. It needs careful planning and appropriate allocation of resources if it is to be achieved successfully.

Above all else, personnel are required who can operate under pressure in difficult situations and yet maintain relationships at the very time when they are under the greatest threat.

11.9 Chapter summary

- Technology transfer is the process of commissioning and installing a new product or process in a manufacturing facility.
- It is a major project activity and should be managed as such.
- There are a variety of reasons why a company might initiate a technology transfer project.
- Scale-up and product launch involves the transfer of technology from R&D to production.
- As a product matures and new markets are reached, the manufacturing base may need to be extended, which will require technology transfer from one factory to another.
- Contracting out or licensing a product to another company is a common option chosen by companies as an alternative to increasing their in-house manufacturing capacity. This will involve technology transfer between two companies.
- When a product nears the end of its lifecycle, it may be discontinued; alternatively, it may be sold to another company if there is a small, ongoing need for the product in some markets. Again, this will involve technology transfer between two companies.
- Factory closures are a factor of the pharmaceutical industry, especially after company mergers. This may involve technology transfer between factories in the same company, or between two or more companies.

- There are a number of factors to be considered when choosing the receiving site for a technology transfer project.
- The receiving site must have sufficient capacity to take on the new product(s) without jeopardizing the supply to the marketplace or the production of its existing products.
- The receiving site must have appropriate quality standards to satisfy the requirements both of the transferring company and of the markets it will serve.
- The cost to produce the product in the receiving site must be appropriate for the markets it will serve.
- There may be geopolitical issues relating to trade agreements, import duties, or regulatory requirements; this is particularly true when technology transfer is proposed across international borders.
- The perception from the marketplace of the quality of product delivered from a particular country is an important consideration and will need to be addressed, even if that perception is no longer valid.
- Factors to be considered when planning a technology transfer project will include not only hardware issues, relating to equipment and facilities; but also software issues relating to people and processes.
- The cost-benefit analysis for any given option must be rigorous enough to consider all costs including those associated with refitting.
- Even where an identical product is supposedly produced in different factories, there is likely to have been processing drift over a period of time. Attention to the detail of the process is important in ensuring all implications of a transfer are identified.
- The knowledge of a product or process will not be contained just in the formal documentation, but also in the experience of the existing production staff. Their help should be sought by the receiving site in order to ensure a smooth transfer.
- Issues such as the logistics software of the receiving site, and the availability of trained production staff, are important to ensure the smooth transfer.
- A technology transfer project will require a varying level of validation depending on the nature of the products and the type of transfer being carried out.
- Registration issues to be addressed will cover both the needs of the new manufacturer and the needs of the markets being served.
- While there are no regulatory guidelines for technology transfer, the ISPE Technology Guide was written in collaboration between industry and regulators; and aims to balance risk management and cost-effectiveness while satisfying regulatory requirements.
- Project planning is an important aspect of successful technology transfers. It should include a detailed training plan and a comprehensive product dossier.
- Where a technology transfer project is associated with a factory closure, there are additional aspects to be considered, particularly relating to personnel issues.

- Three studies are used to review issues observed by the author during factory closure projects.
- It is important to maintain the support of the existing workforce in the closing factory, to maintain the quality of the product and to ensure a smooth transfer.
- The benefits of building stock prior to a closure should be balanced against the benefits of achieving a rapid closure and thus minimizing the adverse effects of the closure on both the workforce and the quality of the product.
- Project management is even more critical in the case of a factory closure than in other types of technology transfer projects.

11.10 Questions/problems

1. List the reasons why a company might wish to carry out a technology transfer project of a single product.
2. List the reasons why a company might wish to carry out a technology transfer project for the whole portfolio of products.
3. What issues might be common in the scenarios in questions 1 and 2? What issues might apply in one, but not in the other?
4. You are the general manager of a factory which is part of a multinational company. You have been told your site will be the main one for supplying a new bulk tablet to markets around the world. Who would you include in your technology transfer project team?
5. You are the general manager of a company with only one factory. You need to release additional manufacturing capacity for new products coming on-line. In your portfolio there are a number of products which have low volume demand, but which are important for a specific tropical disease prevalent in just a couple of countries. What would you do?
6. You are the general manager of a factory which is part of a multinational company, recently formed by merger of two smaller companies. You have been told your factory is to close within a year. What do you need to organize? What factors will affect how you react to the news?

Further reading

International Society for Pharmaceutical Engineering, 2018. *ISPE Good Practice Guide: Technology Transfer* (third ed.).

CHAPTER 12

Water for pharmaceutical use

12.1 Introduction

In the pharmaceutical industry, water is a very important material. It is used in large quantities for cleaning and sanitation purposes. It is used in the manufacture and/or formulation of active pharmaceutical ingredients (APIs). And it is an ingredient in a variety of dosage forms of medicinal products for human and veterinary use, including injections, creams, oral liquid products, and as a granulating solution in dry product manufacture. The preparation of water is a key technology within our factories.

This chapter reviews the international regulations and guidelines for water systems and defines the different grades of water and their uses. It then discusses the design of treatment systems required to produce, distribute, monitor, and control each type. The problems of biofilm, its development, and control are then presented. Common problems of purified water and water for injection (WFI) systems are reviewed, using experience from regulatory inspections. The chapter concludes with an overview of the critical topic of wastewater treatment.

12.2 Reference documentation

There are several national and international guidelines of relevance to this chapter plus industry-produced references.

12.2.1 European Union guidance

The European Medicines Agency recently approved a new reference document: Guidance on the quality of water for pharmaceutical use (EMA, 2020). This document, which came into effect on February 1, 2021, replaced two previous documents dating from 2001 and 2002. The revision relates to changes in the European Pharmacopoeia (Ph. Eur.), including approval of alternative methods for the production of WFIs. The guideline defines four grades of water and references the appropriate monograph:
1. Potable water (Directive 98/83/EC)
2. Water for injections (WFIs) (Ph. Eur. monograph 0169) (European Pharmacopoeia, n.d.)
3. Purified water (Ph. Eur. monograph 0008) (European Pharmacopoeia, n.d.)

Quality
DOI: https://doi.org/10.1016/B978-0-323-90815-3.00004-9

4. Water for preparation of extracts (Ph. Eur. monograph 2249) (European Pharmacopoeia, n.d.)

There is no discussion in the guideline of production and control systems since these are presented in the relevant Ph. Eur. monograph. The guideline identifies three general uses of pharmaceutical waters and presents examples of minimum grades to be used for various product types in each case. The three uses, in descending order of criticality, are:

- Water present as an excipient in the final formulation.
- Water used during the manufacture of active substances and medicinal products excluding water present as an excipient in the final formulation.
- Water used for cleaning/rinsing of equipment, containers and closures.

12.2.2 United States guidance

There are two major references for pharmaceutical water listed by the United States Food and Drug Administration (US FDA), both of which appear in the section on inspections guides. While these are aimed primarily at FDA inspectors, they are public access documents and can be consulted and downloaded by anyone. They are therefore useful documents both in designing a water system and its accompanying quality system and documentation, and in preparing for regulatory inspections.

The inspection technical guide, Water for Pharmaceutical Use, was originally issued in 1986. It was most recently reviewed and confirmed to be current in 2014. It is a short document listing eight grades of water in total:

1. Nonpotable
2. Potable (drinkable) water
3. United States Pharmacopeia (USP) purified water
4. USP WFI
5. USP sterile water for injection
6. LUSP sterile water for inhalation
7. USP bacteriostatic WFI
8. USP sterile water for irrigation

As with the European Union guidance document, there is a reference to the USP monographs which provide full specifications for the different grades. The document goes on to briefly review:

- water production sources
- sources of water contamination
- in-plant water treatment systems

More detailed guidance is provided in The Guide to Inspection of High Purity Water Systems (US FDA 1993), which was reviewed and confirmed as current in 2016. It does not cover the specifications for grades of water but instead deals with system design and validation issues. It discusses microbial limits for a WFI system, then breaks it down into its constituent parts. There are much less detailed sections on purified water systems and process water. The document ends with a brief note on inspection strategy.

12.2.3 Industry-generated guidance

In addition to the pharmacopeia specifications and the regulatory documents, there are several practical guides published by the International Society for Pharmaceutical Engineering (ISPE), which are written collaboratively by teams of industry practitioners. For example, the third edition of the Baseline Guide on Water and Steam Systems (International Society for Pharmaceutical Engineering, 2019) has "a global team of critical utilities experts with a combined experience of more than 500 years. Much of the team responsible for the earlier versions of the Water and Steam Systems Baseline Guide has returned to contribute to the revised Guide, providing continuity and longevity of vision to the Guide's contents." In addition to the baseline guide, there are good practice guides on:

- Ozone Sanitization of Pharmaceutical Water Systems (International Society for Pharmaceutical Engineering, 2012)
- Commissioning and Qualification of Pharmaceutical Water and Steam Systems (International Society for Pharmaceutical Engineering, 2014)
- Sampling for Pharmaceutical Water, Steam, and Process Gases (International Society for Pharmaceutical Engineering, 2016)

12.3 Grades of water

There are several different quality grades of water found in a pharmaceutical factory, which are described below, although, as shown in Section 12.2. Reference document section, terminology varies slightly with different regulatory environments. The grades are defined in terms of the chemical, physical, and microbiological characteristics of the water. The relevant specifications are given in the various pharmacopeias and will provide critical quality attributes (CQAs) for each grade of water. A typical specification would include:

- total organic carbon (TOC)
- conductivity
- microbial levels
- endotoxin levels
- nitrate concentration
- heavy metal concentrations

  (ISPE Commissioning and Qualification of Pharmaceutical Water and Steam Systems).

Since this chapter is a precursor to Chapter 13, reference is primarily made to the microbiological aspects of each grade.

12.3.1 Untreated water

This is the raw water entering the company either from a local source, such as a private bore hole or, possibly, from the metropolitan system. It provides the raw material for the water treatment plants and is also used for nonprocess purposes such as fire-security systems or irrigation.

There is no microbial standard for untreated water. However, it is important that the bioburden is known to ensure appropriate pretreatment and treatment systems are in place to provide the right quality for the higher grades of water. It is also necessary to review the standard of supply over a period of at least 12 months to ensure there are no significant seasonal variations. For example, at times of low water levels, the microbiological contamination levels are likely to be higher than normal.

12.3.2 Potable water

Potable water is either delivered by the metropolitan system or obtained by treatment of raw water. It is used primarily for drinking. It must be of a quality at least as good as one of the international or national standards such as European Council Directive 98/83/EC, the US Environmental Protection Agency Drinking Water Regulations, or the WHO guidelines for drinking water quality. The microbiological standard is typically less than 500 colony forming units (CFU) per milliliter and the complete absence of coliforms.

12.3.3 Process water

As with potable water, process water is either delivered by the metropolitan system or by treatment of raw water. It is used for washing of equipment, cooling of process equipment, manufacture of APIs, and as the feedwater for purified water preparation plants.

Process water must be equal to or better than the standard achieved for potable water. Since one of its uses is in finished bulk APIs, the relevant standard will depend not only on the country in which it is being used but also on any potential export markets.

12.3.4 Purified water

Purified water is the output of water purification plants, using ion exchange, reverse osmosis (RO), or distillation. It is used for the manufacture of nonsterile pharmaceuticals, for preparation of laboratory reagents and test solutions, and as the final rinse water for equipment that will come into contact with nonsterile products.

Once again, the microbiological standard is defined by pharmacopeia. The WHO guideline is 50 CFU/mL with an absence of pathogens. The Ph. Eur quotes an action limit for purified water of 100 CFU/mL. There is no microbiological limit quoted in the USP. However, the FDA reference document "Guide to Inspections of High Purity Water Systems" states that an inspector would find an action limit of more than 100 CFU/mL to be unacceptable.

12.3.5 Water for injections

WFI is officially called Water for Injections in European standards and Water for Injection in the USP. It was traditionally produced by distillation, although the USP has for many years accepted purification methods if proved to be "equivalent or superior to distillation." Similarly, the Japanese pharmacopeia accepted distillation or RO and/or ultrafiltration. The latest revision of EU guidelines, referred to in Section 12.2.1 European guidance, also accepts the use of RO, but with stipulations. WFI is used in the manufacture of parenterals and for the final rinse of equipment that comes into contact with sterile products.

The WHO guideline for WFI is 10 CFU/mL with an absence of pathogens and also an absence of pyrogens. The European pharmacopeia quotes an action limit for WFI of 10 CFU/100 mL. Again, there is no microbiological limit quoted in the USP. However, the same FDA reference document "Guide to Inspections of High Purity Water Systems" states that an inspector would find an action limit of more than 10 CFU/100 mL to be unacceptable. In other words, in the cases of both purified water and WFI the microbiological standards are tacitly, if not officially, the same in Europe and the United States. Both standards require a bacterial endotoxin level of less than 0.25 EU/mL.

All these specifications refer to water in bulk. There are several other specifications for a variety of grades of packaged water, depending on the intended use.

12.3.6 Water for preparation of extracts

Water for preparation of extracts is used for the production of herbal products and will comply as appropriate with the standards for purified water or potable water, depending on the nature of the product.

12.4 Design of water treatment systems

There are many options available to companies wishing to install a water purification plant. The decisions taken on design are based on many variables:
- The specification of the feedwater that has to be treated: This has particular relevance in choosing the pretreatment stages. It is important to consider

information relating to feedwater specification over a 12-month period to ensure any seasonality is recognized.

- The balance between capital investment and ongoing running costs: Some of the methods are capital-intensive to install but can be run cost-effectively; others are low-cost initially but have high running costs.
- The importance of reducing wastewater: This was always particularly relevant in regions that have a shortage of water, such as the Middle East or Africa. However, with the criticality of environmental issues, it has become a major consideration for all companies.
- The grade of water required: Most factories require a mix of grades in varying quantities. In some cases, a single system will satisfy all requirements. However, on other occasions, it may be necessary to install a hybrid system or more than one stand-alone system.
- The demand profile: It is not enough to know how much of each grade of water will be required. It is important to understand the profile of demand; in other words, what will be the daily off-take, and will it be a smooth demand with time (unlikely) or will there be certain times of the days when demand will peak, such as the start of the day, when manufacturing is taking place; or late in a shift, when cleaning is taking place?
- The ability to manage downtime: Most water treatment plants require time off-line for regeneration or backwash. In a one or two-shift factory, these operations could be scheduled outside normal working hours. However, for a factory operating 24 hours per day, as is often the case in API manufacturing facilities, this is not so easy. In this case, continuity of production would require the system design to have extra capacity, duplicate equipment, or buffer storage.

The various stages and types of water treatment are described in the next three sections, with particular reference to microbiological aspects.

12.5 Water pretreatment methods

12.5.1 Filtration

The first step in pretreatment is often one or more coarse filters to remove particulate matter of more than 50 μm and to greatly reduce the level of particulates of more than 10 μm. Sand or multimedia filters are generally used in these stages. It is possible to purchase filters with disposable elements. However, if the raw water is known to have high particulate contamination, which will lead to frequent blocking of filters, it would be better to install a regenerative system.

These filters are susceptible to microbial contamination and the formation of biofilm. If not properly managed, this can lead to higher levels of microorganisms after the filter than before it. Hence, careful monitoring and frequent sanitization are required.

12.5.2 Organic scavengers

Carbon filters are often used in the pretreatment of water to remove organics and oxidizing chemicals. This is particularly important if there are high levels of dissolved organic matter in the raw water supply. If this step in the pretreatment is not effective, the anion resins in the deionizer will quickly become fouled. Once again, microbial growth and biofilm are risks against which precautions have to be taken.

12.5.3 Chemical treatments

During pretreatment, it is also common to add chemicals to the water for several purposes. One of these is the control of microbiological contamination, which is carried out using sodium hypochlorite, chlorine, ozone, or hydrogen peroxide.

In many cases, the municipal supply of water will already have been chlorinated to ensure it achieves potable quality. However, if the residual chlorine level at the point of supply is less than 0.2 ppm, it may be necessary to carry out further chlorination on-site. The effectiveness of the process will be affected by the pH of the water, the concentration of the chlorine, and residual time. It is important to determine the effect, if any, of residual chlorine on the final product and to design the system accordingly.

12.5.4 Water softeners

Water softening is often carried out in hard water areas during pretreatment to reduce the load on the purification units further downstream. This is achieved with base ion exchange, which replaces calcium and magnesium ions with sodium ions. The resins are once again a major source of microbiological contamination and need to be monitored and controlled. As an alternative to putting this process into the main water treatment system, it can be used in specific locations such as the feedwater to boilers or RO units.

12.5.5 Specific treatments

Since all raw water specifications differ, all water treatment systems will also differ. To protect purification equipment or to produce the higher quality treated process water, it may be necessary to target specific contaminants. Treatments required could include clarification, ozone treatment, carbon absorption, organic scavenging, and deionization. Such techniques may be used singly or in combination, to remove specific problem contaminants including organic matter, colloidal particles, and dissolved iron.

12.6 Preparation of purified water

The selection of the appropriate equipment for the preparation of purified water will depend on the quality of the raw water which would normally be fed from the process water plant and on priorities as determined from the issues reviewed in Section 12.4. There are several equipment options available.

12.6.1 Carbon filters

Carbon filters are frequently used to protect deionizers from dissolved chlorine and modest concentrations of dissolved organics.

Where possible, disposable cartridge-type activated carbon filters should be used. These must be regularly discarded and replaced to suppress bacterial growth. In large installations, regenerable carbon beds may be used, provided they are regularly regenerated and sanitized. See Section 12.11.

12.6.2 Reverse osmosis (hyperfiltration)

Where process water contains high levels of dissolved organics, RO is very effective in reducing these, although such plants require careful specification and operation.

Water is fed at high pressure across a semipermeable membrane. Some of the water, the permeate, passes through substantially free from dissolved organics, including pyrogens, and bacteria. Some ionic species are also partially retained by the membrane. The residue, the retentate, is a more concentrated solution of the original contaminants that is flushed continuously to drain.

The feedwater should not contain significant quantities of suspended solid and colloidal matter, also called silt. In some hard water areas, organic species may salt out on the membrane surface. Good pretreatment of the process water supply to capture and remove these organics will help to prevent fouling and consequent performance loss. Even so, membranes will require frequent chemical cleaning and sanitization to restore performance and subdue bacterial growth.

Membrane selection will normally be on the advice of a specialist supplier. It is important to establish operating limits and performance guarantees for the membranes with respect to temperature, pH, chlorine levels, silt, hardness, etc.

Disposal of the retentate stream must also be considered. This can be a significant effluent volume, and there are several ways of dealing with it.

12.6.3 Deionization

Deionization involves passing water over a resin bed, which exchanges metal ions and dissolved salts in the water for hydrogen and hydroxyl ions. The resin has a finite potential for ion removal, which means the performance of a bed will deteriorate. Resins are regenerated chemically using acids and alkalis.

Resin selection will normally be based on vendor recommendations. The possible effect of nonionic contaminants on resins should be examined. The system should also prevent the carryover of resin fines into the output water. The design should ensure that feedwater chlorine levels do not adversely affect resin performance.

Most systems will consist of two ion exchange units used in series as described below, with the first system taking out most of the contaminants and the second system polishing the output of the first.

12.6.3.1 Twin bed deionization units

These units are generally recommended for the initial deionization duty or any application where frequent regeneration is likely to be required. They consist of two columns in series, one removing cationic contaminants and the other removing anionic contaminants.

The conductivity of the output must be measured continuously. During equipment qualification, an appropriate cut-off point must be defined to initiate regeneration of the bed. Microbiological buildup inside the columns can be expected. A maximum safe interval between regenerations must be established. The entire regeneration initiation control should be automatic.

Purified water should be used to flush the resin beds after regeneration. This reduces the time needed to restore good water quality.

Proper consideration must be given to the handling, storage, and use of regeneration chemicals. In particular, the design should ensure the purified water storage and distribution system is suitably isolated from the column while it regenerates.

12.6.3.2 Mixed resin beds

These beds contain both anion and cation resins. They are recommended for polishing applications where the ionic loading of the feedwater is relatively low. Performance is monitored by comparing the conductivity at the outlet with that at the inlet. From a chemical point of view, several months of operation can be expected without regeneration. However, during this time, bacterial growth may be expected. Microbiological monitoring is an essential part of establishing and checking the safe interval between regenerations.

The regeneration of a mixed resin system is more complex than a twin bed system. Cartridge-type systems are recommended. Cartridge exchange must be controlled to avoid the risk of contamination during and after the changeover. *In situ* regeneration should only be considered in large volume systems.

12.6.3.3 Electrodeionization

An alternative to classical ion exchange processes emerged in the 1980s when continuous electrodeinization (CDI) was developed in the United States to produce purified water without the problems or costs of chemical regeneration.

The CDI system uses ion exchange membranes, ion exchange resins, and electricity to produce a consistent quality of purified water. Water enters the unit and flows inside the resin/membrane compartments where the resins capture dissolved ions. By the application of an electrical potential, captured cations are driven through cation membranes and captured anions through anion membranes. The cation permeable membranes transport the cations out of the concentrating compartment but prevent anions from leaving. The anion permeable membranes transport anions out of the concentrating compartment but prevent cations from leaving.

These units are normally used for polishing water supplied from an RO unit, removing carbon dioxide, silica, and total organic carbon. Although there is a waste stream from the unit, the recovery is in the order of 80%—90%

12.6.4 Ultraviolet radiation

Ultraviolet (UV) radiation, predominantly at 254 nm wavelength, has the capability of reducing bacterial loading. Provided bacteria are exposed to sufficient UV energy for a sufficient time, they will be killed. The performance of a UV unit is therefore dependent on the intensity of UV, the residence time of water within the unit, and whether bacteria can be shadowed by other contaminants.

UV lamps are particularly useful for controlling the bacterial loading in cold, recirculating, purified water systems. However, by killing bacteria, the UV process could add to the level of pyrogens in the water and increase the dissolved carbon dioxide levels.

The UV lamp system must be sized to achieve the required residence time at the maximum anticipated flow rate. A UV lamp has a finite life and therefore must be fitted with an intensity meter and subjected to an appropriate monitoring program, to ensure a fall-off in performance is detected before an unacceptably low level is reached.

The use of UV will not alter the need for the system to be periodically sanitized.

12.6.5 Ultrafiltration

This is a mechanical method used primarily to remove bacteria. It is frequently positioned as the final stage of the water treatment plant. Pore sizes vary between 0.22 and 10 μm.

12.7 Preparation of water for injection

The production of WFI and its storage and distribution, which is discussed in Section 12.8, requires careful attention to detail, from design through to performance qualification. In general, the simpler the design concept, the more reliable the resulting system.

WFI will most commonly be produced from purified water using a distillation unit. All the previous methods are part of the process of producing purified water. Distillation is generally used only to produce WFI, although, in some countries, it is a common methodology for producing purified water.

There are three different types of stills available: single effect, double effect, and vapor compression. Each type results in thermal vaporization, mist elimination, and condensation. It is an effective method for the removal of chemicals, bacteria, and pyrogens.

Water stills should be purchased as packaged plant items from vendors with a good track record of supplying such equipment to the pharmaceutical industry. The still should be purchased complete with all associated instrumentation and controls necessary for safe, effective, and reliable operation in accordance with GMP. The design should be assessed paying particular attention to several items as discussed below.

As mentioned previously, WFI can also be produced using RO and/or ultrafiltration, and more details can be found on these types of equipment in Sections 12.6.2 and 12.6.5, respectively.

12.7.1 Feedwater quality requirements

This relates particularly to chloride content and microbiological quality. Purified water should be used. This provides the best means of ensuring consistent production of WFI quality water and protecting the still from corrosion.

12.7.2 Contamination risks

It is important to prevent the carryover of droplets or particles into the WFI condenser. Measures must also be provided to prevent contamination of the WFI by the heating and cooling media. Heat exchangers should be designed to the double tube sheet principle.

12.7.3 Energy efficiency

Multiple effect and vapor compression stills are highly energy efficient. The payback on the higher initial capital cost should be assessed. The WFI should be delivered to hot storage at 80°C minimum, which may require the WFI to be heated between the still and storage tank.

12.7.4 Location

The still and storage tank should be located in a technical area dedicated to manufacturing services. The equipment should be arranged so that WFI flows by gravity from the still to the storage tank. Access must be provided for periodic inspection of the internal condition of the still.

12.7.5 Control system

The control system should be arranged to reject any poor quality water. The initial production should be rejected for a predetermined time at every start-up. Any high conductivity water produced must also be rejected. Ideally, the still should self-drain when not operating, to minimize the potential for bacterial growth. Blow down control should be provided to prevent the accumulation of corrosive contaminants.

12.7.6 Sterilization

Stills with a self-sterilization cycle should be carefully assessed. Some stills are also capable of generating clean steam for sterilizing the storage and distribution system.

12.8 Storage and distribution of process water

Process water distribution systems must not be used to supply water for human consumption. Where raw water is treated on-site for both domestic and process use, the design must ensure there are air breaks between process and domestic systems and all local drinking water regulations are complied with.

The distribution system will typically consist of a storage tank and distribution pipework running at ambient temperature. Distribution can be effected by gravity feed where possible, or by a pumping system. Unless the process water is protected against bacterial growth, frequent draining and sanitization will be necessary.

12.8.1 Storage tanks

Tank volume will be determined by the level and variability of demand, supply security, and any need for treatment system downtime. Tank volume should not grossly exceed that required for normal operation. If possible, the tank working volume should ensure a mean residence time of less than 24 hours to avoid depletion of chlorine levels and resultant microbial contamination and buildup of biofilm. The tank must be capable of complete draining.

Storage tanks must be closed, with vents and overflow protected from ingress of water spray, fumes, insects, birds, and vermin. Any reduction in the vent area caused by such protection should be accounted for when sizing the vent pipework.

Storage tanks must be capable of regular sanitization. Any chemical sanitization operation must be designed to ensure the process water cannot be contaminated by sanitization chemicals.

Process water storage tanks must not be interconnected with other water systems.

It is recommended that storage tanks are constructed from opaque polypropylene, glass-reinforced plastic (GRP), or plastic-lined steel. The tank design should be free from crevices.

12.8.2 Distribution system

All pipework must be capable of sanitization. It must either be self-draining or capable of being flushed to drain. Stagnant areas must be minimized.

Welded polypropylene or high-density polyethylene pipework is preferred for underground systems. This may also be used on pipe-racks or inside buildings provided it is continuously supported. Alternatively, steel pipes with polypropylene or polyethylene lining may be used. Copper tubing may be used for small diameter off-takes within buildings.

Pumps must be of the centrifugal type with single mechanical seals without external seal lubrication.

12.8.3 Use points and sample points

Use points must be designed to minimize any potential for backflow. Where possible there should be an atmospheric break between the distribution system and the point of use. Provision should be made for periodic flushing and sanitization.

Sample points should be provided such that a representative picture of water quality throughout the distribution system may be obtained.

12.8.4 Control system

Generally, water systems are not subject to detailed operator attention. The control system should ensure any out-of-control situations are communicated to system engineers as soon as possible.

Equipment requiring backwashing or regeneration will often be supplied with its own control system. Monitoring and alarming of suitable parameters should be considered, to ensure the correct operation of these functions could be verified. For example, monitoring the pressure drop across a filter will allow verification of the backwashing operation and trending of inlet water particulate loading.

The installation of instrumentation to allow measurement of the facility's usage of process water is recommended. Appropriate monitoring of individual accountability zones is also recommended.

12.9 Storage and distribution of purified water

12.9.1 Storage tank

The tank volume will be determined by operational considerations, that is, the need to buffer against demand fluctuations and regeneration/cleaning of purification equipment. A sterilizing grade hydrophobic vent filter must be fitted, and precautions taken to prevent waterlogging (e.g., heating).

The tank should be designed for full vacuum and overpressure. Sources of overpressure should be evaluated to determine whether a modest design pressure (e.g., up to 4 barg) would be sufficient to avoid the use of an overpressure protection device. If, however, such a device is needed, a bursting disk, not a pressure relief valve, should be used. A stainless steel nonfragmenting disk fitted with an integral rupture detector should be used. Initiation of relief should be alarmed.

The tank design and operation must minimize static areas and cold spots where bacteria can lodge and multiply. Surfaces should either fully drain or be flushed by water reentering the tank from the return loop. The level in the storage tank should be displayed.

12.9.2 Distribution system

Ideally, the distribution loop of the water system should be recirculatory, with a feed pipe back into the storage tank, or even back into one of the units of the purification system. In this way, the water is continuously moving, even when none is being drawn off the system at any of the outlets.

It is even better if the water is circulated at an elevated temperature (75°C−80°C). Some systems circulate at temperatures of between ambient and 60°C, with an occasional increase in temperature to reduce the bioburden.

If circulation is carried out at ambient temperatures, it is necessary to review the pattern of usage of the water. From experience, systems with ambient circulation and relatively low water usage develop problems with heat gain within the system. In such cases, the actual circulation temperature is closer to 37°C, which is an ideal medium for bacterial growth.

All pipework should be sloped to allow self-draining and must be capable of chemical or thermal sanitization. There should be no dead-legs in the system, that is, points where water may be stagnant. These are sometimes found at outlets if the arrangement of valves is not correct. In some texts, it is stated that a dead leg should be no more than six times the diameter of the pipe, and, in the author's experience, some companies believe this applies to all systems. However, this rule is only valid in systems where the water is circulated at an elevated temperature.

Filters should generally not be used in ring systems, as they provide a breeding ground for bacteria and can mask upstream problems.

The recirculation system should achieve a pipe velocity of between 0.6 and 3.0 m/s, under all usage conditions. The flow must be turbulent.

Pumps for purified water recirculation should be of the centrifugal type, of sanitary design, and be drainable. The shaft seal should be of a single mechanical type. External seal lubrication must not be used.

Pipework must be welded in preference to clamped joints. However, pumps, filters, vessel connections, and instruments should be installed using clamp fittings, to allow maintenance.

Heat exchangers for purified water must be constructed so there is no seal with purified water on one side and service fluid on the other. The use of a double tube sheet exchanger, jacketed pipe exchanger, or a plate exchanger with a double gasket arrangement is acceptable when there is a permanent flow. If either seal should fail, it must be readily detectable. It should be noted that the FDA has expressed a marked preference for double tube sheet types and is suspicious of plate exchangers.

If a heat exchanger is sited without a continuous flow of purified water, it should be self-draining and capable of daily sanitization. It is unlikely a plate heat exchanger could meet these criteria.

12.9.3 Use points and sample points

Use points must be designed to minimize any potential for backflow. Where possible there should be an atmospheric break between the distribution ring and the point of use. If this is not possible, then connections must be demountable and capable of regular sanitization. All user points must be capable of being sampled and must be uniquely identified. Additional sample points should be provided as required for water quality checking.

12.9.4 Control system

Most purification equipment items can be purchased with an independent control system. The integration of these systems will generally provide a centralized alarm system and start/stop signals.

The conductivity of water leaving the purification system should be monitored continuously, with a suitable alarm to indicate system problems. The calibration of conductivity meters should be discussed with the suppliers, as this can be problematic.

If UV lamps are in use, their performance should be monitored by a photometer and run time totalizer.

The installation of instrumentation to ascertain the facility's usage of purified water is recommended. To minimize the risk of contamination, this is best achieved by measuring the flow of water into the deionizers.

Sanitary pressure gauges must be installed where appropriate. The gauge side of the diaphragm must be filled with a food-grade substance acceptable to the regulatory authorities.

In hot recirculatory systems, the temperature should be monitored at the coldest point in the system.

12.9.5 Materials of construction

Ideally, purified water should be stored in 316 L stainless steel tanks and distributed in stainless steel pipework. However, because of the high costs involved, companies often prefer alternatives for pipework in particular. In some systems where it has been determined that polypropylene, polyvinylidene fluoride (PVDF), or acrylonitrile butadiene styrene (ABS) are acceptable, they may be used as an alternative. However, it is important to control construction to ensure crevice-free, full bore joints and well-supported sloping pipework.

Polyvinyl chloride (PVC) distribution systems are not recommended. They are difficult to support and deteriorate rapidly. All materials of construction must comply with good manufacturing practice (GMP) requirements for materials of contact and be capable of withstanding repeated sanitization by steam or hot water. Any solvent residues present from the plastic pipe jointing process must be flushed out. If nonmetallic pipework is installed it should be designed for chemical cleaning and sanitization with an appropriate solution such as sodium hypochlorite or hydrogen peroxide. The design must allow complete removal of the cleaning and sanitization chemicals by flushing to the drain.

Valves must be of the polytetrafluoroethylene (PTFE) diaphragm type with crevice-free construction, mounted to ensure complete self-draining.

The process of ion exchange involves the use of acid and alkali regenerants. Most deionizing equipment is supplied in PVC, polypropylene, or ABS. Screw fittings must not be used. Solvent or heat welds should be specified.

Suppliers should be investigated for construction techniques and standards. Sample joints should be requested, to assure the quality of the jointing mechanism. Cleaning operations carried out should be documented by the supplier.

RO systems utilize high pressures to achieve separation. The safety aspects of this should be addressed, and maintenance procedures should ensure safety features are not compromised.

12.9.6 Insulation

Hot purified water systems must be fully insulated to conserve energy and minimize cold spots. The quality of insulation and cladding should align with the company standards and be appropriate to the quality of the area.

12.10 Storage and distribution of water for injection

The production of WFI will generally be achieved by a packaged unit purchased from a specialist supplier. The storage and distribution of WFI demand more detailed investigation and design on the part of the engineer. The design, manufacture, and installation of all elements are of critical importance to the satisfactory performance of the system.

For WFI systems, the storage and distribution system is generally recirculatory and at elevated temperatures, above 80°C, unless the water is going to be freshly made and not stored. A system that operates at less than 80°C will require regular sanitization and will not allow storage of WFI for more than 24 hours. Such a system should only be used in a laboratory application, or for a single isolated manufacturing user.

Water at 80°C represents a potential hazard to operators. The system design should be reviewed to minimize any risk of injury.

The entire system must be equipped for sterilization with steam and must therefore be pressure rated. A clean steam supply should be used to achieve this.

12.10.1 Storage tank

WFI storage tanks must be capable of steam sterilization. This will require the tank to be pressure rated (sterilizing steam pressure plus a design margin, and full vacuum). As with purified water storage tanks, sources of overpressure should be evaluated to determine whether a modest design pressure increase, for example, up to 4 barg, could avoid the use of an overpressure protection device. Tank pressure relief must be installed such that initiation of relief is readily detectable and alarmed. A bursting disk with an integral rupture detector is preferred. Pressure relief valves are not recommended. A stainless steel nonfragmenting disk should be used.

The WFI in the storage tank must be maintained above 80°C. All WFI entering or reentering must also be above 80°C. The operating temperature must be high enough to ensure the coldest point of the recirculation loop will be above 80°C. Heat should be applied either by a heat exchanger in the recirculation loop or via a jacket on the storage tank. The selection should be made after consideration of the operational and design features. Tank jackets are noninvasive but require tanks to remain substantially filled at all times. External heat exchangers are useful when it is necessary to re-heat the water in the recirculation loop.

The tank must have a hydrophobic 0.2 μm vent filter installed. The vent filter must be capable of sterilization when fitted. Precautions should be taken to ensure condensate does not build up in the filter housing (e.g., by heating the filter).

The tank design and operation must eliminate static areas where water can lodge and cool. Bacteria can multiply in such areas. The entry of the recirculation loop to the tank may be fitted with a spray device to continuously flush all parts of the tank above the water level. This will also provide a back-pressure to the recirculation loop.

12.10.2 Distribution system

Filters must not be installed in the WFI recirculation system since they constitute an area where microbiological contamination is concentrated.

Pumps for WFI should be of centrifugal type, of sanitary design, and drainable. The shaft seal should be of the single mechanical type. External seal lubrication must not be used.

A standby pump should be available at all times for key applications. It is recommended that the standby pump is not permanently installed but is kept available for a speedy changeover. If the standby pump is installed, precautions should be taken to ensure there is no danger of contamination or dead-legs resulting. The changeover should be in accordance with written procedures and be fully validated. The pump must be steam sanitized before use.

Pumps and piping must be sized to achieve a pipe velocity of between 0.6 and 3.0 minutes/seconds under all operating conditions. The flow must be turbulent. Calculations and pump performance data must be documented to form part of the specification and installation qualification. It will be necessary to demonstrate these velocities are being achieved in practice during operational qualification. None of the available sanitary designs of flow meters can be used with WFI because of its low conductivity.

The pipework must be sloped to ensure the system can be completely drained. A minimum fall of 1:100 is recommended. Drain points should be provided at sufficient intervals around the ring main. The system must not have any dead-legs.

Sanitary clamped connections should be used to connect pipework to the tank, pump(s), and other major equipment items. Where possible, connections to use points should be physically disconnected when not in use. All other connections must be welded.

The pipework must be equipped for sterilization with clean steam. Consideration should be given to the introduction of adequate steam and the removal of condensate and air, to allow sterilizing conditions to be reached at all points of the system.

Consideration must be given to methods of providing evidence that sterilizing conditions were obtained, for example, systematic identification of cold spots during operational qualification, followed by temperature logging during sterilization.

Problems can be encountered in clean areas with flash steam from condensate removal during steam sterilization. It may be necessary to declassify clean areas during the steam sterilization of the WFI system.

Where flow restrictors are used, it is important that correct installation can be verified, and any failure is readily detectable.

Fixed pipework should be clearly labeled to indicate the contents and direction of flow.

12.10.3 Heat exchangers

The points to be considered for heat exchangers are similar for WFI and purified water. Heat exchangers for WFI must be constructed so there is no seal with WFI on one side and service fluid on the other.

Use of a double tube sheet exchanger, jacketed pipe exchanger, or a plate exchanger with a double gasket arrangement is acceptable when there is a permanent flow. If either seal should fail it must be readily detectable. As for purified water, the FDA has expressed a marked preference for double tube sheet types and is suspicious of plate exchangers.

If a heat exchanger is sited without a continuous flow of WFI, it should be self-draining and capable of daily sanitization. It is unlikely a plate heat exchanger could meet these criteria.

The use of ordinary shell and tube or plate heat exchangers with single seals and monitored pressure differential between the WFI and utility streams is not acceptable.

12.10.4 Use points and sample points

Generally, the greatest potential for contamination of a WFI system is via its use and sample points. Where feasible, there should be an air break between the ring and the equipment requiring water. Where this is not possible, connections must be demountable and self-draining. The connection should be capable of regular sterilization and should eliminate the potential for back-flow into the ring.

Every use point must be capable of being sampled. When equipment is directly connected to the distribution system, a sample point must be provided. All use points must be uniquely identified.

Equipment items such as component washers often have internal valves used to control water flow, which can lead to potential dead-legs when closed. Careful study of the equipment installed at use points is required, to ensure it does not jeopardize the integrity of the ring.

The design and operation of sample points is of critical importance in obtaining a representative sample and avoiding contamination either of the sample or the system. Also, the hazards associated with sampling hot water should be made clear, and appropriate warning signs fitted.

Routine sampling need not be performed aseptically since any airborne bacterial contamination can be identified as such and their presence in the water discounted.

12.10.5 Monitoring and control system

There are a number of critical parameters which must be continuously recorded and alarmed:

- temperature in the storage tank,
- conductivity and temperature of WFI at the still outlet,
- temperature of the recirculation loop at the coldest point,
- conductivity of the still feed water and the return from the WFI.

The distillation unit should have adequate instrumentation to ensure an alarm is raised when the still shuts down abnormally, and basic troubleshooting can be carried out quickly, without the need for additional equipment.

Loss of flow in the recirculation system should be detectable. However, the resulting fall in temperature in the loop is usually a sufficient indicator.

Diaphragm pressure gauges of sanitary design only should be installed on the ring, to ensure pump performance can be determined. The gauge side of the diaphragm should be filled with a food-grade fluid. The diaphragm must be of an approved material such as 316 L stainless steel. The number of gauges should be the minimum necessary for effective operation.

Measurement of the approximate level or weight in the storage tank should be provided.

In instances where heated vent filters are used, it may prove useful to monitor the temperature of the housing to forewarn against condensate buildup that could block the vent.

12.10.6 Materials of construction

All metallic parts coming into contact with WFI must be constructed from 316 L stainless steel or a near equivalent. Valves must be of the diaphragm type with crevice-free construction, mounted to ensure complete self-draining. Gaskets and valve diaphragms etc. must be of materials acceptable to the regulatory authorities, capable of withstanding continuous use at 80°C to 95°C and repeated sterilization at temperatures up to 140°C.

Pipework should be in 316 L stainless steel, internally electropolished. The storage tank, pumps, and any other equipment items should have a finish in keeping with the pipework specification.

12.10.7 Ambient systems

Applications where WFI is required at temperatures below 80°C present additional challenges. In considering potential solutions, it is advisable to retain simplicity as a design concept.

Ideally, WFI should be stored at high temperature and only be cooled as it is used. The location of heat exchangers should ensure the additional potential for bacterial growth is kept to a minimum. WFI should not be allowed to re-enter the storage tank at less than 80°C.

If all use points require ambient WFI, a cooler can be installed in the ring, with a heater on the return leg. The section of line between the two exchangers could then run cold when water is required, returning to above 80°C at all other times. Frequent or protracted cold operation will require careful design and validation.

If there is a variety of temperature requirements, heat exchangers may be installed external to the distribution ring. In these cases, it is important to either keep a permanent flow through the heat exchanger or sanitize the exchanger each time before use.

12.10.8 Insulation

WFI systems must be fully insulated to minimize cold spots, conserve energy and protect personnel. The quality of insulation and cladding should accord with national standards and be appropriate to the quality of the area. A good external finish is an important attribute and of critical importance where pipes pass into clean areas.

12.11 Monitoring and maintenance of pharmaceutical water systems

Once a company has invested significant time and money into the purification of water to the appropriate grades, the quality level must be maintained throughout its period of storage and distribution before use. During validation, a wide range of tests would be carried out to establish the normal profile for the water. These results can then be used to determine what routine tests should be completed.

For potable and processed water, tests are used appropriate to the standard being applied. If the water is potable when it comes from the metropolitan system, it should be possible to get some information from the authorities. If no such information is available, it may be necessary to do testing in-house.

Providing the materials of construction are suitable, there is very little risk of chemical recontamination of purified water or WFI. There are several standard tests carried out for measuring the chemical aspects, which are the same for both grades of water. These are not covered here but may be found in the relevant pharmacopeial monographs.

On the other hand, the possibility of microbiological recontamination is very real, and a great amount of effort goes into preventing this.

For purified water and WFI, there are differences in the microbiological approach, just as there are differences in the standards to be achieved for each grade.

12.11.1 Validation of purified water treatment systems

A water treatment system is different from other equipment used in the manufacture of pharmaceuticals, and there is a significant validation requirement. Due to the seasonality factor of raw water supply, the system cannot be completely validated until twelve months of data is available. Hence, in addition to the installation qualification (IQ) and operational qualification (OQ) stages, there is a 52-week performance qualification (PQ) stage, which can be divided into two phases with different sampling requirements, as shown in Table 12.1.

12.11.2 Sampling of purified water

During Phase I of validation, all points are sampled and tested daily. This phase lasts between 2 and 4 weeks.

During Phase II (weeks 5–52), weekly samples should be taken from the system feedwater, after every stage of the purification system and on the return loop. Daily sampling is required on at least one user point per day, with the whole system being covered weekly. These results can then be used to set routine monitoring schedules.

12.11.3 Sampling of water for injection systems

Since a WFI system operating at elevated temperatures is essentially self-sanitizing, frequent sampling is unnecessary. For points of the system where the temperature is known to be maintained at above 80°C, monthly sampling should be sufficient. Emphasis is placed instead on temperature monitoring and control.

For any points within the system which are subject to reduced temperature, more frequent sampling is recommended.

Samples for endotoxin measurement should be taken from each user point each day batches of the product are being produced.

12.11.4 Microbiological limits

Microbiological limits are indicators of the need for some action to bring the quality of water back under control. They are not intended as accept/reject criteria, either for

Table 12.1 An example of a routine monitoring schedule.

Sample location	Microbiological sampling and testing	
	Phase I weeks 1–4	Phase II weeks 5–52
System feedwater	Daily	Weekly
After each stage of purification	Daily	Weekly
At each point of use	Daily	At least one point daily
Return	Daily	Weekly

the water or for the batches of product produced with that water, so long as all product specifications are met and there is a demonstrated compliance to GMP.

For ease of operation and to ensure a system remains operating at optimal conditions, companies should set three levels of limits:

1. **Target limits:** Limits known to be attainable with the current technology. For example, a much tighter limit could be considered with a hot system than with a cold one.
2. **Alert limits:** Limits which, when exceeded, indicate a process may have drifted from its normal operating range. Contravention of alert levels does not necessarily require corrective action.
3. **Action limits:** Limits which, when exceeded, indicate a process has drifted from its normal operating range. Exceeding these levels indicates prompt corrective action should be taken to bring the process back within its normal operating range. It does NOT indicate the automatic necessity to reject batches of water or finished product.

The action limit will generally be set at the pharmacopeial level. Determination of appropriate target and alert limits should be based on the consideration of several points:

- the process and product specification tolerances;
- susceptibility of the product types (preservative efficacy, pH, etc.) based on the most susceptible product to be made;
- subsequent processing of the finished product;
- equipment design specifications;
- and historical and/or statistically based levels of microbiological contamination.

In practice, this would mean limits for purified water stored in a hot circulating system could be tighter than for an ambient system. Limits for water to be used in the manufacture of a semisolid product without a preservative are likely to be tighter than for water used in the manufacture of semisolid products which all contain preservatives. And limits for WFI used in the manufacture of a parenteral product that is terminally sterilized would not need to be so tight as limits for WFI used to manufacture parenteral products aseptically.

Monitoring data should be analyzed on an ongoing basis to ensure the process continues to perform within acceptable limits. Analysis of data trends may be used to evaluate process performance.

This information may be used to predict departures from established operating parameters, signaling the need for appropriate preventative maintenance.

12.11.5 Methodology

The preferred methodology for analysis of samples is membrane filtration using 0.45-μm filters.

The sample size for WFI is at least 200 mL and for purified water "appropriate to the expected result." In other words, for low levels of contamination, a larger sample is required than for higher levels of contamination.

12.11.6 Monitoring of filters

Vent filters should be integrity tested to ensure they are still intact. It is important to ensure vent filters are not "blinded" by water, for example, condensation getting onto the hydrophobic filter. If this happens, it can cause a rupture of the filter or collapse of the tank.

Other filters, both large pore size, such as sand filters, and microbiological filters should be monitored to ensure they are not blocked. This can be done by measuring the pressure differential across the filter.

For microbiological filters, an alternative method would be to use validation data to determine a time period after which they should be replaced.

UV lamps should also be monitored in terms of their intensity. Manufacturers recommend a number of running hours after which the lamp needs to be replaced. However, it is also possible to measure the intensity of the lamp, using relatively low-cost meters.

12.11.7 Regeneration

Regeneration is an issue for softeners (brine) and twin bed and mixed-bed deionizers (chemicals) only. There is no regeneration required for CDI units. Regeneration is necessary to remove ions from the resin when it becomes saturated. It can also be a method of sanitization of the unit. The process can be automatic or manual and the procedure should be set based on the information obtained during the IQ phase of validation. For mixed-bed units, used as polishers after the RO units, regeneration frequency might be quite low.

Standard regeneration cycles are two to three hours. The problems associated with regeneration are the downtime of the unit, which can be overcome by having dual units in parallel or running the cycle at times when the plant is not running; and the large volumes of chemicals which need to be handled.

It is possible to get rapid regenerating units with an additional cation polisher after the anion resin bed. They have a shorter cycle, 30−40 minutes. The advantages include space-saving, reduction in the need for water storage, energy-saving, and the requirement for less resin. The disadvantages include the fact that they are packed beds that prevent movement of the resin during regeneration and hence the trapped material does not have the same opportunity to wash away. Pretreatment is much more important for this type of unit.

12.11.8 Sanitization

The storage tank and the distribution pipework must be subject to a written program of cleaning and sterilization. The frequency of such activity will be determined by the historical results collected during validation and the ongoing quality control testing.

Sanitization splits into many stages within the system. There is the front-end, pretreatment stage, where chemical means are used. Up to the point of the carbon filter, there will generally be a level of chlorine in the water to prevent contamination buildup. Hence, sanitization of this part of the system will tend to be very rare. However, as discussed in Section 12.12, biofilm can be a problem needing to be dealt with.

The second stage is the deionization plant, RO or EDI, which is generally sanitized chemically, although heat can be used in CDI plants.

The third stage is the WFI plant, which is sanitized by heat. Finally, there is the distribution loop that may be sterilized by either chemicals or heat.

12.11.8.1 Chemical sanitization methods

Chemical sanitizers may be divided into oxidizing and nonoxidizing agents. Of the oxidizers, the most commonly used is chlorine, which is the most effective and least expensive option. It is highly effective against biofilm. The standard dosage is between 50 and 100 mg/L and the exposure time should be 1–2 hours.

A similar effect can be obtained with chlorine dioxide, using the same concentration and exposure time. However, this is a corrosive material, mixed on-site and, hence, should be handled with care.

For chlorine or chlorine dioxide, the main disadvantage is potential problems with contamination of the output water and the finished product. Hence, there needs to be an effective removal process.

An alternative sanitizer is ozone. It is generally dosed at between 10 and 50 mg/L and has an exposure time of less than 1 hour. Under these conditions, it is between 50% and 100% as effective as chlorine. It needs to be produced on-site and dosed continuously due to its instability. The FDA paper on Water Treatment Systems raises the implications for employee health and safety in its use. However, manufacturers and suppliers of ozone generators state the exposure likely from this use of ozone is an order of magnitude lower than the maximum safe limit for humans. Ozone, apart from its rapid degradation to oxygen, can be destroyed by UV, which is frequently found downstream of the point where it would enter the system.

A further alternative in the oxidizing agents is hydrogen peroxide, which is dosed at 10% volume per volume for 2–3 hours. It has no problems with by-products since it degrades to form water and oxygen. However, its effectiveness against biofilm has yet to be proven.

In addition to the oxidizing agents, several nonoxidizing agents are available. Quaternary ammonium compounds are effective as biocides and surfactants. However, there can be problems in removing them from the system. Anionic and nonanionic surfactants are not particularly effective as biocides on their own but can be used in conjunction with other compounds to remove biofilm.

Previously, many companies used formaldehyde as a sanitizing agent. It is relatively noncorrosive to stainless steel and is an effective biocide. However, it is less effective against biofilm and as it is carcinogenic, it presents significant health and safety issues. Its use was thus phased out.

12.11.8.2 Physical methods: heat

Stills supply WFI to the system at temperatures above 95°C. However, this temperature cannot be maintained without a heat exchanger and heat loss within the system will reduce the temperature to around 80°C. Circulation at this temperature will prevent the proliferation of bacteria. However, a paper by Mittelman (1986), shows this will only reduce but not prevent, biofilm development.

Therefore, although such hot circulating systems for WFI are essentially self-sanitizing, it may be necessary to sanitize the entire system periodically. This may be achieved by raising the temperature above 121°C for around 30 minutes. This can be carried out by draining the system contents and injecting pure, clean steam, and pressurizing to around 2 barg. This traditional method is very reliable but has the disadvantages of the direct expense of extending the pure steam system to the WFI system and the indirect expense caused through the downtime incurred in removing air from the system and manually fitting steam-trapping equipment. There are also health and safety issues associated with steam.

An alternative to pure steam is to sterilize the system with high-temperature WFI. The system is drained down and a predetermined quantity of WFI is heated by an in-line heat exchanger. When the vessel temperature has reached 100°C, the vessel vent valve is closed and the system starts to pressurize, allowing heating to 125°C. Water at 125°C is circulated in the system for 25−30 minutes.

Whichever method of sterilization is used, it will be necessary to use thermocouples connected to chart recorders to obtain a record of the process.

Hot water sanitization can also be effective for CDI units. It has been demonstrated that a weekly cycle of 40 minutes warm-up at 25°C−65°C; a hold period of 60 minutes at 65°C; and a cooldown period of 40 minutes, achieves effective sanitization and a 3-year life could be expected from the unit. This work is fully described in the paper by Wood, Hirayama, and Satoh (2000).

12.11.8.3 Physical methods: mechanical scrubbing

Heavy biofilm cannot be removed from storage tank walls by the use of chemicals alone; mechanical scrubbing or scraping, high-pressure spraying, or a combination, is also required. However, mechanical removal of biofilm from distribution systems is impractical.

12.12 Biofilm

Water systems exhibit a particular microbiological problem in the form of biofilm. As well as existing as free organisms within the water, bacteria also become attached to the surfaces of the pipes and tanks. This biofilm will act as a form of protection for the individual organisms; however, periodically sections of the biofilm will slough off and increase the microbial level in the water. As a result, contamination levels will not be uniform throughout the system. Under these circumstances, sample results will not be representative of the type and level of contamination across the entire system. Counts of 10 CFU/mL in one sample and 100 or even 1000 CFU/mL in other samples might easily be observed.

The reason that biofilm is such a problem is that it provides protection to bacteria and hence is much more difficult to remove from the water system. Bacteria in this form may be 150−3000 times more resistant to free chlorine and 2−100 times more resistant to monochloramine than free-floating bacteria.

The development of biofilm is independent of the material of the surface. Biofilm will develop just as easily on stainless steel as on plastic. A major factor aiding the development of biofilm is the large surface area within a water treatment, storage, and distribution system. All the elements of the system including RO membranes, DI resins, storage tanks, cartridge filters, and piping systems provide surfaces suitable for bacterial attachment and growth.

12.12.1 Development of biofilm

As soon as a clean tank or piece of pipework is filled with water, a biofilm may start to form. The development of the biofilm occurs in several steps:

- Surface conditioning: Trace organics are deposited at the interface between the water and the walls of the tank or the pipework. This layer neutralizes surface charges and allows the bacteria to get close enough to become attached to the wall. Additionally, the layer provides a source of nutrients for the bacteria.
- Adhesion of pioneer bacteria: Free-floating bacteria enter the boundary layer area at the wall where the velocity is virtually zero and become adsorbed onto the walls. The attachment is initially due to physical rather than chemical factors.
- Slime formation: The bacteria within the biofilm produce sticky polymers which hold the biofilm together and increase the adhesion to the walls. The strands of polymer also act as a protective barrier and concentrate any nutrients available in the water. The pioneer bacteria start to reproduce and thus increase the surface area of the biofilm.

- Secondary colonizers: The slime will trap other bacteria from the water by physical, electrostatic attraction. These secondary colonizers feed off the waste produced by the primary colonizers and increase the size of the biofilm.
- Fully functioning biofilm: A mature biofilm is living tissue, made up of different bacterial types living as a community. It may even be considered to have a primary circulatory system.

Biofilm continues to develop in two ways. Growth will occur by normal reproduction, which will increase the size of the original community. However, as the thickness of the film increases, it will move out of the boundary layer into areas where the velocity of the water is greater and thus the sloughing off process will occur. Some of these cells will then form other areas of biofilm elsewhere in the tank or the pipework.

The speed of development of the mature biofilm can vary from hours to weeks, depending on a number of variables in the system. Vanhaecke et al. (1990) showed that *Pseudomonas* cells could start to form a biofilm on electropolished stainless steel surfaces, within 30 seconds of exposure.

A smooth surface may delay the early stages of development; however, in the long run, the overall size of the biofilm does not appear to be reduced by smoothness.

12.12.2 Common misconceptions about biofilm

Biofilm was originally thought to be disorganized associations of cells. However, advances in microscopy of biofilm showed they are highly organized, complex structures.

It was originally assumed that biochemically, there was no difference between free-floating bacteria and those in the biofilm. However, it was discovered that although genetically they are the same, due to a change in the genes in use, the biochemical behavior is different.

The biocidal activity of any given disinfectant is expressed as CT, being the product of concentration and time. However, CT values for free-floating bacteria cannot be extrapolated to the bacteria within the biofilm.

12.12.3 Biocorrosion

Biocorrosion occurs on metal surfaces as a result of the presence of biofilm. It is exhibited in several forms, including:

- pitting
- crevice corrosion
- selective de-alloying
- stress corrosion cracking
- underdeposit corrosion

It is caused either by oxygen depletion, leading to a difference in electrical potential between different parts of the surface; or by the destruction of the passivation oxide film. Additionally, anaerobic bacteria such as sulfate-reducing types can flourish in this environment and increase corrosion.

12.12.4 Control of biofilm

The control of biofilm in water treatment systems is very difficult. As free-floating organisms, bacteria do not develop a resistance to biocides, as they do to the antibiotics used in medicine, since there are many potential target sites that can be attacked. However, in the form of a biofilm, there is physical protection from the biocide. If sanitization is not completely carried out, it will only be a short time before the biofilm is fully functional once more.

There are several reasons why control of biofilm is very difficult:

- The nutrient levels required are so low that even purified water can provide sufficient food.
- The sticky polymers form such tight bonds that the turbulence within the pipework is not strong enough to break them.
- Even after smoothing the surfaces and removing all crevices in welds etc., the bacteria are still able to attach themselves.
- The slime forms physical protection of the bacteria from chlorine or other sanitizers.

In conclusion, the methods adopted by companies will tend to involve a number of different measures and it will be accepted that this will tend to control the biofilm, rather than completely eradicate it.

12.13 Common problems and troubleshooting

From a microbiological viewpoint, there are several areas that can cause problems within pharmaceutical water treatment systems. The FDA guideline presents a discussion of some of these areas, quoting cases found during factory inspections. Some of these are briefly reviewed in this section.

12.13.1 Problems with purified water systems

Problems have been observed with RO systems since they operate at ambient temperatures and the filters do not retain bacteria. Suggested solutions include the use of a UV lamp or heat exchangers downstream of the RO unit; in either case, this would reduce the contamination level.

12.13.2 Problems with water for injection systems

Problems have been observed more with endotoxin levels than microbial contamination. These are due to such causes as:

- feedwater droplets being carried into the distillate
- stagnant water in the condenser over the weekend
- insufficient pretreatment of feedwater

Since most stills will only result in fewer than 2.5 log reduction in endotoxin content, a low level in the feedwater is essential.

Observations of a circulatory system when switched off showed contamination developed in less than 24 hours. This resulted in the FDA recommendation that noncirculating systems should be drained at least daily.

12.13.3 Problems with heat exchangers

There is an FDA Inspectors Technical Guide entitled "Heat Exchangers to Avoid Contamination," which discusses design issues and potential problems. Contamination due to leakage can be prevented by using pressure differential monitors to ensure there is always a higher pressure on the clean fluid side. As discussed previously, the use of the double tube sheet type of heat exchanger is also preferable. Problems can also be seen if the cooling water is drained out of the heat exchanger when it is not in use, since corrosion can lead to pinholes being formed.

12.13.4 Problems with pumps

If pumps are not operational continuously, they should be fully drained, to prevent the buildup of contamination in static water within the reservoir.

12.13.5 Problems with the distribution loop

Problems with the distribution loop include the contamination occurring when a user point has a hose connection containing nonsterile air. Depending on the order in which valves are opened, the nonsterile air can contaminates the rest of the system.

The issue of dead-legs is also discussed and the nonvalidity of the "six diameters" rule is emphasized for systems not held at above 80°C.

Problems also relate to the use of bacterial grade filters in the system since they can provide a good environment for growth. In addition, they tend to hide any underlying contamination in the system and do not remove endotoxin. If a filter is unavoidable, there must be a written procedure, including the frequency of changing the filter.

The importance of "cracking" terminal valves during sanitization is stressed, to ensure all parts of the pipework are filled with water and thus exposed to the sanitizer.

The storage tank is one part of the system where it is hard to maintain high turbulence. To minimize the problems, it is recommended that tanks be sized such that the volume change is four to six times per hour.

12.14 Wastewater treatment

The pharmaceutical industry develops products that can have a high degree of potency and toxicity. This has always been an issue from the point of view of the safe disposal of waste. With the growth in the past two decades of worldwide public awareness of the dangers resulting from pollution of the environment, the importance of dealing with waste within the pharmaceutical and chemical industries took on a new urgency. In both Europe and the United States, failure to comply with the regulations will have serious consequences for a company. In the context of this chapter, the discussion will center on the treatment and disposal of wastewater.

The treatment of wastewater dates back to the construction of sewers in the cities of Crete, ancient Assyria, and the areas ruled by the Romans. Towards the end of the middle ages, cesspools and underground systems were constructed to deal with human waste.

As the population grew in the 19th century and cities started to grow in size it was recognized that human health would be improved if human waste could be rapidly removed using storm drains. The significant leap forward in sanitary engineering was the invention of flushing toilets enabling the development of the modern sewerage system.

During the middle of the 20th century, it was realized that flushing ever-increasing quantities of waste into lakes and rivers caused serious health risks, and as a result, governments started to invest in the construction of central sewerage treatment plants for major centers of population. In addition, legislation was enacted to start the control of liquid and gaseous pollutants.

12.14.1 Measurement of water contamination

The composition of wastewater is analyzed using several physical, chemical, and biological measurements. The main ones are as follows:

- Biological oxygen demand: BOD is the amount of oxygen used over a 5-day period by microorganisms as they decompose the organic matter in the effluent at a temperature of 20°C. BOD tests the strength of untreated effluent and biodegradable waste in the water.
- Chemical oxygen demand: COD is the amount of oxygen required to oxidize the organic matter by using dichromate in an acid solution to convert it to carbon dioxide. COD tests the strength of wastewater that is either not biodegradable or contains compounds that inhibit the activities of microorganisms.

The value of COD is always higher than BOD because many organic substances can be oxidized chemically but cannot be oxidized biologically. As their names suggest, BOD and COD combine with free oxygen in the water. In extreme cases, oxygen depletion can cause damage to living creatures in the water.

Other measures include pH and chemical composition.

12.14.2 Treatment of wastewater

A pharmaceutical manufacturing plant will produce a variety of wastewater streams:
- domestic sewage: from toilets, washrooms, and the canteen;
- process wastewater: noncontaminated washing water and process cooling water;
- contaminated wastewater: any effluent contaminated either chemically or biologically during the process;
- and general site drainage: water runoff from the site infrastructure.

There are a number of options that can be incorporated in designing a wastewater treatment system:
- Settle tanks allow the wastewater stream to pass very slowly through a specially designed trough system. Inorganic particles of greater than 0.2 mm fall out of suspension and drop to the bottom of the tank. After removal, these are disposed of in landfill sites or are incinerated.
- Sedimentation is similar in principle to the settling tank and results in between 40% and 60% of the suspended solids being removed. By the addition of chemicals to the sedimentation, coagulation occurs which further increases solids removal.
- Flocculation: With additional treatment, up to 80% of the suspended solids can be removed, reducing up to 40% of the BOD.
- Digestion is an anaerobic microbiological process that converts organic sludge to methane and carbon dioxide.
- Biological treatment is an aerobic process where organic matter is converted to carbon dioxide, water, nitrates, and phosphates. The solid waste generated would go to landfills or be incinerated.
- Filters: Depending on the contaminant to be removed from the effluent stream, the major filter manufacturers have a range of products that will be suitable. However, filtration would normally be only one stage in the treatment of the effluent stream
- Advanced oxidation is a simple but effective way of treating industrial effluent, using the oxidization power of ozone which is enhanced by the catalyzing effect of UV light (producing hydroxyl free radicals) and destroying the chemical demand for oxygen. The system is a very green solution as not only does it treat the contaminants, but it results in a clean discharge stream saturated in oxygen.

- Macroporous polymer extraction is a system developed by Akzo Nobel in the Netherlands using polymer-based technology for the removal of hydrocarbons from water. It has shown excellent performance in the removal of many of the solvents used in the pharmaceutical industry. The manufacturers claim up to 99.99% removal for the system. The waste stream is passed through a specially designed column, which is packed with the macroporous polymer. An extraction fluid, immobilized within the polymer matrix, draws the hydrocarbons out of the water. When the extraction fluid is saturated, the column is regenerated by top feeding the column with low-pressure steam, releasing the hydrocarbons, which can be condensed and collected for reuse or incineration.

12.15 Chapter summary

- Water, in a variety of grades, is a key component of pharmaceutical manufacturing both as a raw material and as a processing element.
- There are several national and international guidelines relating to pharmaceutical water, plus several industry-produced references.
- Although the terminology may differ occasionally between different regulatory systems, there are four main water grades to consider: potable water; process water; purified water; and WFI, standing for Water for Injections (Europe) or Water for Injection (United States).
- The specification for each grade will be found in the relevant pharmacopeia.
- There are many options available for the design of a water treatment system and decisions will be based on a variety of factors both physical and economic.
- Water pretreatment methods available include coarse filtration to remove larger particles; carbon filters to remove organics; chemical treatments to control microbiological contamination; and water softeners.
- Preparation of purified water may be achieved using one or more of the following technologies: RO (hyperfiltration); one of several types of deionization units; ultraviolet radiation; and ultrafiltration.
- Preparation of WFI is most commonly achieved using distillation; there are a number of different types of still available. Additionally, RO and/or ultrafiltration are acceptable methods under certain conditions.
- There are a number of factors to consider in designing a WFI preparation system, including quality of the feedwater, contamination risks, and energy efficiency.
- There are specific requirements for each grade of water in terms of storage tanks; distribution system design and construction; use points and sample points; and the control system.
- Monitoring and maintenance programs are critical in ensuring the quality of each water system is sustained. Chemical recontamination is a low risk, providing the

system has been designed and constructed appropriately. However, the risk of microbiological recontamination is high and significant effort is required to prevent this.

- Validation of purified water treatment systems requires a minimum of a one-year program to ensure any seasonality in the water supply is accounted for.
- Microbiological limits are not intended as accept/reject criteria. Three levels need to be set: target limits, alert limits, and action limits.
- Other key aspects to maintenance programs include monitoring of filters; regeneration; and sanitization, which may be achieved via chemicals, heat, or mechanical scrubbing.
- The formation of biofilm on even smooth surfaces within water treatment systems is a high risk. Biofilm affords protection to individual organisms and increases the overall contamination level as parts of the film slough off.
- There are a number of misconceptions about biofilms that increase the difficulty of prevention. The presence of biofilm can lead to internal biocorrosion.
- Several problems with purified water treatment systems and suggestions for solutions have been presented by regulatory inspectors.
- Wastewater treatment is a major topic for the pharmaceutical industry due to the high levels of toxic chemicals used in the manufacturing process. This issue is of increasing importance because of the growing awareness of risks to the environment.
- Measurement of contamination in wastewater is done both from a biological and chemical point of view.
- A variety of methods are available to the industry to treat wastewater to reduce the risk to the environment,

12.16 Questions/problems

1. You are the engineering manager for a pharmaceutical company producing a mixed range of products: tablets, cream, and ointments. List all the purposes for which water will be used in the factory and identify which grade would be required in each case.
2. You are the design engineer for a company installing a small sterile products facility to produce SVPs (ampules and vials). What issues would you have to consider in designing the water treatment system for the facility?
3. You are the quality assurance manager for the company in the previous question. How would you design the validation plan for the water treatment system?
4. You are the maintenance engineer for an API manufacturing facility. What would you expect to see on the monitoring and maintenance program for the water treatment system?

5. You are the design engineer for the company installing the SVP facility in the second question above. How would you minimize the risk of biofilm becoming a problem in your new water treatment system?
6. You are the new quality assurance manager for the company producing a mixed portfolio of products in the first question. The company has been fined by the local authority for contaminated wastewater. How would you investigate the problem?

References

European Medicines Agency, 2020. EMA/CHMP/CVMP/QWP/496873/2018 guideline on the quality of water for pharmaceutical use. <https://www.ema.europa.eu/en/documents/scientific-guideline/guideline-quality-water-pharmaceutical-use_en.pdf/> (accessed 09.07.21).

European Pharmacopoeia (n.d.) Water for injections (0169).

European Pharmacopoeia (n.d.) Water, purified (0008).

European Pharmacopoeia (n.d.) Water for preparation of extracts (2249).

International Society for Pharmaceutical Engineering, 2012. ISPE good practice guide: ozone sanitization of pharmaceutical water systems.

International Society for Pharmaceutical Engineering, 2014 ISPE good practice guide: commissioning and qualification of pharmaceutical water and steam systems.

International Society for Pharmaceutical Engineering, 2016. ISPE good practice guide: sampling for pharmaceutical water, steam, and process gases.

International Society for Pharmaceutical Engineering, 2019 ISPE baseline guide: volume 4 – water and steam systems (third edition).

Mittelman, M.W., 1986. Biological fouling of purified water systems: part III treatment. microcontamination, January 1986.

Vanhaecke, E. et al. (1990) *Kinetics of* Pseudomonas aeruginosa *adhesion to 304 and 316-L stainless steel: role of cell surface hydrophobicity.* Applied and Environmental Microbiology. Vol 56 No. 3

Wood, J., Hirayama, J., Satoh, S., 2000. Hot water sanitization of continuous electrodeionization systems. Pharm. Eng. 20-6, 34–40.

Further reading

European Council, 2020. DIRECTIVE 98/83/EC on the quality of water intended for human consumption. <https://eur-lex.europa.eu/legal-content/EN/TXT/PDF/?uri = CELEX:01998L008320151027&from = EN> (accessed 10.07.21).

The European Parliament & The Council of the European Union, 2015. Council directive 98/83/EC on the quality of water intended for human consumption (amended). <https://eur-lex.europa.eu/legal-content/EN/TXT/PDF/?uri = CELEX:01998L0083-20151027&from = EN> (accessed 09.07.21).

United States Food and Drug Administration, 2016. High purity water system (7/93) guide to inspections of high purity water systems. <https://www.fda.gov/inspections-compliance-enforcement-and-criminal-investigations/inspection-guides/high-purity-water-system-793> (accessed 09.07.21).

United States Food and Drug Administration, 2014. Inspection Technical Guides 46 water for pharmaceutical use. <https://www.fda.gov/inspections-compliance-enforcement-and-criminal-investigations/inspection-technical-guides/water-pharmacuetical-use> (accessed 09.07.21).

CHAPTER 13

Pharmaceutical microbiology

13.1 Introduction

This chapter covers a variety of topics, which are all connected by microbiology. The association of microorganisms with the pharmaceutical industry can be a positive one, where the microorganism is an integral part of manufacturing the finished product, whether that product is an antibiotic, a vaccine, a hormone, an enzyme, and so on.

However, the association of microorganisms with the pharmaceutical industry can be a negative one, where contamination of the product with viable or nonviable particles can lead to adverse reactions in the patient. It is this aspect that is being addressed in this chapter. As Tim Sandle states in the introduction to his book on Pharmaceutical Microbiology (2016):

> In drawing from risk assessment terminology, pharmaceutical microbiology centers on understanding the likelihood of product contamination arising; understanding the severity of such contamination; considering ways to minimize contamination; and, where contamination cannot be satisfactorily mitigated, using established and developing new methods to detect contamination.

The chapter begins with an overview of basic microbiology, as it relates to the pharmaceutical industry. Next, there is a discussion of the microbiological aspects of raw materials. Although water is a key raw material in the pharmaceutical industry, as well as being a major element in the provision of services and cleaning, it is excluded from the discussions in this chapter, as it is dealt with fully in Chapter 12.

There is a short section on the microbiology of nonsterile products, but the remainder of the chapter deals with the topic of sterile manufacturing. First, there is a review of the main types of sterile products and other items sold in the sterile state. Next, there is a discussion of the manufacturing of sterile products, with particular emphasis on the differences between terminally sterilized products and those that must be manufactured aseptically. There follow discussions on the contamination risks inherent in a pharmaceutical factory and the methods used within the industry to control contamination levels; also the different monitoring programs needed to ensure contamination has been controlled. Finally, there is a brief review of the huge topic of sterilization.

Quality
DOI: https://doi.org/10.1016/B978-0-323-90815-3.00013-X

13.2 Overview of microorganisms

Microorganisms can be subdivided into six main categories: algae, archaea, bacteria, fungi, protozoa, and viruses. In the context of pharmaceutical manufacturing, the main focus is on bacteria, and this will be reflected in this chapter.

13.2.1 Bacteria

Bacteria are unicellular and lack a nucleus. They are found in four basic shapes: round, rod-shaped, spiral, or curved. They range in size from 0.2 to 10 μm and most are less than 5 μm in length; an exception to this being spiral organisms which can grow to 100 μm long. The bacteria most commonly found in our environment are round or rod-shaped.

Round-shaped bacteria are called cocci. Common examples of cocci genus are *Staphylococcus* and *Streptococcus*, both of which are associated with infections. Rod-shaped bacteria are called bacilli. Common examples are *Escherichia coli*, which is associated with intestinal disorders, and *Pseudomonas* genus, which is associated with infections.

Although most living organisms require oxygen to survive, this is not true of all bacteria. Some bacteria exist as aerobes, which means they require oxygen to live. Alternatively, there are other bacteria called anaerobes as they are killed by the presence of oxygen. There are also two intermediate types: aerotolerant anaerobes can exist with or without oxygen, and facultative anaerobes can grow with or without oxygen but develop better in the presence of oxygen.

Bacteria can be divided into pathogenic organisms, the ones that cause disease, and the nonpathogenic organisms which are present in the environment all the time and, in many cases, are necessary for healthy living. All the examples given above are pathogens. However, the vast majority of bacteria are nonpathogenic. In pharmaceutical terms, it is more important to prevent contamination with pathogens. That is why, for example, pharmacopeial monographs for purified water grades quote a maximum level for total bacterial count (which is about particulate reduction as much as anything) but specify the absence of pathogens such as coliforms or pseudomonads.

Bacteria can exist in one of two states, depending on whether conditions are optimal or adverse from the organism's point of view. Under optimal conditions, the organism is in a vegetative state and continues to feed and grow. In this situation, cells are relatively easy to destroy and will tend to be controlled by disinfection and sanitization processes. Cocci only exist in this state and hence are relatively easy to kill. However, they are quite resistant to drying and hence can exist on the skin or dry surfaces or in the air over time.

Under adverse conditions, some bacteria, such as Bacillus species can form spores. These are similar to seeds in that they produce a protective casing and remain dormant until more favorable environmental conditions exist. This will often occur when there is insufficient moisture around. For bacterial spores to be killed, full sterilization conditions need to be achieved.

13.2.2 Fungi

Fungi consist of mushrooms, molds, and yeasts. They are usually multicellular and contain a nucleus. They may be described as decomposers, absorbing organic material from the environment; symbionts, growing through a mutually beneficial relationship with a host; or parasites, where the relationship is harmful to the host. They reproduce by releasing spores.

Fungi are relatively susceptible and will tend to be controlled by the measures in place to control bacteria. There is not generally much emphasis on fungi in the context of pharmaceutical microbiology. However, it is fungi that cause spoilage of raw materials and/or packaging materials under damp conditions and this is one of the reasons it is important to check the condition of all deliveries received in the factory.

13.2.3 Viruses

Viruses are the most common biological microorganism on Earth. A virus cannot capture or store energy and cannot grow or reproduce outside the living cell of its host organism. On this basis, it must be considered as being nonliving. However, within a host, it can reproduce itself. And while many viruses are harmless, some can cause infections of varying severity, up to and including being fatal to humans.

Like fungi, viruses are relatively susceptible outside the host cells and will tend to be controlled by the measures in place to control bacteria.

13.2.4 Pyrogens and endotoxins

Another area of importance about pharmaceutical manufacturing is that of pyrogens, a mixed group of nonviable particles which trigger an immune reaction if injected into the bloodstream. Pyrogens may be bacterial or nonbacterial in origin. However, the main category of pyrogens of concern within pharmaceutical manufacturing is endotoxins. These are toxic substances consisting of lipopolysaccharide and lipoprotein complexes bound to the cell walls of gram-negative bacteria such as E. Coli and Pseudomonas species. When the bacteria rupture or disintegrate, endotoxins are released.

While endotoxins are rarely fatal, they can cause fevers. For all products administered parenterally, there is a requirement not only for sterility but also for the absence of endotoxins.

13.3 The microbiology of raw materials

One of the tests carried out on many raw materials before they are approved for use is an analysis of microbiological content. The specification for the material should contain not only chemical and physical data but also the maximum permitted level of microbial contamination. Where that level should be set will depend on several factors including the following:

- The source of the material: A raw material produced from natural sources such as plant matter will tend to have a higher microbial content than a material produced synthetically.
- The intended use of the material: A raw material to be used in the manufacture of a clean liquid or an ointment without preservative will tend to have a tighter microbial limit than one being used in the manufacture of tablets.

If a raw material is to be used in the aseptic manufacture of a sterile product, it will usually have been purchased ready-sterilized from the supplier. In this case, it is acceptable to delay the sampling and testing of the container until it has been transferred into the sterile area and manufacturing is due to commence. This is because the normal conditions under which samples are taken, while suitable for nonsterile materials, would not provide sufficient protection for a sterile material.

13.4 Nonsterile products

Nonsterile products are those which, while being pharmaceutically clean, do not need to be sterile when they are administered to the patient. They include dry products such as tablets or capsules, oral liquids which may be solutions or suspensions, suppositories, and some ointments and creams. Even though there is no requirement for sterility, it is important to ensure the product is not heavily contaminated and hence many precautions need to be taken.

There are no clear-cut rules for the production of nonsterile products. Companies need to justify to the regulators their chosen approach, and this will be based on a risk assessment, particularly about microbiological contamination. While there are no rules, it is custom and practice within the industry that wherever a raw material, intermediate, or finished product is exposed to the atmosphere, an area classification of at least ISO grade 8 is required. The topic of area classifications is fully discussed in Section 13.6.1.

The conditions under which manufacturing is carried out will increase in stringency if the nature of the product is such that microbial contamination is likely to occur. For example, dry products tend not to support microbial growth. On the other hand, a cream, which is water-based, may be susceptible to contamination, depending on whether the formulation contains a preservative or not.

On occasion, manufacturing requirements may be driven by national regulations. In some countries, the microbial limit for oral suspensions to be given to infants younger than 12 months is much tighter than for the same product if it is for children older than 12 months. Hence, in a facility where products of different specifications are being manufactured, the tighter limit must be included in the design parameters.

The topic of environmental monitoring is covered in detail later in this chapter. In the context of nonsterile manufacturing, it is sufficient to say that monitoring programs should be established to suit the design of the facility and the process, the required results, and the historical profile as obtained during validation.

13.5 Sterile products

Sterile products are those products that need to be free of both microorganisms and nonviable particulates, including endotoxins, due to the method in which they are administered to the patient. The largest class of sterile products are the small volume parenterals (SVPs), which are injectable products. Other types of sterile products include large volume parenterals (LVPs), some ointments and creams, and eye drops. Additionally, there is a wide range of medical devices that need to be sterile when sold.

13.5.1 Small volume parenterals

Primary containers in the case of SVPs are ampules, vials, or prefilled syringes. They may be made of glass or plastic. The fill-volume in an SVP is generally 10 mL or less. In most cases, it is 1 or 2 mL.

Ampules contain single-unit doses. They are more common in Europe than in the United States, where there is concern about the particulate contamination caused by broken glass at the point of opening. They are the cheapest to manufacture and purchase. The product within an ampule will generally be in liquid form.

Vials can either be single or multiunit doses. They have a rubber disk within the seal, below the cap, which can be pierced several times as the doses are taken out. Product within a vial may be liquid, powder, or a freeze-dried pellet. In the latter two cases, the drug is dissolved or reconstituted with a suitable sterile diluent before administration of the injection.

Prefilled syringes are single-unit dosage forms. They are the most convenient to use since the needle is attached to the pack. They are the most expensive to manufacture and purchase. The product is a prefilled syringe will always be liquid.

13.5.2 Large volume parenterals

Primary containers for LVPs are bottles or bags. The former may be made from glass or plastic; the latter tend to be made from plastic. The fill-volume can be anything from 25 mL to 1 L. LVPs are the products associated with the administration of drips, such as blood products or saline, or transfusions.

13.5.3 Ointments and creams

Sterile ointments and creams are normally filled into tubes. These tubes can be made of metal but are more usually made of plastic. The fill-volume is usually 5 mL or less since once the tube is opened, the sterility can no longer be guaranteed.

In some cases, ointments and creams are packed in more novel containers, such as pump dispensers, which allow a measured amount to be dispensed without the risk of the remainder of the product becoming contaminated.

13.5.4 Eye drops

Sterile eye drops are liquids, which are filled into dispensing containers such as dropper bottles. The fill-volume is generally less than 10 mL.

13.5.5 Medical devices

The range of sterile medical devices is very large, and they come in all shapes and sizes, from single injection needles, to multicomponent dialysis kits.

13.6 Sterile manufacturing

The manufacturing of sterile products takes place in stages, and the exact sequence depends on many variables including the nature of the product and the type and material of the primary container.

In general terms, the sequence of events will be as follows:
- the preparation stage for the bulk batch of the drug, the primary packaging components, and ancillary items such as filling machine parts;
- the filling and sealing stage;
- the inspection stage;
- and the final packaging stage.

In addition, there will be the sterilization stage, which will vary in position, as discussed below. For some dosage forms, there will also be a leak-test stage after filling and sealing.

The type of manufacturing that is appropriate will also have implications for the classification of the manufacturing areas.

13.6.1 Reference documents for cleanrooms

Over the years, there have been a variety of standards used across the world for defining the classification of cleanrooms to be used for manufacturing areas of differing purposes. The classification determines the limits for total particulate contamination, both viable and nonviable; and microbiological contamination. It has implications for the quality of air supplied to the cleanroom; the clothing worn by operators; and a wide range of other factors.

Although the industry-specific standards are written about the manufacture of sterile products, custom and practice within the industry has led to appropriate levels of classification being used for nonsterile manufacturing as well.

A number of these reference documents are listed below since in the author's experience, some companies tend to use older and more familiar terminology, even if they are, in practice, working to the most up-to-date standards.

- United States (US) Federal Standard 209D: with the familiar classes of 100, 10,000, and 100,000, this is the terminology that was formerly most commonly used in many countries. It was updated in the 1990s to 209E, with a change to International System of Units (SI) measurements, and then withdrawn in 2001, to be replaced by the International Organization for Standardization (ISO) standard, 14644.

- British Standard (BS) 5295: this was the United Kingdom standard for environmental conditions in enclosed spaces. It was first issued in 1976, was updated in 1989, and withdrawn in 2007. With classifications running from E to K, it tended to be used within the United Kingdom only.

- European Union guidelines, EudraLex Volume 4 Annex 1: with classifications running from A to D, this terminology is commonly used in many countries, not just in Europe.

- Parenteral Society Technical Practice Monograph No 2: an industry-specific guideline on environmental contamination control with particular reference to microbial contamination. It was first written in 1989 and was revised in 2002, taking into account "the publication of new cleanroom standards from CEN and ISO, the developments in the EU GMP, work of the PIC/S, the evolution of requirements from the US FDA, and developments in engineering practice." Originally written in response to requests from within the industry, this monograph is designed as an adjunct to GMP guidelines and international standards.

- Food and Drug Administration (FDA) guideline on Sterile Drug Products: the guideline contains the FDA's current thinking on the topic and contains nonbinding recommendations. It was issued in 1987, was updated in 2004, and was confirmed to be still current in April 2020. It relates primarily to aseptic manufacturing processes and references the international standard discussed below.

From 1992 onward, the authorities and industries in Europe, the United States, and Japan have worked with the European Committee for Standardization (CEN) and the International Organization for Standardization (ISO) to produce a worldwide standard for airborne cleanliness. This was published in May 1999 as EN/ISO 14644 Cleanrooms and associated controlled environments—Part 1: Classification of air cleanliness by particle concentration. As of July 2021, there are a total of fifteen parts in this family of cleanroom standards, as shown in Table 13.1.

ISO 14644 uses classifications from one to nine, based on maximum permitted particle concentration, and defines three occupancy states for the room:

1. As-built: Condition where the cleanroom or clean zone is complete with all services connected and functioning but with no equipment, furniture, materials or personnel present.

2. At-rest: Condition where the cleanroom or clean zone is complete with equipment installed and operating in a manner agreed upon, but with no personnel present.

3. Operational: Condition where the cleanroom or clean zone is functioning in the specified manner, with equipment operating and with the specified number of personnel present (ISO Standard 14644-1:2-15).

Table 13.1 The ISO 14644 family of standards for design and operation of cleanrooms.

Standard	Date	Title
14644-1	2015	Classification of air cleanliness by particle concentration
14644-2	2015	Monitoring to provide evidence of cleanroom performance related to air cleanliness by particle concentration
14644-3	2005	Test methods (note 1)
14644-4	2001	Design, construction, and start-up
14644-5	2004	Operations
14644-7	2004	Separative devices (clean air hoods, gloveboxes, isolators, minienvironments)
14644-8	2013	Classification of air cleanliness by chemical concentration (ACC)
14644-9	2012	Classification of surface particle cleanliness
14644-10	2013	Classification of surface cleanliness by chemical concentrations
14644-12	2018	Specifications for monitoring air cleanliness by nanoscale particle concentration
14644-13	2017	Cleaning of surfaces to achieve defined levels of cleanliness in terms of particle and chemical classifications
14644-14	2016	Assessment of suitability for use of equipment by airborne particle concentration
14644-15	2017	Assessment of suitability for use of equipment and materials by airborne chemical concentration
14644-16	2019	Code of practice for improving energy efficiency in cleanrooms and clean air devices
14644-17	2021	Particle deposition rate applications

Conditions achieved in the as-built or at-rest states will not be achieved during operational conditions when the sources of particle generation are greater, but once operations cease, the at-rest condition should be recovered within a specified time.

Table 13.2 shows the comparison of the different terminology from the main standards used now and previously within the pharmaceutical industry.

For the remainder of this chapter, the ISO terminology will be used both for consistency, and because it represents current best practice.

13.6.2 Terminally sterilized products

Terminally sterilized products are the ones that can be sterilized after filling, in their sealed primary containers. Since the product at this point is fully contained and will not become exposed to the atmosphere until it is administered to the patient, this is the preferred method for manufacture.

For terminally sterilized products, the sequence of events is therefore:
- preparation
- filling and sealing
- sterilization
- inspection
- final packaging

Products coming under this category include ampules and vials containing liquids that are thermostable and can be sterilized by moist heat; ointments and creams that can be sterilized by irradiation; and medical devices that can be sterilized by heat, irradiation, or gases.

Where products are going to be sterilized after filling, it is not necessary to manufacture them under aseptic conditions. The main concern is to minimize the bioburden within the dose unit during the preparation and filling stages, so a greater level of bacterial kill can be obtained during the sterilization phase. For a full discussion on sterilization, see Section 13.9.

Table 13.2 Comparison of terminology in a variety of national and international standards for air classification in cleanrooms.

Approximate Particles per $m^2 > 0.5\ \mu m$	US 209D	EU GMP	BS52995 1989	ISO EN 14644-1
3,520	100	A		4.8
3,520	100	B	E or F	5
35,200	1000		G or H	6
352,000	10,000	C (at rest)	J	7
3,520,000	100,000	C (in operation)	K	8
		D (at rest)		
35,200,000		D (in operation)		9

It is normally acceptable for the preparation of bulk drugs and components to take place in a grade 8 environment. However, there are situations in which the product is considered to be "at risk," in which case, it would be necessary to manufacture the bulk in a grade 7 environment. Such a situation would arise if the product were susceptible to microbial contamination, or if it is likely to be held in the bulk or filled state for a while before it can be sterilized, or if the processing takes place in open vessels.

For filling these products, it is normally acceptable to use a grade 7 environment. However, once again, there are situations in which the product could be considered to be "at risk." In these cases, the filling should take place in a grade 5 environment, with a grade 7 background. Conditions constituting a risk include primary containers with wide necks or filling operations that necessitate the unit being exposed to the atmosphere for a while between filling and sealing.

13.6.3 Aseptic manufacture

Where it is not possible to sterilize the product after filling, it must be manufactured under aseptic conditions. This means all materials and components are sterile at the point when the product is filled and sealed into the primary container.

For aseptic products, the sequence of events is thus:

- preparation
- sterilization
- filling and sealing
- inspection
- final packaging

For bulk products, the method of sterilization will differ, depending on the nature of the drug and its physical form. Liquids may be filtered into the filling room after manufacturing. Powders will tend to be irradiated, double-wrapped, and passed into the filling room via a hatchway, with the outer wrapping being removed at this point.

For components, the method will vary with the material. For glass, the normal method would be dry heat; for plastic components, irradiation or gassing is used; for rubber and metal stoppers, a mixture of methods is used, varying from heat and chemical methods to irradiation.

The classification of the facilities for aseptic manufacturing varies with the activities that take place in them. Glass vials and other components that are washed and then sterilized into the filling suite should be prepared in a grade 8 area. Solutions or other bulk products that can be filtered into the filling room can be manufactured in a grade 7 area. However, if no filtration is possible, for example with biological suspensions, a grade 5 area with a laminar flow, with a grade 7 background, is necessary.

All other activities associated with aseptic manufacturing must be carried out in a grade 5 area with a laminar flow, with a grade 7 background.

13.6.4 Mixed manufacturing

The requirements for area classifications described above should be considered as the minimum acceptable standard. Many companies have a portfolio containing a mixture of products for which terminal sterilization is an option and others for which aseptic manufacture is mandatory.

In these circumstances, it is preferable to have separate facilities for the different types of product, since the controls and requirements for aseptic manufacturing are far more stringent than those required for terminally sterilized products.

However, it is not compulsory to have such an arrangement. It is perfectly acceptable to produce the two types of products within the same facility, providing all products are manufactured to the same (tighter) standards. Once the facility has been validated as acceptable for the manufacture of aseptic products, all products should be produced as such, even if some of them will be terminally sterilized. To attempt to operate two different standards within the same facility, depending on which part of the product range is currently being produced, would be an impossible task.

13.7 Risks of contamination and their control

There are several possible sources of microbiological contamination within the manufacturing environment. Each requires specific measures to minimize or eliminate the risk. The controls can be associated with a number of different aspects of manufacturing:

- personnel working in the cleanrooms
- the design and construction of the facility
- the design and construction of the equipment
- the way the facility is operated
- the programs for cleaning and sanitation

13.7.1 Personnel

The greatest source of contamination within a clean or sterile area comes from the personnel working there. During sterile manufacturing, it is important to keep to a minimum the number of people working in the area, particularly in an aseptic operation. Where possible, in-process controls are performed outside the cleanroom. Alternatively, operators may be trained to carry out tests themselves, to reduce the number of indirect personnel who enter the area.

There should be a regular training program for all personnel who routinely enter the sterile areas, both direct operators, and service personnel such as cleaners and mechanics. This training should not only cover the job itself, but also hygiene and the basics of microbiology.

To avoid cross-contamination, it is important personnel who have worked with animal-tissue material or live microorganisms do not enter the sterile area. If this cannot be avoided, then strict decontamination procedures must be followed in all cases.

High standards of personal hygiene are important for all aspects of pharmaceutical manufacturing. It is even more important in the case of sterile manufacture. Periodic health checks and monitoring by swabs are important in the identification of conditions that can cause contamination. In addition, operators should be trained to report such conditions themselves.

Regarding clothing, some rules are the same in all factories. There should be no outside clothing brought into the area; watches and jewelry should not be worn; and nor should cosmetics since these may shed particles. Some companies insist on the removal of wedding rings. There should be a written procedure for changing and washing.

However, when it comes to the detail of that procedure, there are a variety of approaches that may be taken. In particular, the order in which different pieces of clothing are taken off or put on and the point at which hands are washed will vary between companies. There is no one right answer to this question and the important point is the logic of the approach and the consistency with which it is applied.

In the grade 8 area, a simple coat or another protective garment, hat, and shoe cover is sufficient, although facial hair must also be covered. In the grade 7 area, a one- or two-piece nonshedding trouser suit is preferable. Hair, including facial hair, must be covered. In grade 5 areas, masks and gloves are added to the outfit.

Arrangements must be in place for the laundering and sterilization of cleanroom clothing. This should be carried out in a controlled environment. The use of contract laundries for this requires an audit by the company to ensure appropriate procedures are in place.

It is important to consider visitors to the sterile area, although these should be kept to an absolute minimum. An appropriate procedure for clothing and supervising visitors should be in place. Visitors may need special training before entry to the sterile area is permitted. This special training is necessary to ensure they can conform to entry procedures.

13.7.2 Premises

There are several specific aspects to the design and construction of premises used for the manufacture of sterile products, which are designed to reduce the risk of both microbial and nonviable particulate contamination. Entry to all processing areas is through airlocks. For personnel, these airlocks generally take the form of changing rooms, comprising a variable number of interconnecting rooms, depending on the classification of the area. Separate airlocks must be provided for the entry of materials into the area. The doors at either end of an airlock should be interlocked so they cannot both be opened at the same time; although in some countries, this is not permitted by the fire authorities and alternative solutions may be required, such as visual or audible alarms.

Processing takes place in suites of rooms, with different classifications depending on the activities carried on in them. The classifications relate primarily to the supply of air to the rooms as discussed previously. The rooms are designed to reduce the accumulation of dust, which could be a source of microbial and/or particulate contamination, with all exposed surfaces being smooth and unbroken. Ideally, there will be false ceilings, which are sealed so nothing can fall from the void above. This also permits access to light fittings from above, allowing maintenance without stopping production. Wherever possible, pipes and ductwork should be outside the area or boxed in. Sinks and drains should be avoided if possible and must not be installed in aseptic areas. Drains should have cleanable traps and air breaks to prevent backflow. Floor channels must be open and easy to clean.

13.7.3 Equipment

13.7.3.1 Design

Equipment for use in the sterile area should be designed to achieve the following objectives:

- It can be operated with the minimum of personnel interference, thus reducing the possibility of contaminating the product.
- It can be easily sterilized by moist or dry heat sterilization.
- It should be easy to install change parts for different pack sizes.

Sterilizers should be designed with a door at each end, known as double-door autoclaves or double-ended autoclaves, to eliminate the possibility of mixing up sterile and nonsterile materials. This is particularly important when sterilizing components into the filling room. They are loaded in the preparation area and unloaded in the sterile area, although preferably in a buffer room rather than directly in the filling room.

The zone in which the product is to be exposed must be protected to the maximum extent possible. This requires the installation of laminar flow cabinets over the piece of equipment, to provide a grade 5 environment and to ensure a supply of filtered air flowing with positive pressure towards the surrounding areas.

It is also necessary to ensure the relative locations of the equipment and the operators do not cause a risk to the product by interrupting the flow of filtered air. There should be a warning system to indicate a failure in air supply, such as a manometer measuring pressure differentials, or an audible alarm.

13.7.3.2 Maintenance

Where possible, maintenance of equipment should take place outside the area. However, if this is impossible, it should be done when there is no work going on and should be followed by a complete clean down and disinfection. Tools for such work should be sterilized before being taken into the area. It is even better if a full set of sterilized tools can be stored in the area specifically for this purpose. After maintenance has been completed, there should be a documented procedure for obtaining approval to resume operations in the area.

It is permissible to have transport systems to take the product from the filling room to the sterilization/finishing area, but there must be a dead-plate across the interface between the two areas. There should be no conveyor belt passing between two areas of differing classification unless that belt is continuously sterilized, as is the case in a sterilizing tunnel.

13.7.3.3 Alternative technology

Increasingly, isolator technology is being installed within pharmaceutical manufacturing areas as a means of reducing the potential for microbial contamination within an aseptic processing area. While there are many different designs, the basic concept is to minimize the amount of human intervention in the process by the use of some type of "glove-box" arrangement. Apart from reducing the possibility of microbial contamination, it can be a lower cost option since the background environment can be as low as grade 8.

The points of transfer of material into and out of the isolator are the key risk areas and must be carefully controlled. Validation of an isolator must also pay close attention to the quality of air achieved and the airflow patterns, the procedure for sanitization, and the problems associated with rupture or leakage.

One specialized piece of equipment used in some manufacturing areas is the blow/fill/seal technology used to form plastic containers from thermoplastic granulate and to fill and seal them in an in-line continuous process. Such technology can be used for the manufacture of aseptic products or terminally sterilized products. In both cases, a grade 5 laminar flow air shower is required, with a grade 7 background in the former case or a grade 8 background in the latter case.

Key issues to be considered in using such technology include the design of the equipment, the clean-in-place (CIP) and steam-in-place (SIP) systems, and any manual operations that need to be carried out before filling.

13.7.4 Operation of the facility

At all times, there should be measures to ensure contamination is minimized. The processing of preparations containing live microorganisms is not allowed in the same facility as other pharmaceuticals. Inactivated products can be processed in the same facility providing validated procedures are used.

During processing in sterile areas, the level of activity must be kept to a minimum. As discussed above, the greatest source of contamination in a sterile area is the personnel. Hence, the more automated the process and the fewer people in the area the better. These areas should be built with plenty of internal, nonopening windows or glass panels to increase the visibility and remove the need for extra people to enter the room during processing.

No unsuitable materials should be used in the areas. All furniture and fittings should be of metal or plastic rather than wood. Paper may need to be used in the area, for example for batch documentation, but this should be kept to a minimum. Bonded paper or lint-free paper is available. Paper should not be used in a class A area at all. Alternatives include plastic sheets and permanent markers. It should go without saying that extras such as calendars and notices must be excluded.

The microbiological contamination load or bioburden for both raw materials and products before sterilization should be kept to a minimum. There should be documented limits in all cases.

Extreme care must be taken with materials that have been sterilized into the area for use in aseptic production, such as primary containers and filling machine parts. After removal from the sterilizer, they are stored under a laminar flow cabinet until used. All packs must be marked with the date of sterilization and there must be a procedure stating how long an item can remain in the area before it needs to be resterilized. There must also be a validated maximum storage period that is allowed between the manufacture of bulk products and filling into primary containers. This will depend on the nature of the product and whether it has been sterilized into the area or is going to be terminally sterilized.

13.7.5 Cleaning and sanitation

Clean and sterile areas must have a documented and planned program of sanitation. Procedures must include details of who is responsible and the frequency of cleaning in each area; this will vary for different rooms, depending on the activities and the risk to the product. There should also be details of the methodology, including the preparation of cleaning materials.

All cleaning materials should be evaluated and approved by the quality control (QC) department. For disinfection, there should be rotation between different chemicals to prevent the build up of microbial resistance. Dilutions should be prepared with purified water and should only be stored for a short period, as specified by QC or the manufacturer. The use of freshly prepared dilutions is by far the best approach. They should be sterilized before use in the sterile area.

The fumigation of the area, for example with formaldehyde, to decontaminate it, used to be a very common practice. It is an effective method but requires careful use and adequate "degassing" afterward. With effective ventilation systems, it should be possible to eliminate the need to carry out this process or at least to reduce its frequency.

13.8 Validation and environmental monitoring

In a factory producing sterile products, the level of QC requirements is higher than in any other factory. In particular, there is a very high level of environmental monitoring required. This monitoring covers not only microbiological contamination but nonviable particulates as well.

13.8.1 Monitoring of the air

The first aspect of monitoring the environment relates to the air supplied to the rooms. This is carried out in two ways:
- by monitoring the operation of the ventilation system (the inputs),
- by checking the quality of the resulting air (the outputs).

The number of air changes within a room is calculated from the air volumes supplied to the room. This will be carried out at validation and regularly thereafter.

The high efficiency particulate air (HEPA) filter integrity is tested by many means. An aerosol generator can be used to send an aerosol across the filter and a photometer used to view the amount of aerosol that passes downstream. This will show if there is any damage to the filter. Additionally, a manometer can be used to measure the pressure differential across the filter. These tests will be carried out when filters are installed and should be repeated at least annually.

A number of the environmental parameters can be monitored automatically, and new factories should have building management systems not only monitoring, but also making adjustments if required. However, if a factory does have such a system, it is important to ensure personnel looking after the system fully understand it. In the author's experience, it can be all too easy to assume everything is under control and not notice when something goes wrong. An important element of the original validation work is to ensure all the controls are working as intended

In terms of measuring the outputs, there are several methods for taking microbiological samples, but the simplest and most widely used is to place open settle plates of growth medium on the floor for around 4 hours; the exact period has to be developed to suit local conditions. The number of plates required depends on the classification and use of the room and can be determined from international standards, such as ISO 14644 Part 1. The locations of the plates will have been determined during validation and will be based on the risk to the product and the level of activity in the area. It is not necessary to obtain zero-growth results from these plates, but a validated pattern of likely contamination must be established, and significant deviations need to be investigated. If zero growth is observed, then low levels of bacteria are inoculated onto the plate to demonstrate it will support growth.

Measurement of particulate contamination is carried out using "a discrete-particle-counting instrument to determine the concentration of airborne particles equal to and greater than the specified sizes, at designated sampling locations" (ISO Standard No. 14644-1:2015).

13.8.2 Monitoring of surfaces

Monitoring of surfaces is generally carried out using swabs. Emphasis should be placed on the areas coming into contact with the product and in these areas, zero-growth results are expected. This method of monitoring, carried out before and after cleaning and disinfection, can be used to validate the methods of sanitation being used.

13.8.3 Monitoring of personnel

Finally, it is necessary to monitor the microorganisms arising from the personnel in the cleanrooms, since these are the greatest source of contamination. Samples are generally taken by swabs from clothing and by "finger-dabs" onto plates. Sampling must be representative of the situation during operations, hence if the operator normally wears gloves and disinfects them before use, the samples should be taken after that process has been carried out.

13.8.4 Media trials

A media trial, also known as an aseptic process simulation (APS), is an important part of validating an aseptic filling process. It involves filling a growth medium into primary containers and incubating them to see if any are contaminated. There are several factors to be taken into account when reviewing a media trial program:

- First, it is important the trial accurately reflects the true situation during filling. Operators normally working in the area, behaving in the same way they always do, should carry out the media trial.
- Second, the medium used must be capable of supporting the growth of a wide range of microorganisms, including those likely to be found in the filling room. Negative controls must be carried out to prove the medium is sterile before use and positive controls to prove it will support growth.
- Third, it is important to fill sufficient units to ensure low levels of contamination will be picked up. This should be at least 3000 units. However, for trials involving small batch operations, where a small batch is defined as one of less than 3000 units, the trial size should be at least as big as a normal batch. If there is usually a pause for a break during normal operations, this should be simulated.

The objective is for zero growth in the containers. However, a pass level of less than 0.1% contamination with a 95% confidence level is considered acceptable. Any contaminants should be isolated and identified.

The media trial should be repeated at regular intervals; between quarterly and six-monthly is likely to be the standard. However, it is important to carry out full cleaning, to remove all growth medium from the area before filling starts again.

The above is only a brief overview of the topic of media trials. A full discussion is presented in the PIC/S document "Validation of Aseptic Processes."

13.9 Sterilization

This section deals with sterilization, with particular reference to sterilization of products, although other items are referred to as well. There are several available methods, each of which has advantages and disadvantages. In each situation, consideration needs to be given to which is the most appropriate one to use. However, in general terms, heat sterilization should always be the preferred method if it can be used.

The most appropriate method of sterilization for a product will have been identified at the time it was developed. A useful decision tree for the choice of method of sterilization can be found in CPMP/QWP/054/98 Corr, which was produced by the European Union's Committee for Proprietary Medicinal Products.

13.9.1 Sterilization by heat

Heat sterilization may be carried out in one of two ways:
- Moist heat sterilization uses an autoclave and either a porous load or fluid load cycle, depending on the type of material being sterilized. Both types of cycle can be carried out in the same autoclave.
- Dry heat sterilization, where either an oven or a sterilizing tunnel is used.

13.9.1.1 Moist heat sterilization

Moist heat sterilization is a combination of temperature, time and pressure. Hence, all parameters must be recorded and shown to achieve minimum conditions. Porous load cycles are used for sterilizing components such as stoppers for vials, clean area clothing or machine parts, and other ancillary items. Removal of all air from the chamber and replacement with steam is a key characteristic of this type of cycle. In the case of components, they must be wrapped in material allowing removal of air and entry of steam, but not allowing recontamination afterward. All parts of the load must be in contact with water or water vapor throughout the cycle. The quality of the steam is also critical; the use of a clean steam generator is recommended.

Fluid load cycles are used for the sterilization of filled containers of product. They are based on saturated steam, which is used for glass containers such as ampules or vials; steam and air, which is used for LVP bags or blow/fill/seal containers; or hot water, which is used when the product or container will not withstand exposure to steam. Although it is important to ensure there are no pockets of air left in the chamber, the complete removal of air is less important.

13.9.1.2 Dry heat sterilization

Dry heat sterilization is the method used to remove pyrogens or endotoxins as well as viable microorganisms. It takes place in an oven or sterilizing tunnel and uses a combination of temperature and time only. However, the temperature is much higher than for moist heat. This method can be used for dry components such as empty ampules and vials. There should be air circulation within the chamber and a positive pressure to prevent ingress of nonsterile air. The air should be circulated through HEPA filters.

13.9.2 Irradiation

There are a number of different types of irradiation, but the three most commonly used for sterilization are gamma, electron beam, or X-ray.

This method of sterilization generally takes place in a stand-alone, dedicated facility. It is very rare for a pharmaceutical company to have its own irradiation plant. A company that did have such a facility would be unlikely to have sufficient demand to keep it operating full-time and hence would be able to offer a contract sterilization service to other companies in the region or the country.

Radiation sterilization is used primarily for heat-sensitive materials and products, such as ointments, and for plastic components before filling. However, care must be taken to ensure the materials are compatible and not radiation-sensitive. This would form part of the original validation work.

In some countries, ultraviolet radiation is used as a "sterilizer." This should be treated with care. Ultraviolet irradiation is not a very effective method of sterilization, although it can be useful in maintaining a low level of microorganisms once obtained, for example in purified water systems. Its use requires careful validation.

As with heat sterilization, it is important to monitor the effectiveness of the sterilization cycle. In the case of radiation, dosimeters are used which provide a quantitative measure of the dose received. These are inserted within the load in sufficient numbers to ensure there is always one in the chamber. Radiation-sensitive disks on the outside of packs are used to prove the load has passed through the chamber. Like autoclave tape, they do not prove sterility.

13.9.3 Ethylene oxide sterilization

Ethylene oxide gas (ETO) is only to be used as a sterilant if no other method is available. The gas is explosive in air at relatively low concentrations and leaves behind significant residues in the product which need to be removed before the batch can be inspected, packaged, and released for sale into the marketplace. This method is used for plastic items such as medical devices if they are both heat and radiation-sensitive. The cycle is a combination of time, temperature, humidity, and gas concentration. The first three parameters are generally recorded directly while the last is recorded indirectly. The usage of gas is calculated by weighing the cylinders before and after the cycle to crosscheck the gas usage is as expected.

Direct contact between the gas and any microorganisms on the product is essential. Additionally, it is necessary for any microorganisms to be in a moist environment since the rate of kill is inversely proportional to the dryness of the surroundings. Hence the packaging must be suitable to allow ingress of both moisture and gas.

ETO sterilization uses biological indicators to routinely measure the effectiveness of the cycle. Their use should be controlled, and positive controls employed to ensure they are still viable.

As mentioned earlier, one of the problems with ETO is the residues left behind at the end of the cycle. The processing cycle must include a validated degassing period, where the load is stored in a suitably ventilated room under quarantine.

13.9.4 Filtration

It has already been discussed above that terminal sterilization is the preferred method for the product as it reduces the risk of recontamination. However, this is not possible for some products, such as vaccines and insulin. In this case, sterilization by filtration into a sterilized container is required. The filter should have a nominal pore size of no more than 0.22 μm. However, viruses and mycoplasmas might not be removed by this method. EU GMP Annex 1 recommends the use of an element of heat treatment in addition to filtration to overcome this risk.

To reduce the risks associated with the filtration method, double filtration is recommended. There is usually a prefilter before the main one anyway, but in addition, a final filter, just before filling, should also be used, if possible. Where double filtration is not practiced, then further monitoring is required. Media fill validation trials and presterilization bioburden counts are two possible methods. See Section 13.8.4 for a discussion on media fills.

Filters should be integrity-tested after use and in some cases are also tested before use. This requires the use of equipment such as a bubble-point tester. In addition, validation of the method will have produced standard times and pressure differentials for a given volume of liquid. Any variations from this should be noted and investigated.

Filters should not be used for more than one working day unless longer use has been validated. Reusable filters are permissible, but there must be validated methods of cleaning, resterilization, and storage.

13.9.5 Validation and monitoring of sterilization cycles

Validation of the method of sterilization is essential, particularly as sterility testing is always a destructive test and can only be carried out on a sample of the batch. A regulatory inspector would be particularly interested in validation results for any methods not according to national standards, or for materials other than solutions. It is also important that the method of sterilization being used is the one originally validated for the process or product.

Biological indicators can be considered as part of the monitoring of the sterilization process. Their use should always be controlled to prevent contamination of the facility and product with live microorganisms.

It is very important for a company to have effective methods for the separation of sterilized and unsterilized materials. Ideally, sterilizers are double-ended, so there is no cross-flow of materials with the consequent risk of mixing. Containers must be clearly labeled and indicators such as autoclave tape or irradiation disks used to show a particular load has passed through the sterilizer. However, it is important to remember that an indicator can only prove whether a particular load has passed through the sterilizer or not. It is not sensitive enough to assure sterility.

All sterilization cycles are monitored using appropriate recording equipment. This will provide a record of all the cycle parameters. For heat sterilization, probes are located at the coolest part of the chamber, so they are recording the worst-case situation. The charts taken from these recorders will form part of the batch processing records.

For any given cycle and load within a moist or dry heat sterilizer, there will be a period when the sterilizer is heating up before the correct temperature is reached. The recording of the cycle time should not commence until this heating period has been completed. Similarly, there will be a cool-down period at the end of the cycle. Any liquid or gas used to cool the load must be sterile so that it cannot cause recontamination.

13.9.6 Sterility testing

Sterility testing is required as part of the process for batch release for all sterile products. It is important to take representative samples from the batch. For aseptic production, this would be the start and finish of the batch and after any major breaks in work. For terminally sterilized products, the coolest part of the load should be sampled. If a batch is sterilized in more than one load, then samples should be tested from each load.

However, sterility testing will only be a part of the quality assurance for the batch, and results should be considered in the context of all other tests and monitoring carried out during production.

If a test fails, it could be a production problem or a laboratory problem. If a test is to be repeated as allowed by the national drug regulatory authority, it should be conducted in strict conformance to the pharmacopeial method in force.

Batches that fail the initial sterility test, but pass a second one, should only be released for sale if a full evaluation of the production record and environmental monitoring proves the original test was invalid.

13.9.7 Real-time release testing and parametric release

Recognizing the shortcomings of finished product testing as a means of assurance of the quality of a batch of product, and in line with the risk assessment and quality management system approaches discussed elsewhere in this book, there is a growing interest in the topic of Real-Time Release Testing (RTRT). As stated in EU GMP Annex 17:

> *"Advances in the application of process analytical technology (PAT), quality by design (QbD) and quality risk management (QRM) principles to pharmaceutical development and manufacturing have shown that an appropriate combination of process controls together with timely monitoring and verification of preestablished material attributes provides greater assurance of product quality than finished product testing (conventionally regarded as the end-product testing) alone."*

In the context of sterile manufacturing, parametric release, which is a form of RTRT, may be permissible for terminally sterilized products. It is based on reviewing critical process parameters. Before permission is granted for a switch to parametric release, the manufacturer must demonstrate: "a history of acceptable GMP compliance and a robust sterility assurance program in place to demonstrate consistent process control and process understanding." (EU GMP Annex 17.)

13.10 Chapter summary

- Microorganisms can have both a positive and a negative effect on the pharmaceutical industry. This chapter concentrates on the negative aspects of microbiological contamination and how risks are mitigated.
- There are six main categories of microorganisms. However, in the context of pharmaceutical manufacturing, the main focus is on bacteria.
- Bacteria are unicellular microorganisms that are present in a variety of shapes and sizes. The most common types in our environment are round or rod-shaped. They can be pathogenic or harmless. It is the former which are of most concern in pharmaceutical manufacturing. They can exist in two states, vegetative, which are easy to kill; or spores, which require the most stringent measures.
- Fungi are mushrooms, molds, and yeasts. They are relatively susceptible and will tend to be controlled by the measures in place to control bacteria. However, fungi

can be a factor in the spoilage of raw and/or packaging materials under damp conditions.

- Viruses are nonliving organisms that can only survive within the cells of their hosts. Some can be highly pathogenic. However, they are relatively susceptible outside their hosts and tend to be controlled by the measures in place to control bacteria.
- Pyrogens are nonviable particles that can trigger immune reactions if present in the bloodstream. A major class of pyrogens is the bacterial endotoxins which can cause fever. Measures must be in place to minimize endotoxin contamination in injectable products in particular.
- Raw material specifications will contain limits not only for physical and chemical parameters but also for microbiological content. The limits will depend on the source of the material and its intended use. Materials for use in aseptic processing will tend to be received from the supplier already sterilized.
- Nonsterile products are produced under clean conditions but are not sterile at the point of administration to the patient. There are no clear-cut rules for manufacturing conditions, but custom and practice dictates a certain level of control. Additionally, some products in some countries will be subject to specific requirements.
- Sterile products may be injectables, infusions, ointments, creams, or eye drops. They are produced in a variety of forms.
- SVPs are filled into ampules, vials, or prefilled syringes. They are commonly in liquid form but can also be powders or freeze-dried pellets.
- LVPs are filled into bottles or bags. They are always in liquid form.
- Ointments and creams, if administered as sterile products, are usually filled into tubes, which may be glass or plastic. They may also be delivered in novel containers such as pump packs.
- Eye drops are liquids and are generally filled into dropper bottles.
- Medical devices cover a huge range of products, shapes, and sizes.
- Sterile manufacturing takes place in several stages. The exact order of those stages will depend on the nature of the product and, primarily, the method of sterilization.
- Historically, there are many reference documents relating to area classification and air supply to cleanrooms. They each have specific terminology for different classes of cleanroom and this terminology may still be in use, even if more modern standards are being used for design and monitoring.
- In recent years, airborne cleanliness has been standardized around the ISO 14644 family of standards, particularly ISO 14644-1:2015. This standard uses classifications 1−9 and defines three occupancy states: as-built, at-rest, and operational.
- Terminally sterilized products are ones where sterilization takes place once the product has been filled and sealed into its primary containers. It is the process that most assures sterility and should be the method of choice if the nature of the product permits it.

- Aseptic manufacturing is where all components and materials are presterilized before being assembled under aseptic conditions.
- In the case where a company has a mixed portfolio of terminally sterilized and aseptic products, it is preferable to have separate facilities for each type of process. If this is not possible, then all products should be produced under aseptic conditions, even if some will subsequently undergo sterilization.
- There are many potential sources of microbiological contamination within the manufacturing environment.
- Personnel constitute the greatest risk and should be subject to appropriate training, high standards of personal hygiene, and appropriate clothing procedures.
- Premises must be designed to reduce the risks both of microbiological and nonviable particulate contamination. Processing rooms will be supplied with the classification of air appropriate to the activities taking place.
- Equipment should be designed for operation with a minimum of personnel interference, easy sterilization, and easy installation of change parts. Maintenance should take place outside of the cleanroom wherever possible.
- Alternative technologies such as isolators or blow/fill/seal equipment are increasingly being employed to minimize the risks associated with more traditional designs of equipment and facilities.
- Operation of the facility should be according to procedures aimed at reducing the risk of contamination, including minimizing the number of personnel present, banning all unsuitable and/or unnecessary materials, and stringent controls to prevent the mixing of sterilized and unsterilized materials.
- Cleaning and sanitation must be according to planned and documented programs, with controls on the use and storage of cleaning materials. While fumigation of cleanrooms is an option, it should be minimized by other control methods due to safety issues.
- Monitoring of air quality covers both microbiological and nonviable particulate contamination and addresses both the operation of the ventilation system and the quality of the air in the cleanroom. A variety of physical tests and biological tests are used.
- Microbiological monitoring of surfaces is carried out using swabs, with emphasis on areas of high risk.
- Microbiological monitoring of personnel involves swabs and/or finger-dabs.
- The use of media trials is a key part of validating and monitoring the aseptic filling process. There are clear guidelines on the choice of media and the size of the trial. It should be carried out under normal operating procedures.
- Heat sterilization may be via moist or dry heat. The former takes place in an autoclave and is a function of time, temperature and pressure. The latter takes place in an oven or sterilizing tunnel, via a combination of time and temperature.

- Irradiation is appropriate for products and materials that are not thermostable. This is a large-scale process and is usually carried out in a stand-alone contract facility. Common sources of irradiation are gamma, electron beam, or X-ray. Ultraviolet is suitable for disinfection but is not an effective method of sterilization.
- Ethylene oxide sterilization is the method of last resort when neither heat nor irradiation is appropriate. It has safety issues and requires a validated degassing period under quarantine to ensure the removal of all residues.
- Filtration is used where possible for liquids that are to be aseptically filled and sealed. It may not be effective against viruses, and some level of heat treatment may be necessary as well. Filters should be integrity-tested. The length of time they can be in use, and any resterilization and reuse must be fully validated.
- All sterilization cycles must be fully validated and monitored. A distinction must be made between parameters indicative of sterilization, such as temperature or pressure, and mere measures of presence in the sterilizer, such as autoclave tape or irradiation disks.
- Sterility testing is a regulatory requirement in many countries but is only one part of assuring the quality of the batch. Results should be taken in the context of all other tests and monitoring.
- Parametric release, as an alternative to sterility testing, may be permissible for terminally sterilized products only, but an agreement to use this approach will require demonstration of appropriate quality systems by the manufacturing company.

13.11 Questions/problems

1. List the different types of contaminants that might be found in a pharmaceutical manufacturing facility. What are the principal sources of those contaminants?
2. You are the design engineer for a new manufacturing facility. The product portfolio will include a cough suspension for children; a freeze-dried antibiotic; the sterile diluent for reconstitution of the antibiotic; and a saline infusion solution. List the areas you would need to include in your design and the likely classification of each one.
3. You are the quality manager for the new manufacturing facility in the previous question. You have been asked to advise the human resources department on the training needs for the new personnel. What would your advice be?
4. You are the engineering manager for the new manufacturing facility. List ten examples of regular monitoring you would expect to carry out once the facility is fully validated and operational.
5. You are the leader of the project team responsible for introducing a new product into the manufacturing facility. The product is a thermostable liquid that will be

filled into single-dose vials. List all the materials that will need to be sterilized and suggest the most appropriate method in each case.

6. How would your answer differ if the product in the previous question was a soluble compound whose effectiveness was shown to be destroyed at temperatures significantly above ambient?

Further reading

British Standard 5295, 1989. Environmental cleanliness in enclosed spaces.

European Commission, 2008. EudraLex. The rules governing medicinal products in the European Union. Volume 4. EU guidelines to good manufacturing practice medicinal products for human and veterinary use. Annex 1 Manufacture of Sterile Medicinal Products (corrected version). <https://ec. europa.eu/health/sites/default/files/files/eudralex/vol-4/2008_11_25_gmp-an1_en.pdf> (accessed 30.07.21).

European Commission, 2018. EudraLex. The rules governing medicinal products in the European Union. Volume 4. EU guidelines to good manufacturing practice medicinal products for human and veterinary use. Annex 17 Real Time Release Testing and Parametric Release. <https://ec.europa. eu/health/sites/default/files/files/eudralex/vol-4/pdfs-en/2018_annex17_en.pdf> (accessed 31.07.21)

International Organization for Standardization, 2015. EN/ISO 14644 Cleanrooms and associated controlled environments. Part 1: classification of air cleanliness by particle concentration (ISO Standard No. 14644-1:2015).

International Organization for Standardization, 2015. EN/ISO 14644 Cleanrooms and associated controlled environments. Part 2: monitoring to provide evidence of cleanroom performance related to air cleanliness by particle concentration (ISO Standard No. 14644-2:2015).

International Organization for Standardization, 2005. EN/ISO 14644 Cleanrooms and associated controlled environments. Part 3: test methods (ISO Standard No. 14644-3:2005).

International Organization for Standardization. 2001. EN/ISO 14644 Cleanrooms and associated controlled environments. Part 4: design, construction, and start-up (ISO Standard No. 14644-4:2001).

International Organization for Standardization, 2004. EN/ISO 14644 Cleanrooms and associated controlled environments. Part 5: operations (ISO Standard No. 14644-5:2004).

International Organization for Standardization, 2004. EN/ISO 14644 Cleanrooms and associated controlled environments. Part 7: separative devices (clean air hoods, gloveboxes, isolators, minienvironments) (ISO Standard No. 14644-7:2004).

International Organization for Standardization, 2013. EN/ISO 14644 Cleanrooms and associated controlled environments. Part 8: classification of air cleanliness by chemical concentration (ACC) (ISO Standard No. 14644-8:2013).

International Organization for Standardization, 2012. EN/ISO 14644 Cleanrooms and associated controlled environments. Part 9: classification of surface particle cleanliness (ISO Standard No. 14644-9:2012).

International Organization for Standardization, 2013. EN/ISO 14644 Cleanrooms and associated controlled environments. Part 10: classification of surface cleanliness by chemical concentrations (ISO Standard No. 14644-10:2013).

International Organization for Standardization, 2018. EN/ISO 14644 Cleanrooms and associated controlled environments. Part 12: specifications for monitoring air cleanliness by nanoscale particle concentration (ISO Standard No. 14644-12:2018).

International Organization for Standardization, 2017. EN/ISO 14644 Cleanrooms and associated controlled environments. Part 13: cleaning of surfaces to achieve defined levels of cleanliness in terms of particle and chemical classifications (ISO Standard No. 14644-13:2017).

International Organization for Standardization, 2016. EN/ISO 14644 Cleanrooms and associated controlled environments. Part 14: assessment of suitability for use of equipment by airborne particle concentration (ISO Standard No. 14644-14:2016).

International Organization for Standardization, 2017. EN/ISO 14644 Cleanrooms and associated controlled environments. Part 15: assessment of suitability for use of equipment and materials by airborne chemical concentration (ISO Standard No. 14644-15:2017).

International Organization for Standardization, 2019. EN/ISO 14644 Cleanrooms and associated controlled environments. Part 16: code of practice for improving energy efficiency in cleanrooms and clean air devices (ISO Standard No. 14644-16:2019).

International Organization for Standardization, 2021. EN/ISO 14644 Cleanrooms and associated controlled environments. Part 17: particle deposition rate applications (ISO Standard No. 14644-17:2021).

Parenteral Society, 2002. Technical practice monograph no. 2: environmental contamination control practice.

Pharmaceutical Inspection Convention/Pharmaceutical Inspection Co-operation Scheme, 2011. Recommendation on the validation of aseptic processes. <https://picscheme.org/docview/3446> (accessed 31.07.21).

Sandle, T., 2016. Pharmaceutical Microbiology. Essentials for Quality Assurance and Quality Control. Woodhead Publishing Limited, Cambridge.

The European Agency for the Evaluation of Medicinal Products, Committee for Proprietary Medicinal Products, 2000. Decision trees for the selection of sterilisation methods. <https://www.ema.europa.eu/en/documents/scientific-guideline/superseded-annex-note-guidance-development-pharmaceutics-decision-trees-selection-sterilisation_en.pdf> (accessed 31.07.21).

US Federal Standard 209D, 1988. Cleanroom and Work Station Requirements, Controlled Environments. Institute of Environmental Sciences and Technology.

US Federal Standard 209E, 1992. Cleanroom and Work Station Requirements, Controlled Environments. Institute of Environmental Sciences and Technology.

US Food and Drug Administration, 1987. Guidance on sterile drug products produced by aseptic processing.

CHAPTER 14

Good distribution practice

14.1 Introduction

The World Health Organization (WHO) defines good distribution practice (GDP) as

That part of quality assurance that ensures that the quality of a pharmaceutical product is maintained by means of adequate control of the numerous activities which occur during the distribution process as well as providing a tool to secure the distribution system from counterfeits, unapproved, illegally imported, stolen, counterfeit, substandard, adulterated, and/or misbranded pharmaceutical products.

Additionally, distribution is defined as "The procuring, purchasing, holding, storing, selling, supplying, importing, exporting, or movement of pharmaceutical products, with the exception of the dispensing or providing pharmaceutical products directly to a patient or his or her agent."

In general, GDP refers to the guidelines for ensuring that the quality of pharmaceutical products is maintained throughout the distribution chain. The goal of the guidelines is to ensure that there is no change in the quality of the product from the point that it leaves the factory until the point at which it is used by the patients. This is irrespective of the setting in which it is used.

Worldwide, there are many GDP guidelines. The next section will list several national and regional guidelines. It is followed by a section that compares and contrasts the different guidelines.

14.2 National and regional good distribution practice guidelines

14.2.1 Good distribution practice guideline of WHO

As noted earlier the WHO has published a guideline for GDP (Annex 5 WHO Good Distribution Practices for Pharmaceutical Products). This guideline contains 22 sections and provides guidance on the distribution of pharmaceutical products. It covers products for which a prescription is required, products which may be provided to a patient without a prescription, biologicals, and vaccines.

14.2.2 Pharmaceutical Inspection Co-operation Scheme good distribution practice guideline

The Pharmaceutical Inspection Co-operation Scheme (PIC/S) guide is based on the European Union (EU) Guidelines on GDP of Medicinal Products for Human Use

Quality
DOI: https://doi.org/10.1016/B978-0-323-90815-3.00016-5

(2013/C 343/01) and has been adopted by PIC/S as a guidance document. The document notes that it is up to each PIC/S participating authority to decide whether it should become a legally-binding standard.

The document states:

To ensure the maintaining of high standards of quality assurance and the integrity of the distribution processes of medicinal products, to promote uniformity in licensing of wholesaling of medicinal products and to further facilitate the removal of barriers to trade in medicinal products, the following Guide to Good Distribution Practice (GDP) for Medicinal Products has been adopted.

The standards contained in the document apply to medicines and similar products intended for human use. There are nine chapters in the guideline.

14.2.3 European Union good distribution practice guideline

Within Europe, the overriding documents that relate to logistics and distribution are the national regulations. In the United Kingdom, these are The Medicines (Standard Provisions for Wholesale Dealer's Licenses) Regulations, first published in 1971, and subsequently amended several times. However, these are legal documents written in a form that is supposedly beyond question in terms of the legal process. As a result, they are fairly unreadable and are not particularly useful as reference documents.

Resulting from this directive, a guidance document was issued in 1994: Guidelines on Good Distribution Practice of Medicinal Products for Human Use (94/C63/03). This guideline was revised to the current version 2013/C 343/01. This is the key reference document that should be used as the basis for developing or checking for compliance.

The guidelines states: "lay down appropriate tools to assist wholesale distributors in conducting their activities and to prevent falsified medicines from entering the legal supply chain. Compliance with these Guidelines will ensure control of the distribution chain and consequently maintain the quality and the integrity of medicinal products."

In the guideline wholesale distribution is defined as:

All activities consisting of procuring, holding, supplying or exporting medicinal products, apart from supplying medicinal products to the public. Such activities are carried out with manufacturers or their depositories, importers, other wholesale distributors or with pharmacists and persons authorized or entitled to supply medicinal products to the public in the Member State concerned.

There are 11 chapters in this guideline.

14.2.4 US good distribution practice guidelines

GDP is briefly mentioned in the Title 21 of the United States (US) Code of Federal Regulations (CFR). Subpart H (Holding and Distribution) of Part 211 of the CFR discusses things that should be included in procedures for warehousing and the distribution of drug products. Subpart J (Records and Reports) provides details for the information required in distribution records.

14.2.5 Health Canada good distribution practice guidelines

Health Canada's GDP guidelines are contained in the "Guidelines for Environmental Control of Drugs During Storage and Transportation." The guidelines apply to: "all persons (individuals and companies) involved in the storage and transportation of drugs." The guidance contains five chapters and the specific principles for GDP are contained in Chapter 5.

14.3 Comparison of good distribution practice guidelines

As noted earlier and described in Section 14.2, there are many different GDP guidelines. These guidelines require that any distribution company has a quality system in place. Additionally, most of the guidelines contain similar content although it may be listed in different sections and in a different order. Table 14.1 shows a comparison of the contents

Table 14.1 Comparison of good distribution practice guidelines.

World Health Organization	Pharmaceutical Inspection Co-operation Scheme	European Union	Health Canada
1. Introduction	Chapter 1. Quality management	Chapter 1. Quality management	1. Purpose
2. Scope of the document	Chapter 2. Personnel	Chapter 2. Personnel	2. Scope
3. Glossary	Chapter 3. Premises and equipment	Chapter 3. Premises and equipment	3. Introduction
4. General principles	Chapter 4. Documentation	Chapter 4. Documentation	4. Principles
5. Regulation of the distribution of pharmaceutical products	Chapter 5. Operations	Chapter 5. Operations	5. Interpretation
6. Organization and management	Chapter 6. Complaints, returns, suspected falsified medical products and medical products Recall	Chapter 6. Complaints, returns, suspected falsified medical products and medical products Recall	

(Continued)

Table 14.1 (Continued)

World Health Organization	Pharmaceutical Inspection Co-operation Scheme	European Union	Health Canada
7. Personnel	Chapter 7. Outsourced activities	Chapter 7. Outsourced activities	
8. Quality system	Chapter 8. Self-inspections	Chapter 8. Self-inspections	
9. Premises, warehousing and storage	Chapter 9. Transportation	Chapter 9. Transportation	
10. Vehicles and equipment		Chapter 10. Specific provisions for brokers	
11. Shipment containers and container labeling		Chapter 11. Final Provisions	
12. Dispatch and receipt			
13. Transportation and products in transit			
14. Documentation			
15. Repackaging and relabeling			
16. Complaints			
17. Recalls			
18. Returned products			
19. Counterfeit pharmaceutical products			
20. Importation			
21. Contract activities			
22. Self-inspection			

of GDP guidelines from the more advanced countries and international organizations. The table shows that the sections for the PIC/S and EU guidelines are virtually identical. The WHO guidelines contain significantly more sections than the other guidelines; however, this is primarily because this guideline listed each subject in its own section. The other guidelines listed much of the same content under subsections.

14.4 Principles of good distribution practice

Since the WHO guideline contains the most details and is most inclusive of the principles stated in the other guidelines, this section will discuss the principles of GDP as it relates to pharmaceutical distribution as outlined by the WHO guidance. For instances, where the EU guidance includes additional options or clarification, references to that guidance were also included. The discussion of the GDP principles begins with Chapter 4 of the guideline.

14.4.1 General principles

The guidance states:

> *All parties involved in the distribution of pharmaceutical products have a responsibility to ensure that the quality of pharmaceutical products and the integrity of the distribution chain is maintained throughout the distribution process from the site of the manufacturer to the entity responsible for dispensing or providing the product to the patient or his or her agent.*

Additionally, the guidance states that the principles of GDP "should be included in national legislation and guidelines for the distribution of pharmaceutical products, in a country or region as applicable, as a means of establishing minimum standards." These principles are applicable to both product moving forward in the distribution chain from the manufacturer to the dispenser of product to patients and backwards in the chain as a result of a return or recall.

14.4.2 Regulation of the distribution of pharmaceutical products

This principle states: "National legislation should be in place to regulate the activities of persons or entities involved in the distribution of pharmaceutical products." The guidance further states that the distributor or the organization to which the distributor belongs should be an entity that is appropriately authorized to perform the function(s) that it intends to perform.

Similarly, the distributors or their agents should "supply pharmaceutical products only to persons or entities which are themselves authorized to acquire such products." Some of the distribution duties and responsibilities can be delegated or contracted out but only to agents that are authorized in line with national legislation.

14.4.3 Organization and management

This principle states that there should be an adequate organization structure for each entity. The duties and responsibility (as detailed in written job descriptions) for the entities should be clearly defined and understood by the applicable individuals.

"At every level of the supply chain, employees should be fully informed and trained in their duties and responsibilities." Also, a designated person should be appointed within the organization with "defined authority and responsibility for ensuring that a quality system is implemented and maintained."

14.4.4 Personnel

All personnel involved in distribution activities should be trained and qualified both in the responsibilities of their jobs and in the general principles of GDP. "Training should be based on written standard operating procedures (SOPs)."

All training should be recorded, both at the organizational level (to provide information about the overall pool of resources) and at the individual level. These records are useful as an internal document but are also a requirement for external inspections. Personnel should receive initial training, continuing training on relevant tasks, and assessment in accordance with a written training program.

GDP refers to key personnel within the company having the appropriate levels of training, qualifications, and experience. However, there is no statement as to which are the key personnel. In pharmaceutical manufacturing, key personnel are defined as the head of production, the head of QC, and the qualified person (QP). They are required to be full-time employees, independent of one another, but having the authority to delegate their responsibilities if the size of the company requires it. In the context of distribution therefore, the key personnel can be defined as the decision makers who may have any affect on the quality of the product. This would include the head of warehousing and the people responsible for identifying and dealing with suppliers and customers.

Additionally, there should be: "an adequate number of competent personnel involved in all stages of the distribution of pharmaceutical products" with national regulations relating to qualifications and experience adhered to.

Personnel should wear garments suitable for the activities they perform and appropriate procedures relating to personnel hygiene, relevant to the activities performed, should be established and observed.

In the EU guideline, there is a requirement that a management representative be appointed at each distribution point, with the authority and responsibility to ensure that the quality system is implemented and maintained. The term management representative is only used in the GDP guidelines and not in the preceding documents. However, in the directive and the national regulations, this position is referred to as the responsible person (RP). This is the distribution equivalent of the QP within pharmaceutical manufacturing. This representative should carry out the role personally, in other words, delegation is not permitted. An appropriate qualification is required. Ideally, this would be pharmacy but will vary with national regulations.

14.4.5 Quality system

The principle states:

> There should be a documented quality policy describing the overall intentions and requirements of the distributor regarding quality, as formally expressed and authorized by management. The quality system should include an appropriate organizational structure,

procedure, processes and resources and systematic actions necessary to ensure adequate confidence that a product or service and its documentation will satisfy given requirements for quality. The totality of these actions are described as the quality system.

Authorized procurement and release procedures should be in place to ensure that appropriate pharmaceutical products are sourced from approved suppliers and distributed by approved entities.

Inspection, auditing, and certification of compliance by an external certification body is recommended but should not be seen as a substitute for compliance with the GDP guidelines.

"If measures to ensure the integrity of the pharmaceutical products in transit are in place, they should be managed properly." In situations where pharmaceutical products are suspected of being or are found to be, counterfeit, written procedures should be in place for how these products must be handled.

The distributor should periodically conduct risk assessments to determine the potential risk to the quality and integrity of pharmaceutical products. The quality system should be developed in such a way to address any potential risks identified.

The distribution system should include product traceability throughout the supply chain with procedures in place to ensure traceability of received and distributed products. All parties involved in the supply chain should be identified according to the type of product and national policies. Records that include the expiry dates and batch numbers should be part of the secure distribution documentation.

When dealing with potentially counterfeit products, provision should be made for a visual and/or analytical identification of the products.

The procedure to be followed when a suspected product is identified should include provisions for notification, as appropriate, of the holder of the marketing authorization, entity identified on the label (if different from the manufacturer), the appropriate national and/or international regulatory bodies, as well as other relevant competent authorities.

To ensure traceability, a suitable and, where possible, internationally compatible product coding, identification system should be in place and developed in collaboration with the various parties involved in the supply chain.

14.4.6 Premises, warehousing, and storage

Good storage practices (GSP) should be followed throughout the distribution process and in all circumstances where pharmaceutical products are stored. There are a number of specific requirements related to GSP that should be followed. Some of them include:

- Caution must be taken to prevent unauthorized persons from entering storage areas.
- Storage areas should be of adequate capacity to allow the orderly storage of the different categories of pharmaceutical products.

- Storage areas should be clean and dry and maintained within acceptable temperature limits designed to ensure good storage conditions.
- Storage areas should be clean and free of accumulated waste and pests. There should be a written pest control procedure in place using agents with no risk of contamination of pharmaceutical products.
- All possibilities of cross-contamination must be avoided, both during storage and transport and when sampling is conducted. This includes not only cross-contamination between materials but also mix-ups between different products or materials or between different batches of the same products or materials.
- The quarantined products should be stored in separate areas that are clearly marked with access restricted to authorized personnel.
- Physical or another equivalent validated segregation, such as electronic segregation, should be provided for the storage of rejected, expired, recalled, or returned products and suspected counterfeits.
- A system should be in place to ensure that all products are subjected to an appropriate stock-rotation system. Pharmaceutical products due to expire first should be sold and/or distributed first (first expiry/first-out (FEFO)). Exceptions may be permitted provided adequate controls are in place to prevent the distribution of expired products.
- Broken or damaged items should be withdrawn from usable stock and stored in a separate location.
- Storage and handling conditions should comply with applicable national and local regulations and be in compliance with the manufacturer's recommendations.
- Temperature monitoring data and records should be available for review.
- Equipment used for monitoring of storage conditions should be calibrated at defined intervals.
- Periodic stock reconciliation, at defined intervals, should be performed to compare the actual inventory with the recorded inventory. Any stock discrepancies should be investigated.

14.4.7 Vehicles and equipment

The following are some of the principles that apply to vehicles and equipment:
- Vehicles and equipment used for the distribution, storage, or handling of pharmaceutical products should be suitable for their purpose and appropriately equipped to prevent exposure of the products to conditions that could affect their stability and packaging integrity. The vehicles and equipment should also prevent contamination of any kind.
- Dedicated vehicles and equipment should be used where possible. When nondedicated vehicles and equipment are used, procedures should be implemented

to ensure that the quality of the pharmaceutical product will not be compromised. This should include appropriate cleaning.

- Where feasible, additional technologies, such as global positioning system (GPS) electronic tracking devices, and engine-kill buttons, should be added to vehicles to enhance the security of pharmaceutical products while in the vehicle.
- When third-party carriers are used for transportation, distributors should develop written agreements with carriers to ensure that appropriate measures are taken to safeguard pharmaceutical products.
- Procedures that address the operation and maintenance of all vehicles and equipment involved in the distribution process should be in place.
- Vehicles, containers, and equipment should be kept clean and dry and free from accumulated waste and free from rodents, vermin, birds, and other pests.
- When controlled storage conditions (e.g., temperature and/or relative humidity) are required during transportation, the conditions should be provided, checked, monitored, and recorded. All monitoring records should be kept for a minimum of the shelf life of the product distributed plus 1 year or as required by national legislation and made available for inspection by the regulatory or oversight body.
- Equipment used for monitoring conditions, for example, temperature and humidity, in the vehicles and containers should be calibrated at scheduled intervals.
- Vehicles and containers should be of sufficient capacity to allow orderly storage of various categories of pharmaceutical products during transportation.
- Where possible, during transit, mechanisms should be available to allow for the segregation of rejected, recalled, returned, and suspected counterfeit pharmaceutical products. This product should be securely packaged, clearly labeled, and be accompanied by appropriate supporting documentation.

14.4.8 Shipment containers and container labeling

This principle states that: "Pharmaceutical products should be stored and distributed in shipment containers that have no adverse effect on the quality of the products, and that offer adequate protection from external influences, including contamination."

Shipping containers should contain labels that provide sufficient information on the storage and handling conditions as well as precautions to ensure that the products are properly handled and secure at all times. Any special transport and/or storage conditions should be included on the container label.

Written procedures should be provided for the handling of damaged and/or broken shipment containers, particularly those containing potentially toxic and hazardous products.

14.4.9 Dispatch and receipt

This principle states: "Pharmaceutical products should only be sold and/or distributed to persons or entities that are authorized to acquire such products in accordance with the applicable national, regional and international legislation. Written proof of such authority must be obtained prior to the distribution of products to such persons or entities."

Prior to dispatching pharmaceutical products, the supplier should ensure that the person or entity, for example, the contract acceptor for transportation of the pharmaceutical products, is aware of the pharmaceutical products to be distributed and complies with the appropriate storage and transport conditions. Also, the dispatch and transportation of the product should commence only after the receipt of a documented valid delivery order or material replenishment plan.

Written procedures that take into account the nature of the product as well as any special precautions to be observed for the dispatch of pharmaceutical products should be established.

Records for the dispatch of pharmaceutical products should be prepared and include the specific information noted in the guidance. The records should contain enough information to enable traceability of the product. Additionally, to facilitate traceability, the assigned batch number and expiry date of the products should be recorded at the point of receipt.

Realistic delivery schedules should be established, and routes planned, taking into account any security risks and care should be taken to ensure that the volume of pharmaceutical products ordered does not exceed the storage capacity at the destination facility.

Pharmaceutical products should not be supplied or received after their expiry date, or so close to the expiry date that the product will likely expire before the products are used by the consumer.

Companies that deal only with other wholesalers or with larger customers have the opportunity to sell products in whole cases only. This makes the product security issues slightly easier to deal with.

However, when a company deals with smaller companies, such as individual retail pharmacies, orders will frequently include quantities of the product less than a whole case. In these circumstances, the company will be left with open cases on its shelves. This means that there will be a mix of sealed and open cases being stored together and it may be possible to find individual sales packs being stored on open shelves. This is not only a nightmare from the point of view of stocktaking but increases the security risks within the warehouse.

One solution to this problem is to decouple the storage of sealed and open cases. All sealed cases are stored in the main warehouse and orders for multiple cases are serviced from here. However, smaller storage spaces, using pigeonholes or plastic boxes, are used for open cases. Orders for smaller quantities are serviced from this area. This ensures that different storage conditions can be provided for the different circumstances and product security is thus reinforced.

14.4.10 Transportation and products in transit

Product and shipment containers should be secured to prevent unauthorized access. Additional security, as appropriate, should be provided to prevent theft and/or misappropriation of products during transportation. The shipments should be secured and include the appropriate documentation needed to facilitate identification and verification of regulatory compliance.

There is a requirement that pharmaceutical products in transit are accompanied by the appropriate documentation.

The people responsible for the transportation of pharmaceutical products should be informed about all relevant conditions for storage and transportation and these requirements should be adhered to throughout transportation and at any intermediate storage stages.

Pharmaceutical products should be stored and transported in accordance with procedures that will prevent the loss of identity of the product; prevent contamination; provide adequate precautions against spillage, breakage, misappropriation, or theft; and ensure that appropriate environmental conditions are maintained.

The required storage conditions, within acceptable limits, for pharmaceutical products should be maintained throughout transit. If a deviation is noticed during transit by the person or entity responsible for transportation, this should be reported to the distributor and recipient. Any special conditions required during transportation should be monitored and recorded and provided by the manufacturer on the labels. There should be written procedures for investigating and responding to any failure to comply with storage requirements.

The transport and storage of pharmaceutical products that contain hazardous substances, that is, toxic, radioactive material, or other dangerous pharmaceutical products presenting special risks of abuse, fire, or explosion (e.g., combustible or flammable liquids, solids, and pressurized gases) should be completed in a safe, dedicated and secure area, and suitably safe and secure containers and vehicles.

Products that contain narcotics and other dependence-producing substances should be transported in safe and secure containers and vehicles and stored in safe and secure areas.

Physical or other equivalent validated segregation, such as electronic segregation, should be provided for the storage of rejected, expired, recalled, or returned products, and suspected counterfeit products. The product should be appropriately identified, securely packaged, clearly labeled, and be accompanied by appropriate supporting documentation.

The packaging materials and shipment containers should be of suitable design to prevent damage to the pharmaceutical products during transport.

Any damage to the container and any other event or problem that occurs during transit must be recorded, investigated, and reported to the relevant department, entity, or authority.

14.4.11 Documentation

Written instructions, all applicable receipts, invoices, and other records which document all activities relating to the distribution of pharmaceutical products should be available for review. Unless otherwise specified in national or regional regulations, records should be kept for seven years.

"Distributors should keep documentation on all pharmaceutical products received. The documentation, for example, records, should contain at least the following information:

- date;
- name of the pharmaceutical product;
- quantity received, or supplied; and
- name and address of the supplier."

Procedures should be developed and maintained for the preparation, review, approval, use of, and control of changes to all documents that relate to distribution processes. Documents, particularly instructions and procedures relating to any activity that could impact the quality of pharmaceutical products should be designed, completed, reviewed, and distributed with care.

The title, nature, and purpose of each document should be clearly stated, and the contents should be clear and unambiguous. The distributor must develop and maintain procedures for the identification, collection, indexing, retrieval, storage, maintenance, disposal, and access to all applicable documentation.

Documents should be completed, approved, signed (as required), and dated by an appropriate authorized person(s) and should not be changed without the approved authorization. The nature, content, and retention of documentation should comply with national legislative requirements. If there are no such requirements in place, the documents should be retained for at least one year after the expiry date of the product concerned.

All records must be easily retrievable, stored, and retained using facilities that are safeguarded against unauthorized modification, damage, deterioration, and/or loss of documentation. They should be readily available upon request.

Documents should be reviewed regularly and kept up to date. If a document is revised, a system should exist to prevent inadvertent use of the superseded version.

Mechanisms should be in place to permit the transfer of information, including quality or regulatory information, between a manufacturer and a customer, as well as the transfer of required information to relevant regulatory authorities.

Permanent documentation, written or electronic, should exist for each stored product. The documentation, that is, records should indicate recommended storage conditions, precautions to be observed, and retest dates. Back-ups should be maintained of any records generated or kept in electronic form.

14.4.12 Repackaging and relabeling

Repackaging and relabeling of pharmaceutical products should be limited because these practices may present a risk to the safety and security of the supply chain. If they do occur, these activities should only be performed by appropriately authorized entities and in compliance with the applicable national, regional and international guidelines and good manufacturing practice (GMP) principles.

14.4.13 Complaints

There should be a written procedure in place to address complaints; however, a clear distinction should be made between complaints about a product or its packaging and those relating to distribution. A complaint about the quality of a product or its packaging should be forwarded to the original manufacturer and/or marketing authorization holder.

Written procedures should be in place to carefully review complaints and other information concerning potentially defective and potentially counterfeit pharmaceutical products. The procedure should describe the action to be taken, including the need to consider a recall where appropriate.

Any complaint about a material defect should be recorded and thoroughly investigated to identify the origin or type of the complaint (e.g., repackaging procedure or original manufacturing process). If a defect relating to a pharmaceutical product is discovered or suspected, the decision to check other batches of the product should be considered.

"Where necessary, appropriate follow-up action should be taken after investigation and evaluation of the complaint. There should be a system in place to ensure that the complaint, the response received from the original product manufacturer, or the results of the investigation of the complaint, are shared with all the relevant parties."

All product quality problems or suspected cases of counterfeit products should be documented, and the information should be shared with the appropriate national and/or regional regulatory authorities.

14.4.14 Recalls

There should be a written procedure and system in place, with a designated person(s), to effectively and promptly recall pharmaceutical products known or suspected to be defective or counterfeit. The recall system should comply with the guidance issued by the national or regional regulatory authority.

In the event of a recall, the original manufacturer and/or marketing authorization holder should be informed. If the recall is initiated by an entity other than the original manufacturer and/or marketing authorization holder, consultation with these entities should take place before the recall is instituted.

Information about a recall should be shared with the appropriate national or regional regulatory authority. If a recall of the original product is necessary because of a counterfeited product that is not easily distinguishable from the original product, the manufacturer of the original product and the relevant health authority should be informed.

Pending appropriate action, all recalled pharmaceutical products should be stored in a secure, segregated area. Also, any recalled product should be clearly labeled and segregated during transit.

Until a decision is made regarding the fate of a product which is subject to recall, the particular storage conditions applicable to the pharmaceutical product should be maintained during storage and transit.

If a product is suspected to be defective or counterfeit, all customers and competent authorities of all countries to which the pharmaceutical product may have been distributed should be informed promptly of any intention to recall the product.

All records should be readily available to the designated person(s) responsible for a recall. These records should contain sufficient information about the pharmaceutical products supplied to the customers (including exported products).

If necessary, emergency recall procedures can be implemented.

14.4.15 Returned products

"A distributor should receive pharmaceutical product returns or exchanges pursuant to the terms and conditions of the agreement between the distributor and the recipient. Both distributors and recipients should be accountable for administering their returns process and ensuring that the aspects of this operation are secure and do not permit the entry of counterfeit products."

A suitably authorized person will make the necessary assessment and decision regarding the disposition of returned products. If there is any doubt about the quality of a pharmaceutical product, it should not be considered suitable for reissue or reuse.

Provision should be made for the appropriate and safe transport of returned products in accordance with the relevant storage and other requirements and for rejected pharmaceutical products prior to their disposal.

Rejected pharmaceutical products and those returned to a distributor should be appropriately identified and physically or electronically segregated. The particular storage conditions applicable to a pharmaceutical product that is rejected or returned should be maintained during storage and transit until a final decision has been made regarding the product in question.

Destruction of any pharmaceutical products must follow the international, national, and local requirements in regard to the disposal of such products, including consideration for the protection of the environment.

Documentation of all returned, rejected, and/or destroyed pharmaceutical products should be kept for a predetermined period.

14.4.16 European Union approach to returned product

Since the EU GDP guidance on this topic is somewhat different from the WHO guidance, this section is included to show the European Union's approach to returned product.

There are two types of returns that a distributor must deal with. These are discussed separately in the following sections.

14.4.16.1 Returns of nondefective product

Depending on the terms of agreements between distributors and their customers, there may be occasions when nondefective products are returned to the warehouse. Such material should be segregated from saleable material, pending a decision on how it should be treated.

There are only three possible routes for a returned material. It can be reapproved and put back into stock for sale; it can be returned to the manufacturer; or it can be destroyed.

Before a material can be returned to stock, it must undergo some rigorous checks. First of all, it must be in the original, unopened containers and must all be in a good condition. The history of handling and storage of the material since it originally left the distributor's premises must be known with certainty. There must be an acceptable shelf life remaining.

Assuming the returns satisfy all the above conditions, they must be examined and assessed by QC as though it was a new delivery. Considerations would include the nature of the product, any special conditions that the product is subject to, and the duration of time that has elapsed since the product was sold. If in doubt, advice should be sought from the original supplier or manufacturer.

If the returns are judged to be suitable for resale, they are formally released back into stock and entered into the FIFO system at an appropriate point. Full records must be kept of this process.

14.4.16.2 Returns of defective product

There are a few specific points to be noted in relation to recalls within distribution. There is a distinction made between urgent recalls, for which an emergency plan is required, and nonurgent recalls, which can be managed via a recall procedure. However, in either case, there must be a responsible person appointed to coordinate the activities.

Distributors will always be involved in recalls, and on occasion, it will be a distributor who will discover the problem that leads to a manufacturer triggering a recall. However, it is rare for the distributor to be the cause of a recall. They will generally be merely a part of the chain. Depending on the reason for the recall and its severity, a decision will be taken by the manufacturer as to whether the recall will take place at a wholesale level or it will extend to the retail sector. In this case, it is critical that the distributor can easily access the records kept of all deliveries of the batch of product in question.

14.4.17 Counterfeit pharmaceutical products

Counterfeit pharmaceutical products found in the distribution chain should be segregated from other pharmaceutical products to avoid any confusion. They should be clearly labeled as "not for sale." Also, the national regulatory authorities and the holder of the marketing authorization for the original product should be immediately informed.

The sale and distribution of a suspected counterfeit pharmaceutical product should be suspended, and the national regulatory authority notified immediately. Upon confirmation of the product being counterfeit, a formal decision will be made about its disposal, ensuring that it does not reenter the market. The final decision will be recorded.

14.4.18 Importation

Several aspects about import procedures are listed in the WHO guidance. The aspects include:

- The number of ports of entry into a country responsible for handling imports of pharmaceutical products should be limited by appropriate legislation.
- The port(s) of entry should be those most appropriately located and best equipped to handle imports of pharmaceutical products.
- At the port of entry, shipments of pharmaceutical products should be stored under suitable conditions for the shortest time as possible.
- All reasonable steps should be taken by importers to ensure that products are not mishandled or exposed to adverse storage conditions at piers or airports.
- Where necessary, persons with pharmaceutical training should be involved with the customs actions or they should be readily available.

Customs, enforcement agencies, and regulatory agencies responsible for the supervision of pharmaceutical products should establish means of cooperation and information exchange to prevent the importation of counterfeit pharmaceutical products.

14.4.19 Contract activities

Any activity relating to the distribution of a pharmaceutical product that is delegated to another person or entity should be performed by persons who are authorized for that function and in accordance with the terms of a written contract.

The contract should define the responsibilities of each party including the observance of the principles of GDP. Also, the contractor must accept the responsibility to include measures that avoid the entry of counterfeit medicines into the distribution chain.

Contractors should be audited periodically.

Under certain conditions, subcontracting may be permissible, with the written approval of the contract giver.

14.4.20 Self-inspection

Self-inspections of the quality system should be conducted to monitor implementation and compliance with GDP principles. If necessary, corrective and preventive measures should be taken.

Self-inspections should be conducted in an independent and detailed manner by a competent designated person.

The results of all self-inspection should be recorded, and the reports should include all observations made during the inspection and any proposed corrective measures.

14.5 Chapter summary

- GDP is defined as the part of quality assurance that ensures that the quality of a pharmaceutical product is maintained by means of adequate control of the numerous activities which occur during the distribution process as well as providing a tool to secure the distribution system from counterfeits, unapproved, illegally imported, stolen, counterfeit, substandard, adulterated, and/or misbranded pharmaceutical products.
- Distribution is defined as the procuring, purchasing, holding, storing, selling, supplying, importing, exporting, or movement of pharmaceutical products, with the exception of the dispensing or providing pharmaceutical products directly to a patient or his or her agent.
- There are many different national versions of GDP.
- The WHO and PIC/S published GDP guidelines.

14.6 Questions/problems

1. What is the acronym for good distribution practice?
2. Which countries have established GDP guidelines?

3. How are the GDP guidelines for the United States, the European Union, and Canada similar? How are they different?

4. How are the GDP guidelines published by the WHO and PIC/S similar? How are they different?

Further reading

European Commission, 2013. Guidelines on good distribution practice of medicinal products for human use.

Health Canada, 2020. Guidelines for environmental control of drugs during storage and transportation.

Jeong, S., Ji, E., 2018. Global perspectives on ensuring the safety of pharmaceutical products in the distribution process. Int. J. Clin. Pharm. g Ther. 56 (1), 12–23. Vol.

McCormick, K., 2002. Quality. Butterworth Heinemann, Oxford.

Pharmaceutical Inspection Co-Operation Scheme, 2014. PIC/S guide to good distribution practice for medicinal products.

US FDA. Title 21 of the United States (US) Code of Federal Regulations (CFR).

World Health Organization, 2010. Annex 5 WHO Good Distribution Practices for Pharmaceutical Products. WHO Technical Report Series, No. 957.

Index

Note: Page numbers followed by "*f*" and "*t*" refer to figures and tables, respectively.